PRISMA

Program on Research for Integrating Services
for the Maintenance of Autonomy

Volume II

Integration of Services for Disabled People: Research Leading to Action

Edited by

RÉJEAN HÉBERT
ANDRÉ TOURIGNY
MICHEL RAÎCHE

EDISEM

Edisem, Québec, ISBN 978-2-89130-215-9, 2008; 560 p.

Legal deposit – 1st quarter, 2008
Bibliothèque nationale du Québec
National Library of Canada

ISBN 978-2-89130-215-9

Table of Contents

PREFACES
by the Honorable Philippe Couillard, Minister of Health and Social
Services, Quebec, and Minister responsible for the Capitale-Nationale
Region xv

by Jonathan Lomas, Chief Executive Officer, Canadian Health Services
Research Foundation (CHSRF) xvi

INTRODUCTION
by Réjean Hébert 1

Implementation of Integrated Service Delivery Networks for the Elderly

1 *Louis Demers and Judith Lavoie*
Integrating Services for Frail Elderly People: the Role of Local, Regional,
and Departmental Actors 5

2. *Anne Veil and Réjean Hébert*
Assessment of the Degree of Implementation of Integrated Services
Networks in the Three Estrie Experimental Sites 23

3. *Anne Veil and Réjean Hébert*
Results of Service Integration: Perceptions of Managers and Service
Providers 33

4. *Anne Veil and Réjean Hébert*
Measuring the Integration of Services between Stakeholders in the
Continuum of Services for the Elderly in Three Territories 71

5. *Yves Couturier, Sébastien Carrier, Dominique Gagnon, and
Isabelle Chouinard*
Local Ownership of Case Management and Its Lessons for Implementing
Case Management in Other Settings 109

6. *Anne Veil and Réjean Hébert*
Perceived Self-Efficacy of Case Managers 125

7. *Anne Veil, Lynne Michaud, and Réjean Hébert*
Perceptions of Service Continuity among Case Managed Recipients of
Services for Frail Elders during Implementation of the Integrated Services
Network 149

8. *Louis Voyer and Réjean Hébert*
Family Physicians' Perceptions of the Integrated Services Network and
Case Managers 167

9. *Dominique Somme, Réjean Hébert, Gina Bravo, François Blanchard,
and Olivier Saint-Jean*
The Individualized Service Plan as a Clinical Integration Tool: Qualitative
Analysis in the Quebec PRISMA Experiment 179

10. *Suzanne Durand, Danièle Blanchette, and Réjean Hébert*
Implementation and Operation Costs for an Integrated Service Delivery
Network for the Frail Elderly in Estrie 199

Impacts of an Integrated Service Delivery Network

11. *Réjean Hébert, Marie-France Dubois, Michel Raîche, Nicole Dubuc,
and the PRISMA-Estrie Group*
The Effectiveness of the PRISMA Integrated Service Delivery Network:
Preliminary Report on Methods and Baseline Data 213

12. *Réjean Hébert, Michel Raîche, Marie-France Dubois, Nicole Dubuc,
Michel Tousignant, N'Deye Rokhaya Gueye, and the PRISMA-Estrie
Group*
Impact of the PRISMA-Estrie Integrated Service Delivery Network
on the Elderly and their Informal Caregivers 237

13. *Michel Raîche, Réjean Hébert, Danièle Blanchette, Suzanne Durand,
Marie-France Dubois, N'Deye Rokhaya Gueye, and the PRISMA-
Estrie Group*
RISPA Overall Performance: Impacts on the Use of Health Services,
Their Costs and Efficiency under the PRISMA-Estrie Study 265

Integration, Quality Assessment, and Service-Planning Tools

14. *Diane Morin, André Tourigny, Line Robichaud, Daniel Pelletier,
Lucie Bonin, Aline Vézina, Luc Mathieu and Martin Buteau*
Evaluation of an Information System within an Integrated Services
Network for Frail Seniors: Its Use and User Perception of Usefulness
and Impact 289

15. *Diane Morin, André Tourigny, Daniel Pelletier, Line Robichaud,
Luc Mathieu, Aline Vézina, Lucie Bonin, and Martin Buteau*
Seniors' Views on the Use of an Electronic Health Record 305

16. *André Tourigny, Diane Morin, Marie-Jeanne Kergoat, Nicole Dubuc,*
    Line Robichaud, Jacques Morin, Lise Côté, Paule Lebel, René Verreault,
    Edeltraut Kröger, Zohra Benounissa, and Solange Proulx
    Measuring and Improving the Quality and Continuity of Health Care and
    Services Delivered to Vulnerable Elders: Pilot Project for People with
    Cognitive Impairments or Dementia 319

17. *Edeltraut Kröger, André Tourigny, Diane Morin, Lise Côté,*
    Marie-Jeanne Kergoat, Paule Lebel, Line Robichaud, Shirley Imbeault,
    and Solange Proulx
    Validation of Process Quality Indicators for the Integrated Care of Frail
    Older Adults 337

18. *Nathalie Delli-Colli, Nicole Dubuc, Réjean Hébert, and Catherine Lestage*
    The Selection of Essential Variables to Establish the Psychological
    and Social Needs of Residents and the Social Service Workload in
    Long-Term Care Hospital Centers..,...... 361

19. *Danielle Benoît, Michel Tousignant, Guylaine Allard, Myriam Bergeron,*
    Nicole Dubuc, and Rejean Hébert
    Assessment of the Adequacy of the Home Support Program's Services
    Offered Versus User Needs: Bridging the Gap between a Research Project
    and the Harnessing of Administratively Valuable Data 383

20. *Pauline Gervais, Réjean Hébert, and Michel Tousignant*
    Profiles of the Functional Independence of the Clientele in Private
    Residences for the Elderly in Estrie.. 393

21. *Danièle Blanchette, Suzanne Durand, and Réjean Hébert*
    The PRISMA-Estrie Study: Determining the Cost of Health
    Services 407

22. *Michel Raîche, Réjean Hébert, Marie-France Dubois, Johanne Bolduc,*
    Maryse Grégoire, Celine Bureau, and Anne Veil
    Case-Finding of Older Persons with Moderate to Severe Disabilities
    by means of PRISMA-7 Questionnaire: A Presentation of the
    Instrument, Its Implementation, and Its Use 435

23. *Anne Veil and Réjean Hébert*
    Estimating a Territory's Case-Management Resources 451

24. *Linda Dieleman, Pierre Richard, Céline Bureau, and Johanne Bolduc*
    The Use of Research Data for Management Purposes 485

Transfer and Application to Other Patients and Countries

25. *Nicole Dubuc, Michel Tousignant, Danielle Benoit, Guylaine Allard, Myriam Bergeron, Lise Trottier, and Réjean Hébert*
    Physically and Intellectually Disabled Target Groups Served by CLSCs: Representing Their Functional-Autonomy Needs Using Classification by Iso-SMAF Profiles.. 497

26. *Dominique Somme, Hélène Trouvé, Yves Couturier, Sébastien Carrier, Dominique Gagnon, Benoît Lavallart, Réjean Hébert, Carole Crétin, and Olivier St-Jean*
    PRISMA France: Adapting the PRISMA Integration Model to the French Health and Social Services System 511

27. *Pauline Gervais, Michel Tousignant, Réjean Hébert, and Sylvain Connangle*
    Classifying the Frail Elderly: A Comparison of Iso-SMAF Profile Assignment with AGGIR-based Classification into GIRs (Iso-Ressources Groups) 527

ASSISTANCE IN PUBLISHING THIS BOOK 541

FUNDING OF THE PRISMA PROGRAM 541

ACKNOWLEDGMENTS.. 542

Authors and Contributors

Acronyms for Host Institutions
CHA: Affiliated hospital center
CHU: University hospital
CSSS: Centre de santé et de services sociaux (health and social services center)
IUG: Institut universitaire de gériatrie (university geriatrics institute)
MSSS: Ministère de la Santé et des Services sociaux

Allard, Guylaine, Medical Archivist
Consultant, Archives and Information Systems, Agence de la santé et
des services sociaux de la Montérégie

Bédard, Mariette, RN
Head, Administration of Home-Care Programs, Granit CSSS

Bellefleur, Robert, MA
Human Relations Officer, Elderly Sector, Granit CSSS

Benoit, Danielle, MAP
Planning Officer; Planning, Programming, and Research, Agence de la santé et
des services sociaux de la Montérégie

Benounissa, Zohra, MSc
Biostatistician, Laval University Geriatric Research Unit, Centre de recherche
du CHA universitaire de Québec

Bergeron, Myriam, BSc
Database Manager, Research Centre on Aging, CSSS–IUG of Sherbrooke

Blanchard, François, MD, PhD
Service de médecine interne et gériatrie, CHU Sébastopol, Reims, France

Blanchette, Danièle, CA, PhD
Researcher, Research Centre on Aging, CSSS–IUG of Sherbrooke
Professor, Faculty of Business Administration, Université de Sherbrooke

Boissé, Marie-Claude, MA
Research Officer, Research Centre on Aging, CSSS–IUG of Sherbrooke

Bolduc, Johanne, RN, MSc
Program Director, CSSS, MRC-de-Coaticook

Bonin, Lucie, MD, MSc
Researcher, Laval University Geriatric Research Unit, Centre de recherche,
CHA universitaire de Québec
Agence de la santé et des services sociaux de la Mauricie-Centre-du-Québec
Institut national de santé publique du Québec

Bravo, Gina, PhD
Researcher, Research Centre on Aging, CSSS–IUG of Sherbrooke
Professor, Faculty of Medicine and Health Sciences, Université de Sherbrooke

Bureau, Céline, RN, MSc
Director, Clinical, Public-Health, and Community Development Program,
CSSS–IUG of Sherbrooke

Buteau, Martin, PhD
Vice Rector, Information Resources, Université de Sherbrooke

Caron, Chantal, RN, PhD
Researcher, Research Centre on Aging, CSSS–IUG of Sherbrooke
Professor, Faculty of Medicine and Health Sciences, Université de Sherbrooke

Carrier, Sébastien, BSS, PhD (candidate)
Research Officer, PRISMA
Student, Doctorate in Gerontology, Faculty of Letters and Humanities,
Université de Sherbrooke

Chouinard, Isabelle, MSS, PhD (candidate)
Research Officer, PRISMA
Student, Doctorate in Education, Faculty of Letters and Humanities,
Université de Sherbrooke

Connangle, Sylvain, CAF, D.E.S.
Director, Établissement d'hébergement pour personnes âgées dépendantes
(EHPAD) La Madeleine, Bergerac, France

Côté, Lise, RN, MSc
Research Professional, Organisation des services et évaluation,
Direction régionale santé publique de la Capitale-Nationale

Couturier, Yves, PhD
Researcher, Research Centre on Aging, CSSS–IUG of Sherbrooke
Professor, Faculty of Letters and Humanities, Université de Sherbrooke

Crétin, Carole, MD
Direction générale de la Santé, Ministère de la santé et des solidarités,
Sous-direction Pathologies et santé, Paris, France

Delli-Colli, Nathalie, SW, MSS, PhD (candidate)
Consultant, Iso-SMAF Profiles, Centre d'expertise en santé de Sherbrooke
Student, Doctorate of Clinical Science, Faculty of Medicine and Health Sciences,
Université de Sherbrooke

Demers, Louis, PhD
Professor, École nationale d'administration publique

Desrosiers, Johanne, OT, PhD
Researcher, Research Centre on Aging, CSSS–IUG of Sherbrooke
Director, School of Rehabilitation, Faculty of Medicine and Health Sciences,
Université de Sherbrooke

Dieleman, Linda, MSc
Planning, Programming, and Research Officer, Service Organization,
Agence de la santé et des services sociaux de l'Estrie

Dubois, Marie-France, PhD
Researcher, Research Centre on Aging, CSSS–IUG of Sherbrooke
Professor, Faculty of Medicine and Health Sciences, Université de Sherbrooke

Dubuc, Nicole, RN, PhD
Researcher, Research Centre on Aging, CSSS–IUG of Sherbrooke
Professor, Faculty of Medicine and Health Sciences, Université de Sherbrooke

Durand, Pierre, MD
Researcher, Laval University Geriatric Research Unit, CHA,
Hôpital Saint-Sacrement
Dean, Faculty of Medicine, Université Laval

Durand, Suzanne, CGA, DBA (candidate)
Research Officer, Research Centre on Aging, CSSS–IUG of Sherbrooke
Professor, Teaching and Research Unit, Management Science,
Université du Québec en Abitibi-Témiscamingue

Gagnon, Dominique, BSS, PhD (candidate)
Research Officer, PRISMA
Student, Doctorate in Gerontology, Faculty of Letters and Humanities,
Université de Sherbrooke

Gagnon, Maxime, PhD
Research Officer, Research Centre on Aging, CSSS–IUG of Sherbrooke

Gervais, Pauline, MA, PhD (candidate)
Research Officer, Research Centre on Aging, CSSS–IUG of Sherbrooke
Student, Doctorate in Gerontology, Faculty of Letters and Humanities,
Université de Sherbrooke

Grégoire, Maryse, RN, BSc, MA (candidate)
Clinical Consultant, General and Emergency Medicine, Direction des Soins
Infirmiers et de la Qualité, CHU de Sherbrooke

Gueye, N'Deye Rokhaya, PhD
Statistician, Research Centre on Aging, CSSS–IUG of Sherbrooke

Guillot, Valérie, MA
Research Officer, Research Centre on Aging, CSSS–IUG of Sherbrooke

Hébert, Réjean, MD, MPhil
Researcher, Research Centre on Aging, CSSS–IUG of Sherbrooke
Dean, Faculty of Medicine and Health Sciences, Université de Sherbrooke

Imbeault, Shirley, DPsy
Research Professional, Laval University Geriatric Research Unit,
Centre de recherche, CHA universitaire de Québec

Joly, Nathalie-Audrey, MA
Research Officer, Research Centre on Aging, CSSS–IUG of Sherbrooke

Kergoat, Marie-Jeanne, MD, Geriatrician
Researcher, Institut universitaire de gériatrie de Montréal
Professor, Université de Montréal

Kröger, Edeltraut, Pharm., MSc, PhD (candidate)
Research Professional, Laval University Geriatric Research Unit,
Centre de recherche, CHA universitaire de Québec
Student, Doctorate in Epidemiology, Université Laval

Labrecque, Isabelle, MA (candidate)
Research Officer, Research Centre on Aging, CSSS–IUG of Sherbrooke

Lavallart, Benoît, MD
Direction générale de la Santé, Ministère de la santé et des solidarités,
Sous-direction Pathologies et santé, Paris, France

Lavoie, Judith, MSc
Research Professional, École nationale d'administration publique

Lebel, Paule, MD
Researcher, McGill University–Université de Montréal Research Group on
Integrated Services for Older Persons
Professor, Faculty of Medicine, Université de Montréal
Director of Teaching, Institut universitaire de gériatrie de Montréal

Lestage, Catherine, MPs, PhD (candidate)
Research Officer, Research Centre on Aging, CSSS–IUG of Sherbrooke
Student, Master of Clinical Science, Faculty of Medicine and Health Sciences,
Université de Sherbrooke

Mathieu, Luc, RN, D.B.A.
Researcher, Research Centre on Aging, CSSS–IUG of Sherbrooke
Director, School of Nursing, Faculty of Medicine and Health Sciences,
Université de Sherbrooke

Michaud, Lynne, SW, MSs
CSSS, MRC-de-Coaticook

Morin, Diane, RN, PhD
Researcher, Laval University Geriatric Research Unit, Centre de recherche,
CHA universitaire de Québec
Dean, Faculty of Nursing, Université Laval

Morin, Jacques, MD, Geriatrician
Researcher, Laval University Geriatric Research Unit, Centre de recherche,
CHA universitaire de Québec
Professor, Faculty of Medicine, Université Laval

Murray, William, MA
Direction de l'évaluation, Planification stratégique, évaluation et qualité,
MSSS du Québec

Pelletier, Daniel, MPs
Research Professional, Laval University Geriatric Research Unit,
Centre de recherche, CHA universitaire de Québec

Proulx, Solange, MA
Research Professional, Laval University Geriatric Research Unit,
Centre de recherche, CHA universitaire de Québec

Raîche, Michel, MSc, PhD (candidate)
Research Coordinator, Research Centre on Aging, CSSS–IUG of Sherbrooke
Student, Doctorate of Clinical Science, Faculty of Medicine and Health Sciences,
Université de Sherbrooke

Richard, Pierre, MSS
Director, Programs for Clienteles in the Community, Granit CSSS
Consultant, Clinical Projects, Agence de la santé et des services sociaux de l'Estrie

Robichaud, Line, OT, PhD
Researcher, Laval University Geriatric Research Unit, Centre de recherche,
CHA universitaire de Québec
Professor, Department of Rehabilitation, Université Laval

Simard, Dany, MA
Research Officer, Research Centre on Aging, CSSS–IUG of Sherbrooke

Somme, Dominique, MD
PRISMA-France, Service de gériatrie-Pôle urgence réseaux Hôpital Européen
Georges Pompidou, Paris, France

St-Jean, Olivier, MD, PhD
Service de gériatrie-Pôle urgence réseaux, Hôpital Européen
Georges Pompidou, Paris, France

Tourigny, André, MD, MBA
Scientific Director and Researcher, Centre d'excellence sur le vieillissement,
Hôpital du Saint-Sacrement, Québec
Professor, Faculty of Medicine, Université Laval
Institut national de santé publique du Québec
Direction régionale de santé publique de la Capitale-Nationale

Tousignant, Michel, PT, PhD
Researcher, Research Centre on Aging, CSSS–IUG of Sherbrooke
Professor, Faculty of Medicine and Health Sciences, Université de Sherbrooke

Trahan, Lysette, PhD
Direction de l'évaluation, Planification stratégique, évaluation et qualité,
MSSS du Québec

Trottier, Lise, MSc
Statistician, Research Centre on Aging, CSSS–IUG of Sherbrooke

Trouvé, Hélène, PhD (candidate)
PRISMA-France, Hôpital Européen Georges Pompidou, Paris, France

Veil, Anne, MSs
Research Officer, Research Centre on Aging, CSSS–IUG of Sherbrooke

Veilleux, Karine, MA
Research Officer, Research Centre on Aging, CSSS–IUG of Sherbrooke

Verreault, René, MD, PhD
Director and Researcher, Laval University Geriatric Research Unit, CHA,
Hôpital Saint-Sacrement
Professor, Faculty of Medicine, Université Laval

Vézina, Aline, Psy., PhD
Researcher, Laval University Geriatric Research Unit, Centre de recherche,
CHA universitaire de Québec
Professor, School of Social Services, Université Laval

Voyer, Louis, MPs
PRISMA Coordinator, Research Centre on Aging, CSSS–IUG of Sherbrooke

The PRISMA-Estrie Group referred to as authors in chapters 11, 12, and 13 includes the following:
Mariette Bédard, Robert Bellefleur, Myriam Bergeron, Danièle Blanchette, Marie-Claude Boissé, Johanne Bolduc, Lucie Bonin, Gina Bravo, Céline Bureau, Chantal Caron, Johanne Desrosiers, Linda Dieleman, Marie-France Dubois, Nicole Dubuc, Pierre Durand, Suzanne Durand, Maxime Gagnon, N'Deye Rokhaya Gueye, Valérie Guillot, Réjean Hébert, Nathalie-Audrey Joly, Isabelle Labrecque, William Murray, Michel Raîche, Pierre Richard, Dany Simard, André Tourigny, Michel Tousignant, Lysette Trahan, Anne Veil, and Karine Veilleux.

Prefaces

Dear Reader:

When the theme of integrating services is the focal point of a research project, it is not surprising that, in my role as Minister of Health and Social Services, I have associated myself with the presentation of the second volume of the Program of Research on the Integration of Services for the Maintenance of Autonomy or PRISMA.

Service integration has been the central theme of the actions that we have taken in our health and social services system in recent years, especially the networking of the different caregivers and institutions serving the same population. The creation of health and social services centres (French acronym: CSSS) aims specifically at having the general public benefit from better coordination and greater cooperation between the individuals who ensure the deliver of health care and social services.

As we all know, Québec's society will undergo rapid aging. While we should be delighted that our society's social and economic development is translating into increased longevity and improved health for the population, we also bear the responsibility for seeing that the network adapts to offer solutions that better respond to the needs of the elderly. As a government, we have set a course in this direction and we will continue to devote significant energy and resources into it.

In today's context, which calls on us to adapt our approaches to new realities, the work of the PRISMA team takes on even greater value. This initiative enables us to rely on research as a factor in continuously improving practices insofar as we are able to use the successes of some as a springboard to success for others. This guarantees improved quality and accessibility of the care that we provide to the general public.

I would like to particularly salute the efforts deployed within the framework of PRISMA to put a clearly human face on this enormous amount of work in which the daily realities, the individuals receiving services, and those delivering them, serve as central reference points.

As the title of this book so aptly indicates, there is no doubt that the research outcomes will lead to action.

I hope that you will find reading it both enjoyable and profitable.

Sincerely,

Philippe Couillard
Minister of Health and Social Services
and Minister responsible for the Capitale-Nationale Region
July 2007

All too often valuable research is done by those who are detached from the systems it can influence. Not surprisingly it usually goes unused, despite its clear potential to improve the health of patients and/or the effectiveness of the delivery and management of the services they receive. Our investment in this type of health services research is well-intentioned but often poorly designed to actually have an impact on the area being studied. What follows shows that it does not have to be that way. It is a testament to what can be achieved when investigators such as Réjean Hébert and his colleagues embrace the challenge of getting research used.

The assumption that good research "speaks for itself" is just that – an assumption, unsupported by the experience of the last twenty years in health services research. After nearly a quarter of a century of study we have learned that the way to get valuable research used is to do what the researchers in this book did – involve those who can implement their results from the start.

Doing research in splendid isolation from the system to which it pertains may lead to pristine methods and publishable papers, but it leaves the investigators removed from reality. Under this detached model of health research, which has dominated university-based investigation for the last half century, the researchers are left marketing their results after the fact to busy, preoccupied, and often uninterested clinicians and managers. The researchers find themselves competing for the attention of these decision makers with drug companies, provider associations, consultants and many others who have access to far more resources and persuasive skills than they will ever have.

This book recounts the adventure that followed when a group of Quebec researchers decided to do it differently – the PRISMA project. My own foundation has been a major sponsor and supporter of this project precisely because it is such a good example of the new "linkage and exchange" model for applied research, wherein researchers become co-investigators with those in the system.

Their first choice was to focus on the needs of the whole patient in the context of the entire system of potential services – not a particular disease, a specific body part, a unique treatment, or a sector of service carefully isolated in a "university laboratory" from its overall context. For them the important motivation was to focus the efforts of the health system on how best to address the needs of the frail elderly with compromised independence and chronic disease. They saw the importance of integrating all health and social services to the benefit of this population by overcoming the tendency of policy and management to fragment services and the organizations delivering them into self-perpetuating, sometimes competing and always separate institutions.

Second, they realized that to do this they not only needed to identify through research what that integration looked like, but they also needed the cooperation of all those whose lives would be affected by the research – the clinicians and managers working in the institutions. They systematically went about the task of gaining that cooperation by recruiting all the relevant stakeholders in Quebec regions as co-investigators on the PRISMA project. Thus general practitioners, community services agencies, system managers and others became as important to the project as were the researchers.

Finally, as they went along their journey they found out what true "linkage and exchange" means – not only did they recruit those in the system to the research but in turn they were recruited from research into the implementation of findings by those working in the system. New measurement and monitoring tools were needed by the managers and clinicians as they started to see what the research meant for them and so the researchers got pulled further and further into the implementation and spread of their health service innovation.

The results of this adventure recounted in this book cover an impressive landscape of investigation. Those working on PRISMA found themselves engaged in a breathtaking scope of work from service perceptions and need assessments, through personnel training and development, on to tool development and outcomes measurement, through electronic information systems and economics, finally to change management and innovation diffusion.

The Canadian Health Services Research Foundation is proud to have been a sponsor and supporter of this work. It serves as a great example of how to do research that makes a difference. It also shows how big the pay-off is from investments in well designed applied research. Not only are tens of thousands of vulnerable elderly who previously received poorly integrated support now getting the services they need, but also the costs and satisfaction of those delivering and managing those services have improved. It is no wonder that the PRISMA project has had such a positive influence on the network delivery model now adopted by Quebec, and that this influence is fast spreading well beyond care for the frail elderly and well beyond the borders of Quebec.

Jonathan Lomas
Chief Executive Officer
Canadian Health Services Research Foundation
March 2007

Introduction

by Réjean Hébert

This book brings together the results of the final years of the PRISMA group. Whereas the first PRISMA book, *Integrated Service Delivery to Ensure Persons' Functional Autonomy*[1] presented the principles of integration, the PRISMA coordination model, and the preliminary assessment of its implementation, this second volume pulls together the outcomes produced by network researchers and partners at the end of many studies carried out on the model over the last three years. We have called the second PRISMA book *Integration of Services for Disabled People: Research Leading to Action* to emphasize the efforts made to transfer research results into better health and social-services policies and services.

The PRISMA partnership was distinctive for the close cooperation between researchers, policy makers, managers, and clinicians, as reflected by the book's 68 contributors and where they work. This collaboration, stimulated through the support of the Canadian Health Services Research Foundation (CHSRF), generated pertinent, applied research questions as well as a constant concern to rapid transfer research results to partners and the entire Canadian and Quebec health and social services network. The Canadian Institutes of Health Research (CIHR) took note of and called attention to this knowledge transfer by bestowing the Knowledge Translation Award on November 2005, which, moreover, provided funding for this book. PRISMA work was also analyzed in the Knowledge Translation casebooks published by the CIHR Institute of Health Services and Policy Research.[2]

The coordination model developed, implemented, and assessed by the PRISMA group is the only of its kind in the world.[3] The other experiments with integration carried out up to now referred to two other forms of integration according to Leutz's taxonomy,[4] either liaison or full integration. The PRISMA coordination model aims primarily at making optimal, rational use of the services in a locality or region. It targets improving the efficient use of existing services. Consequently, it fits into the current network, instead of lying on its periphery. This, without a doubt, explains why it is easier to implement in a public and universal health and social services system. PRISMA model was first initiated and tested in Bois-Francs[5] before being developed, implemented, and assessed in Estrie and Montérégie.

We have collated the PRISMA findings in four sections in this book: model implementation, assessment of model impact, instruments supporting model implementation, and transfer and application to other target groups and countries. The implementation of the PRISMA model in Estrie was assessed at all levels in minute details. On the macroscopic level, a sociopolitical analysis of service integration is provided. On the mesoscopic level, a summative assessment of implementation reports on monitoring the degree of implementation as well as the opinions of managers, clinicians, the older people, and their caregivers. On the microscopic level, we performed in-depth analysis of the roles of case managers as well as their perception of effectiveness. We also measured the costs of implementing and operating an integrated service network, and more carefully examined one of the model's components that has been neglected up until now: the individualized service plan.

The impacts of the integrated services delivery (ISD) network for the elderly were examined during a quasi-experimental longitudinal study lasting four years and funded by a major CIHR grant. The impacts on the older people themselves and their caregivers as well as on the use and cost of services were measured and are presented in the section on ISD impacts. The ISD was also assessed in economic and efficiency terms.

Putting an integrated network into place requires integration and planning tools. The section on integration, assessment, and assistance tools for planning services provides a number of applied responses in this regard. The use of the computerized clinical chart is described, along with its impacts and how the older people perceive it. Quality measurement and indicator validation among the vulnerable older people are also presented. The service needs of the older people are measured from different viewpoints: psychosocial needs in placement centers, adequacy of the service offer and the needs of users of the home-care program, and functional profiles of the older people living in private nursing homes. Determining the costs of health-care services is not only useful in research. It can be valuable to managers in making their decisions. Implementation of a process for finding cases of the older people with disabilities is presented. One chapter makes it possible to estimate the case-management resources required in a territory, while, in another, managers explain how they use research data for management purposes.

The final section reveals PRISMA spin-offs, with the model being exported to France as well as to other target groups. Iso-SMAF profiles are used in Montérégie to measure physical and intellectual disabilities. How these profiles are used in a residential institution for disabled older persons in France is presented as well as how the PRISMA integration model is adapted to the French health and social services system.

Now that the PRISMA model has demonstrated its feasibility and positive impacts both in terms of clients and services, it is ready for generalization. In Quebec, the Minister of Health and Social Services made it a major element in his *Orientations ministérielles sur les services offerts aux personnes âgées en perte d'autonomie*.[6] The reform he conducted in recent years by integrating home-care structures (CLSC), hospitals, and hursing homes through the creation of health and social services centers (CSSS) is similar to the service integration advocated under the PRISMA model. This structural integration, however, must translate into functional integration within institutions and into effective coordination of CSSSs with the network's private and volunteer stakeholders. The creation of local services networks and the development of clinical projects are the mechanisms provided to achieve this functional integration. These mechanisms can be based, to a large degree, on PRISMA work.

Other provinces and countries are looking at the coordination model developed and proven by the PRISMA team. The model was recommended by a group of independent researchers for its relevance and evidence of its impact.[7, 8]

We want to express our appreciation to funding organizations (CIHR, CHSRF, Fonds de la recherche en santé du Québec, Réseau québécois de recherche sur le vieillissement), public health and social services organizations (Ministère de la Santé et des Services sociaux, Institut national de santé publique du Québec, Health and Social Services Agencies of Estrie, Montérégie, Mauricie-Centre-du-Québec, Laval, and Québec, Centre de santé et de services sociaux – Institut Universitaire de Gériatrie de Sherbrooke), and Université de Sherbrooke for their financial support of PRISMA. Our thanks go out to all the older people who took part in our projects. Without them, we would not have been able to collect all the information revealing their state of independence, their perceptions, and their satisfaction. We also thank their caregivers. We are grateful to the managers, policy makers, and clinicians who collaborated in implementing the ISDs and who agreed to be questioned and observed throughout the process. Without them, we would not have known if the ISDs should be generalized across Quebec. Thanks to all the research teams, research officers, evaluators, and statisticians, for whom research is part of their daily lives. Clinicians, researchers, managers, and even the policy makers interested in service integration will find this book quite illuminating. Integrating services for the elderly represents a formidable challenge and, as we now know, unavoidable in improving services.

References

1. Hébert R, Tourigny A, Gagnon M. *Integrated service delivery to ensure persons' functional autonomy.* Québec: Edisem; 2005.

2. Institute of Health Services and Policy Research. *Evidence in Action, Acting on Evidence: A casebook of health services and policy research knowledge translation stories.* Ottawa: Canadian Institutes of Health Research; 2006.

3. Leutz W. Reflections on Integrating Medical and Social Care: Five Laws Revisited. *Journal of Integrated Care* 2005; 13(5):3-14.

4. Leutz WN. Five laws for integrating medical and social services: Lessons from the United States and the United Kingdom. *Milbank Quarterly* 1999; 77(1):77-110.

5. Tourigny A. Durand P. Bonin L. Hébert R. Rochette L. Quasi-experimental Study of the Effectiveness of an Integrated Service Delivery Network for the Frail Elderly. *Canadian Journal on Aging* 2004; 23(3):231-46.

6. Ministère de la santé et des services sociaux. *Orientations ministérielles sur les services offerts aux personnes âgées en perte d'autonomie.* Québec: MSSS; 2001.

7. Hollander MJ, Cherry L, MacAdam M, Pallan P, Ritter R. *Development of a strategic framework for continuing care services. Continuing care service delivery systems: Case Studies of current models.* Nova Scotia Department of Health, Continuing Care Branch; 2007.

8. Hollander MJ, Chappell NL, Prince MJ, Shapiro E. Providing care and support for an aging population: Briefing notes on key policy issues. *Health Care Quarterly 2007;* 10(3):34-45.

Chapter 1
Integrating Services for Frail Elderly People: the Role of Local, Regional, and Departmental Actors[1]

Louis Demers and Judith Lavoie

Highlights

- The establishment of an integrated services network:
  - Centers above all on the involvement of competent, credible, and dedicated individuals who will demonstrate the practicality and relevance of the new services co-ordination system.
  - Requires the support of senior executives of organizations involved with the selected co-ordination model.
  - Must appear to these executives as an appropriate solution to problems related to setting up services they feel are a priority.
  - Takes time so that managers and practitioners affected by the change can establish collaborative ties and adopt the selected coordination model.
- The effectiveness of an integrated services network depends on the use of a shareable clinical information system that is both interdisciplinary and inter-institutional.
- The organizational aspect of establishing an integrated services network implies the introduction of governance and coordination procedures based on trust and mutual respect.
- Departmental actors can contribute to the enhanced integration of services:
  - By adopting policies that are both clear and flexible, allowing local actors to choose the specific methods of implementing their selected integration model.
  - By adopting measures in accordance with these policies, particularly in terms of information systems.
  - By strengthening the internal coordination mechanisms used by the ministry to improve the consistency and timing of its actions.

- Regional actors can also promote service integration by setting out their own policies in this area and by supporting desired changes rather than unilaterally imposing them.
- Researchers and research professionals can also contribute to the integration of services by providing a different perspective of the type of problems involved in setting up services for frail elderly people and by offering solutions. To become true agents of change, researchers and research professionals must not only impart knowledge, but establish their credibility among the actors they are looking to support.

Introduction: Issues and Challenges in the Integration of Services for Frail Elderly People

Disabilities and loss of functional independence represent major health problems for the elderly and their families. Dealing with this problem represents a major challenge for health-care systems. On one hand, the number of frail elderly people will increase substantially in the years to come.[2] On the other, for decades, health-care systems have been structured primarily to respond to episodic health problems of young people and adults. In such a system, which is dominated by a silo approach,[3] individuals requiring continuing services over a long period of time are poorly served. Major services are missing; existing services either lack coordination or are poorly coordinated, so that the elderly and their families are left to their own devices in obtaining the appropriate service. As a result, many people felt that better service coordination would provide a generic solution to the discontinuity of services for the frail elderly and other vulnerable groups.[4-9]

Integration occurs when a comprehensive range of services is coordinated so that each user receives "the right service at the right time by the right person" without having to find it by him- or herself.
Coordination refers to the mechanisms and actions that must be put into play to make integration a reality.
Continuity "is how a patient experiences care over time as coherent and linked."[10]

Many experiences[4, 5, 6, 11, 12] demonstrate that lack of coordination among local organizations cannot be held solely accountable for the discontinuity of services. Indeed, the interdependent nature of actions taken by actors at different levels of the health system and their relative lack of knowledge of the context in which other levels of actors operate. Therefore, even though government, regional, and local actors all want to improve services to frail elders, their respective actions are not necessarily in step. Therefore, it is just as important for policymakers as the managers responsible for organizing services for the frail elderly to more clearly understand the factors that strengthen or weaken the synergy of actions taken by and within the three tiers of the health-care system. Taking these factors into account will enable these actors to act and interact more effectively. We examined this question in a recent research project[1].

After describing the project's objectives and methodology, we will present the outcomes by first giving the role of local actors and then the roles of regional and departmental actors. The conclusion brings out a series of lessons that could prove useful in the context of implementing the current reform of Quebec's health and social services system. The chapter is dotted with excerpts from interviews that we carried out during the project.

Research Project

This project aimed at better understanding the respective impact of the three levels of intervention —departmental, regional, and local—on the implementation of mechanisms and practices for coordinating services for the frail elderly. We adopted three general objectives:

- Understand how the actions of the MSSS, regional agencies/boards, and local actors affect five dimensions of integration.
- Bring to light the means used by local actors to coordinate services to the frail elderly.
- Draw out the conditions that promote or impede the implementation of mechanisms and practices for coordinating services.

We adopted a sociopolitical perspective in carrying out this research.[13, 14, 15]. According to this perspective, pursuing a more effective integration of services derives from the issues, which vary according to actor values and interests and depending on the context in which they operate. This is why we are interested in the nature of the linkages between the actors taking part in this innovation and in how they influence service integration. Integration involves a number of elements, which we have broken down into five dimensions, as defined in Table 1.1.

Table 1.1
Five dimensions of services organization

Dimension	Definition
Clinical	Availability of a comprehensive range of services and adoption of common coordination tools and practices that vary in intensity according to user needs.
Informational	Use of information systems and tools to facilitate clinical exchanges and ongoing feedback.
Normative	Understanding and adhering to the integration model.
Organizational	Creation of intra- and interorganizational coordination mechanisms.
Financial	Adoption of means for financing services and allocating budgets that promote the management of target groups.

Making these distinctions is important because different actors are involved in each of these dimensions. The process of translating each one into concrete action does not follow the same logic nor does it proceed at the same pace, which creates consistency and timing problems that must be dealt with. To illustrate, updating a shareable patient record falls under the general development of information systems within a health-care system. Record availability depends on the budgets for information systems allocated by each tier and how important competent authorities view the application with respect to other projects deemed priorities.

We studied seven analysis units on three levels: the MSSS (health and social services department), three regional agencies/boards, and a subregion within each of these regions. The regions are Mauricie and Centre-du-Québec, Estrie, and Chaudière-Appalaches. The three subregions are Bois-Francs, Sherbrooke, and Desjardins (Lévis). These subregions were selected for the following reasons: 1) They are comparable in that they are urbanized and have a full range of public institutions: general and specialized hospital center (hereafter, hospital), CLSC (local community service center), and RLTCC (residential and long-term care center). 2) They differ in the deployment of the mechanisms for coordinating services for the frail elderly: in Bois-Francs, an integrated services network was implemented in 1997. In Sherbrooke, implementation of this type of system has been underway since 2001, while none was in use in Desjardins in 2004.

Most of the material we collected was qualitative. Table 1.2 presents the breakdown of the 66 people that we interviewed according to tier and job category. At the local tier, there were four heads of community organizations and four physicians.

Table 1.2
Breakdown of respondents according to tier and job category

Job/Tier	Central	Regional	Local	Total
Senior management	–	7	11	18
Managers	5	–	11	16
Professionals	4	8	17	29
Researchers	–	1	2	3
Total	9	16	41	66

We also studied a massive amount of official records, reports, and minutes in each of our analysis units. On two occasions, we resorted to direct observation to better understand the dynamics of local cooperation.

Collection was carried out from fall 2002 to spring 2004 in the following sequence: Bois-Francs / Mauricie and Centre-du-Québec regional boards (fall 2002 and winter 2003), Sherbrooke / Estrie regional board (spring and summer 2003), Desjardins / Chaudière-Appalaches regional board (winter 2004 and spring 2004). We conducted interviews at the MSSS at different times (fall 2002, fall 2003, and spring 2004).

This material was analyzed according to three intersecting approaches. We began in each of the seven analysis units by reconstituting the context and chronology of the events related to integrating services for the frail elderly. In the case of the three local units, we also documented the type and operating method of the existing service integration system. We then categorized the material to bring out the overall nature of relations between the actors. Lastly, we broke down these materials according to integration dimension, which enabled us to highlight the focus of each.

Results

This section begins by presenting a summary of our observations on the local level. This is followed by a summary of our results pertaining to relations between the MSSS, the three regional agencies/boards, and organizations in the three subregions.

Subregion Dynamics

As for me, I think that all policies start at the grassroots level.

A professional with a regional board

In the mid 1990s, the three subregions offered a broad range of services for the frail elderly: long-term care, home care, short-term geriatrics unit (STGU), intensive functional rehabilitation unit, and others. Mechanisms for interorganizational liaison were also in effect at that time. These mechanisms aimed primarily at admission in RLTCC of patients who were hospitalized or living at home and at planning the return home of an elderly person. In the latter case, a hospital liaison officer (nurse or social worker) phoned or faxed information about the person's situation to a CLSC caregiver.

This coordination system entails some well-known limitations: the elderly must repeat their case histories to different practitioners, who change from one episode to the next. This negatively impacts on continuity of services, resulting in a person "dropping through the cracks," which means that the appropriate link between the two was not established. This often happens, for example, when a frail elderly person is staying in the emergency room. Nonetheless, this liaison model is suitable for individuals whose conditions do not require continuous care.

The three subregions approached improvement to the liaison model in two different ways: an enhanced liaison model (Desjardins) and an integrated services network (Bois-Francs, Sherbrooke). We will present both models; table three provides their main characteristics. It is important to realize that these two coordination systems are not mutually exclusive. Indeed, the integrated services network takes in the liaison model to which intensive coordination services are added and delivered by a case manager in the case of the elderly residing at home.

Enhanced Liaison Model

> *The CLSC [Desjardins] here is just great. The practitioners there see things like we do. They work fast, using the means they have, but they deliver good service at Desjardins.*
>
> A hospital social worker

The innovation at Desjardins consisted in improving the existing liaison system, either within an institution or between two partners.

CLINICAL INTEGRATION The manager at CLSC Desjardins responsible for home-care services divided his or her staff into multidisciplinary teams across four subterritories. At Hôtel-Dieu-de-Lévis, a new geriatrician set up a multidisciplinary team in the STGU. In both cases, these changes improved the management of the frail elderly, either in their homes or during their hospital stays. Good cooperation was also noted between CLSC staff and local partners: general practitioners in private practice, community organizations offering home-care services, and hospital liaison staff.

INFORMATIONAL INTEGRATION Information about an elderly person's situation is unidirectional from the hospital to the CLSC over an electronic interinstitutional services request system (DSIE).

Table 1.3
Two coordination systems for services to the frail elderly

Enhanced Liaison Model	Integrated Services Network
Clinical Integration	
Multidisciplinary home-care teams	Single entry point
CLSC and hospital liaison nurses	Team of case managers
Good collaboration with physicians	ISP use
	Relations between case managers and physicians
Informational Integration	
DSIE	SIGG
Normative Integration	
Within organizations (CLSC, hospital)	Consensus of executive directors on:
Leadership within organizations	• Prioritizing improvement of services to the elderly
	• Acting jointly in producing a solution
	Presence of visionary leaders
	Presence of researchers
Organizational Integration	
Formal hospital–CLSC and CLSC cooperative agreements	Directors' governing board
Unsystematic contact with executive directors	Horizontal and vertical coordination mechanisms connecting directors, managers, and the team of case managers
Financial Integration	**Intégration financière**
None	Financial agreements
	Common envelope for case management

Note: To make the table more user-friendly, the column describing the integrated services network does not duplicate the characteristics shared with the enhanced liaison model (such as multidisciplinary teams, STGU).

The CLSCs prioritize our systematic follow-up. [...] We always do it that way. There's no problem at all. Except the man who didn't break his hip and needs physiotherapy, because he won't be a priority. It could take 3 to 4 weeks. Sometimes they call back and say they've got no one, so it'll be 6 to 8 weeks before services can be provided. We see that as a break in continuity.

A hospital nurse

NORMATIVE INTEGRATION Except for certain problems with access to services at the CLSC-RLTCC Desjardins, our respondents stated that they were overall satisfied with the current method for delivering services to the elderly. As a result, the response to replacing the existing system with an integrated services network was lukewarm.

ORGANIZATIONAL INTEGRATION. In Desjardins, there is no executive directors' governing table. There are, however, protocols linking the CLSC and hospital for transferring clients to the CLSC for the systematic management of certain client groups and for the DSIE. Another protocol links the CLSC and cooperative that provides home-help services.

FINANCIAL INTEGRATION There are no formal agreements linking organizations in the territory.

Integrated Services Network

A more radical reform in organization of services for the frail elderly took place first in Bois-Francs and then in Sherbrooke. It consisted in setting up an integrated services network with the characteristics provided in Table 1.3 and described in greater detail elsewhere.[16, 17].

CLINICAL INTEGRATION Clinically, the creation of an integrated services network involves changing how services are coordinated. Indeed, it requires that an intraorganizational perspective to subordinate to an interorganizational and territorial perspective. Setting up a single-entry-point approach to take in requests from the elderly and their close relations, entrusting case managers to coordinate services provided to the frail elderly in the territory, progressive recourse to common assessment and planning instruments such as the individualized service plan (ISP) and the Multiclientele Assessment Tool (MAT) are means that affect, as a whole, the practitioners that provide services to the elderly.

In order for case managers to be able to play their role properly, it must be clearly defined and understood by the other practitioners, including physicians. Even if cooperation with general practitioners cannot be taken for granted, case managers have begun to forge links with some of them.

INFORMATIONAL INTEGRATION Operational efficacy of the integrated services network depends on the real-time availability of the user's clinical record. Doing so means implementing a computer system containing information about the individual's condition, the services received, and the medication taken that can be accessed by all authorized professionals. Designed with relatively modest means, the initial version of the gerontogeriatric computerized clinical chart (Système d'information géronto-gériatrique – SIGG) used in Bois-Francs was launched in 1998 and has been continually improved since then.[18] A more recent version of the SIGG was used when implementing the integrated services network in Sherbrooke.

NORMATIVE INTEGRATION How did these changes come about? Both in Bois-Francs and Sherbrooke, designing and implementing the integrated services network called for sustained coordination on the part of the heads of partner organizations and the intervention of agents of change capable of explaining the nature of such a network and convincing doubtful administrative and clinical stakeholders of its efficacy and feasibility. Understanding and buying into the integration model have indeed proven to be essential conditions of success in both subregions.

Given the scope of the changes entailed and the fact that they affect many organizations, their senior executives had to 1) assume collective responsibility for the service-organization issues in their territory, 2) recognize the shortcomings in the organization of services for the frail elderly, 3) make improving these services a priority, 4) have an overall solution to the problem, namely, an integrated services network, 5) take the time to adjust to and adapt the model, and 6) agree upon the model and accept to support the changes it entails in how their organizations operate.

> *The research yielded some sound practices that enabled us to develop a shared vision that broke down corporatism and individualism. [...] Once we committed to a shared vision supported by the researchers, it was like we were committed through somebody from outside who knew what to do, who wanted to support us, and that opened up some attractive possibilities for us.*
>
> An institutional executive director

The presence of agents of change appeared to be a determining factor in bringing about these conditions. These individuals, whether researchers, managers, or professionals, were able to directly change the perceptions of the other actors by 1) presenting research findings and experiences from other countries around the world, elsewhere in Quebec, or in the region and 2) guiding the change in a way that brought local actors to reflect upon what was happening.

ORGANIZATIONAL INTEGRATION

> *The challenge is joint responsibility, that is, joining the clinical with the administrative. Well, I am willing to be responsible, but, if a larger problem crops up, I just want some authority to be there to handle it. That would sure make things easier for me to provoke changes.*
>
> A case manager

If, in Bois-Francs and Sherbrooke, the consensus of the senior management of the institutions proved necessary to implement an integrated services network, these experiences also indicate that managers and caregivers must also offer their input. They also must have the time needed to buy into the model and to mold it to the actual conditions under which it would be used. Moreover, one of the keys to success of such undertakings lies with using vertical and horizontal coordination mechanisms that link the executive directors, middle managers, and case managers. Involving the caregivers and managers in the design and implementation of the integrated services network yielded a more robust system.

Dialogue is easy when money is not on the table.
Consensus of the members of an governing board for executive directors

FINANCIAL INTEGRATION At the time of the study, neither Bois-Francs nor Sherbrooke had financial integration for services for the frail elderly. In other words, there was no dedicated budget for this population segment administered by a single authority. In both these territories, however, interinstitutional financial agreements had been negotiated but not always without difficulty. The purpose of these agreements was primarily to entrust the case-management budget to a fiduciary institution. Yet, in the end, service integration took place without having to modify the rules for allocating budgets to the institutions.

The Role of Departmental and Regional Actors

This section begins with an outline of the context in which actors from the department and the regional agencies/boards operate. Then descriptions of their respective roles will be given according to five dimensions of integration.

MSSS CONTEXT

We're often not necessarily consistent across departments on how things are done or consistent from one case to the next.
An MSSS manager

MSSS actors work in a context that is both complex and changeable. The MSSS acts in multiple ways aimed at a large number of targets. In the case of services to the frail elderly alone, we can point to *Orientations ministérielles* (departmental policy directions), the creation of family-practice groups, home-care policy,[19] generalization of the MCAT, and policy directives on information systems and computerized clinical charts. These decisions must, in turn, fit into more general decisions about service organization and budget allocations within Quebec's health and social services system.

Beyond the intrinsic complexity in governing a vast health and social services system, however, there is a range of disturbances due to the system's public nature: Minister of Health and Social Service's dependancy on its party's commitments and government directions; vagaries of the economy and agreements with the federal government impacting on the province's revenue and, indirectly, on health-care budgets; sudden changes in priorities resulting from sporadic problems that make the headlines; lobbying by interest groups; criticism by the opposition; and so on. In addition, many changes in the department's leadership in the early 2000s and the fact that the leadership has to deal with other institutional actors from the central tier such as the Commission d'accès à l'information (access to information commission: confidentiality of clinical records), the Régie de l'assurance-maladie du Québec et Sogique (information systems and databases), and the Conseil du trésor (treasury board: budget authorizations) affect continuity in the department's actions.

Local and regional actors often reproached the department for its long response time, which also stem from two other phenomena: the most influential decisions in structuring the health-care system often take the form of a new bill or amendments to existing legislation. Recourse to legislative machinery requires considerable time and, as a result of its scope of action, always carried with it the risk of imposing changes that are inappropriate for certain contexts. Moreover, it must be noted that certain local or regional innovations overstep existing rules by the very fact of their novelty. In the long run, MSSS authorities must amend certain laws to accommodate these experiences and provide for them to be generalized. This is specifically the case when the purpose is to share the information in a patient's clinical record with caregivers working for different institutions or organizations.

Lastly, it would be misleading to view the department as a single institutional actor. The problems of compartmentalization and discontinuity of interventions occur not only between the MSSS and the institutional actors mentioned above, but also within the department itself. Despite the creation of departmental committees comprising representatives of the various administrative units, MSSS interventions often turn out to be inconsistent. This can be explained in part by the fact that these interventions arise from different branches, each of which with their own priorities and own means for carrying them out. This division of work within the department immediately gives rise to problems when implementing horizontal objectives such as integrating services for the frail elderly.

Context of the regional boards and agencies

When things are too top-down, you can't work with people.

A professional with a regional agency

Regional authorities find themselves in the awkward position of intermediary. As a result, they must deal concurrently with departmental expectations and requests from the institutions, community organizations, and physicians in their territories. Of course, the boards and agencies have planning and budget-allocation powers provided for in the Act respecting Health Services and Social Services. These powers, however, operate under institutional logic, making them subordinate to the Minister of Health and Social Services' authority. Moreover, while the boards and agencies have real financial means to support certain regional priorities, the funding remains limited because the lion share of their budgets goes to existing services.

In addition, the delegation of ministerial authority can fluctuate significantly depending on the management style of the incumbent. Since the turn of the century, the department has been recentralizing power following the adoption of the *Public Administration Act* and the so-called governance bill, which gives the minister the power to appoint the executive director of the regional board as well as most of the members of its board of directors. These legislative changes, inspired by the new public management, require the institutions and agencies/boards to give an accounting of the objectives stated in management agreements. In addition, the agencies/boards must be prepared to immediately respond to a significant number of demands by the MSSS for "states of the situation" about events that have captured media attention.

Given this context, management of the boards and agencies have a limited number of strategies to promote service integration once they have adopted this direction: impose a model for an integrated services network; provide economic incentives for local directors to put a certain integration of services model into place; support actors in each subregion in their territory in pursuing this objective; and adopt a laissez-faire position with respect to local actors. The support strategy predominated in our three agencies/boards, followed by the laissez-faire approach. While the second option opens the way to local innovation (Bois-Francs), the first one appeared to be the most appropriate for fostering change.

> *[Our position at the board was to say]: "Everyone can take whatever approach they want to implement the integrated services network as long as they take into consideration these major guidelines that experience has brought out."*

A professional from a regional agency

CLINICAL INTEGRATION We observed that departmental and regional actors intervened by creating and progressively implementing family-practice groups and by implementing a provincial training program on the multiclientele assessment tool.

INFORMATIONAL INTEGRATION The regulation of information systems in health and social services is strictly anarchistic. In other words, neither the MSSS nor any actor or group of actors can win acceptance of their concept of the instruments and information systems to be deployed. While the MSSS presented its policy directives on this topic[20] in 2001, for the most part, they have not been applied. On the one hand, rapidly changing technology, including widespread use of the Internet, has left some MSSS choices outmoded. On the other, the department is far from having the means needed to make its plans reality. Indeed, the issue for the MSSS is to put into place tools and information systems that 1) are highly secure, 2) are robust enough to be used on the provincial scale and for the largest number of user groups possible, and 3) achieve the dual outcome of facilitating clinician teamwork and yielding management data.

Since the MSSS does not have the means to deploy such systems, its fall-back strategy has mainly consisted in developing the health-care system's technological infrastructure—the health and social services telecommunications network (RTSS)—and to support (or tolerate, depending on the case) the various demonstration projects run by local "entrepreneurs." The SIGG—put into place in Bois-Francs—ranks among these local innovations. From the department's point of view, letting such projects flourish is a rational strategy because it enables its agents to have a better grasp of the conditions for success and usefulness of these experiences.

We're just stuck in a spiral where we can only say "Well, yes, it makes sense to carry out this experiment." But, we don't have money. Even for operating, do you think that we have the money to anticipate where we're coming down? So, we're captive to the dynamics of decision-making that is just simply beyond us. All we can do is look on intelligently.

An informant from the department

The MSSS's inability to tangibly follow through with its policy directives generates deep dissatisfaction among local actors, who want to improve SIGG functionality (Bois-Francs, Estrie) and regional actors who want to deploy it across their territory (Mauricie and Centre-du-Québec, Estrie). The department's wait-and-see policy is deemed in consistent with the priority given to integrating services in *Orientations ministérielles*. Paradoxically, local innovations related to the information system would undoubtedly never had seen the light of day if the MSSS had been able to implement a consistent province-wide information system.

NORMATIVE INTEGRATION The dissemination of *Orientations ministérielles* promoted implementation of integrated services networks, on the one hand, because the document offered a well-supported diagnosis of the issues related to organizing services for the frail elderly and outlined a logical solution for dealing with them. On the other hand, *Orientations ministérielles* gave a clear signal as to departmental priorities, prompting regional and local actors to make integration of services for the elderly a priority.

According to Kingdon,[15] three streams—problems, solutions, and policy—must be coupled for public problems to be put by authorities on their agenda. Recognition of the problem, the availability of an appropriate solution, and the political will of competent authorities to implement it must come together. The fact that the MSSS committed to integrated services networks was taken into account by regional and local directors. The signal influences each stream at the local and regional levels alike.

The impetus to set in motion integrated services networks can come from the local (Bois-Francs[17]), regional (Estrie[21]), or departmental (Chaudière-Appalaches[22]) levels. Certain local actors will innovate when there are no clear policy directives. These directives will nevertheless reassure them about their choices and encourage who have yet to act to modify their practices.

ORGANIZATIONAL INTEGRATION During the observation period, regional and departmental authorities promoted but did not impose a reduction in the number of institutions.

FINANCIAL INTEGRATION The prevailing trend at the MSSS and regional boards regarding funding is to increase budget equity between the regions and subregions. A method of allocation by client program[23] was progressively implemented. In recent years, the MSSS has also tended to specify how development budgets would be used.

Conclusion: Gleanings from Research and the Reform Underway

Since the data collection ended, MSSS authorities have launched a new reform of Quebec's health and social services system. Beyond the transformation of the regional boards into agencies, the reform made mandatory the creation of a new category of institutions vested with populational responsibility: the health and social services center (CSSS). This includes CLSCs, RLTCCs and, in many cases, a subregion hospital. This reform must pave the way to create local services networks linking CSSSs and public, private, and community partners. Moreover, it includes development of clinical projects, a dramatic reduction in the number of union certification units in each institution, and implementation of integrated university health networks.

It is still too early to form a clear idea of how these organizational modifications impact on the integration services for vulnerable groups, including the frail elderly. Yet, in the light of our study, we can draw certain lessons that would be useful in implementing the current reform in Quebec's health and social services sector.

GENERAL MESSAGE. Enhancing the integration of services for frail elderly people is an innovation that must be brought about locally. The success of this complex undertaking is not only contingent upon the willingness of local actors to collaborate but also upon the structuring decisions made at the regional and provincial levels. These decisions each deal with one of five dimensions of integration: normative, clinical, informational, organizational, and financial.

NORMATIVE INTEGRATION (NI) To achieve service integration, it is essential that affected actors understand and accept the integration model. Actors at all levels can help promote this model and change the way other actors view its practicality and relevance. This way, the involvement of credible and dedicated individuals (including researchers), the prioritization of service integration by senior executives, and the allocation of budgets by these executives to facilitate experimentation will make integration easier.

CLINICAL INTEGRATION (CI) This is the rationale for the other dimensions, as well as the dimension over which local actors have the most control. It is essential that actors at other levels allow them to adapt the service integration model to their specific context.

INFORMATIONAL INTEGRATION (II) is essential if the integrated services system is to operate smoothly. It is vital that the varying concerns of local and ministerial actors in this area be reconciled to build on experiments conducted in the field. It is also crucial that clinical concerns be taken into consideration when designing information systems and tools.

ORGANIZATIONAL INTEGRATION (OI). The integration of services according to territory requires a subregional governing body as well as vertical and horizontal coordination mechanisms linking senior executives, managers, and practitioners in partner organizations.

FINANCIAL INTEGRATION (FI) The shift from an institution-based approach to a population-based approach can be achieved more easily by combining the budgets required for coordination activities.

INTEGRATING DIMENSIONS As a rule, setting up a shareable clinical file (II), merging institutions, and the signing of protocols (OI), and budgeting based on client programs (FI) are conducive to clinical integration (CI). The effect of these measures, however, depends on the affected actors buying into them (NI). From this point of view, the current reform must not fall victim to a bureaucratic-based approach that would undermine the willingness of local actors to achieve this integration.

References

1. This chapter is a reworking of the research report by: Demers L, St-Pierre M, Tourigny A, Bonin L, Bergeron P, Rancourt P, Dieleman L, Trahan L, Caris P, Barrette H, Hébert A, Lavoie J. The Role of Local, Regional, and Ministerial Actors in the Integration of Services for Frail Elderly People. Research report. Canadian Health Services Research Foundation. 2005. This report is available at www.chsrf.ca/final_research/ogc/index_f.php.

2. Ministère de la Santé et des Services sociaux. Plan d'action 2005-2010 sur les services aux aînés en perte d'autonomie: Un défi de solidarité, Québec;2005.

3. Commission d'étude sur les services de santé et les services sociaux. Les solutions émergentes, Rapport et recommandations. Ministère de la Santé et des Services sociaux;2000.

4. Heenan D, Birrell D. The Integration of Health and Social Care: The Lessons from Northern Ireland. Social Policy & Administration. 2006;40 (1): 47-66.

5. Pineault R, Tousignant P, Roberge D. et coll. Collectif de recherche sur l'organisation des services de santé de première ligne au Québec: Rapport

synthèse. Direction de santé publique. Agence de développement de réseaux locaux de services de santé et de services sociaux de Montréal, Montréal;2005.

6. Leatt P, Pink G, Guerriere M. Towards a Canadian Model of Integrated Healthcare. Healthcare Papers. 2000;1 (2): 13-35.

7. Ministère de la Santé et des Services sociaux. Orientations ministérielles sur les services offerts aux personnes âgées en perte d'autonomie. Québec: 2001.

8. Contandriopoulos A P, Denis J L, Touati N. Intégration des soins: concepts et mise en œuvre. 2001. http://www.santemontreal.qc.ca/fr/observatoire/, site visited February 6, 2002.

9. Boelen C. Vers l'unité pour la santé, Défis et opportunités des partenariats pour le développement de la santé. Document de travail. Genève: Organisation mondiale de la santé;2001.

10. Reid R, Haggerty J, McKendry R. Defusing the Confusion: Concepts and Measures of Continuity of Healthcare. Final Report. Ottawa: Canadian Health Services Research Foundation ;2002: p. i.

11. Langlois A M, St-Pierre M, Bégin C. Les réseaux de services intégrés: possibilités, limites et enjeux. Dans: Lemieux V, Bergeron P, Bégin C, Bélanger G, ed. Le système de santé au Québec, organisation, acteurs et enjeux. Sainte-Foy: Les Presses de l'Université Laval;2003: 145-174.

12. Plochg T, Klazinga N S. Community-based Integrated Care: Myth or Must?. International Journal for Quality in Health Care. 2002;14 (2): 91-101.

13. Giddens A. La constitution de la société. Paris: PUF;1987.

14. Lemieux V. Les réseaux sociaux, Paris: PUF;1999.

15. Kingdon J W. Agendas, alternatives, and public policies. New-York: Harper Collins;1984.

16. Paradis M et al. Réseau de services intégrés aux aînés des Bois-Francs: Mécanisme de coordination des services géronto-gériatriques. Rapport de l'évaluation d'implantation et de processus. Québec;2001.

17. Tourigny A et al. Évaluation d'implantation d'une expérience novatrice: le réseau intégré de services aux aînés des Bois-Francs. Santé mentale au Québec. 2002;28(2): 109-135.

18. Tourigny A et al. Système d'information géronto-gériatrique interdisciplinaire et interétablissements: L'utilité perçue et utilisation en temps réel. Rapport de recherche. Québec: Unité de recherche en gériatrie de l'Université Laval;2003.

19. Ministère de la Santé et des Services sociaux. Chez soi: La politique de soutien à domicile. Québec;2003.

20. Ministère de la Santé et des Services sociaux. Orientations technologiques du réseau sociosanitaire. Document synthèse. Québec;2001.

21. Régie régionale de la santé et des services sociaux de l'Estrie. Réseau de services intégrés, ses principes, concepts et composantes. Document de travail. Sherbrooke: Direction de la santé publique et de l'évaluation;2001.

22. Régie régionale de la santé et des services sociaux de Chaudière-Appalaches. Illustration d'une diversité de conditions d'implantation d'un réseau de services intégrés (RSI) pour les personnes en perte d'autonomie (RSI-PPA), de cinq expériences diversifiées à un référentiel régional pour la région de la Chaudière-Appalaches. Direction de l'organisation des services, des affaires médicales et universitaires (DSAMU);2003.

23. Ministère de la Santé et des Services sociaux. L'architecture des services de santé et des services sociaux, les programmes-services et les programmes-soutien. Québec; 2004

Chapter 2
Assessment of the Degree of Implementation of Integrated Services Networks in the Three Estrie Experimental Sites

Anne Veil and Réjean Hébert

Hightlights

There are two benefits to designing and applying a method for measuring the implementation of the integrated services network's six components. First, it allows for ensuring that the results achieved are genuinely the product of a true and adequate implementation of the network's components. Second, it allows us to convey to managers and caregivers a picture of the progress made in their territories.

The monitoring grid was administered every six months and interim findings were published twice, the first time 18 months into the implementation process and the second time after three years. When the process was complete, Sherbrooke had a score of 85.2 %, Granit 77.6 %, and Coaticook 69.3 %. The overall score for the experimental zone thus stood at 77.6 %. The components with the highest results (90 % and over) were coordination, the single-entry point, and use of the SMAF and Iso-SMAF instruments, all of which attained excellent rates of implementation in Sherbrooke; and use of the CCC-SIGG in Granit. In Coaticook, no component had results higher than 90 %. The components that ran into difficulty, with results falling below 70 %, were ISP use and coordination in Granit and case management and ISP use in Coaticook.

Introduction

In conducting the implementation study on the integrated services network, we considered it of interest to specify the degree of implementation in the three regional municipal counties (MRCs) where implementation was regularly monitored. Monitoring the degree of implementation is important because the study on the impact of integrated networks on the health of the elderly must be able to ensure that the effects measured are the genuine results of a true and adequate implementation of each component. As well, the assessment grid makes it possible to routinely determine the progress of implementation activities and allows for the establishment of useful parameters for comparing the three experimental territories.

As a preliminary to measuring the degree of implementation, we postulated that implementation of the six components of the integrated services network would allow us to perceive tangible alterations in the supply of services to the elderly (as manifested in accessibility, continuity, and satisfaction with services), as well as in factors affecting the health of the elderly or their informal caregivers (functional autonomy, empowerment, work burden, and so on). Since the various components were not put into effect in the different territories at the same pace, and given the difficulty of implementing all of them at once, we viewed an overall result of 75 % as sufficient to produce a measurable impact on the elderly population.

Recall the six components of the PRISMA model: 1) coordination, 2) single entry point, 3) case management, 4) use of a shared assessment instrument for functional autonomy (SMAF [Système de mesure de l'autonomie fonctionnelle – functional autonomy measurement system], along with its companion instrument for comparing the profiles of the elderly with resource-intake profiles (Iso-SMAF Profiles), 5) use of the individualized service plan, and 6) the Computerized Clinical Chart (CCC).Measurement of the degree of implementation is thus based on indicators of implementation of these six components.

Method

We relied on relevant theories, those of program implementation and multiple-case study, to underpin the assessment procedure. Assessment of the degree of implementation was based exclusively on quantitative methods (statistics on target groups, patient records, instrument/tool use, and so on). The implementation study allowed for monitoring of the constituent elements of an integrated services network with a reference period of six months. Since the components were not implemented concomitantly with each other within territories and the three territories did not begin implementation at the same time, we deemed the date that case management, which stood in a central relationship to the other components, was put into effect to be the departure point for implementation. The comparability of the data across the three territories is thus subject to standardization of the time elapsed between data collections. A schedule for data collection was devised and was made known to the contact people in the three territories.

The resulting strategy for measuring implementation was put before a group consisting of experts in elder health, caregivers, managers, and research professionals. These individuals discussed, critiqued, and proposed improvements to the planned process, the assessment grid, and the weighting of the elements examined. [1-2]

The grid for measuring the degree of implementation was required to clear three hurdles:

1. Consensus must be reached on the components to be measured, which were to be described in terms of observable indicators subject to objectification; and consensus must be reached on their functional description.
2. Consensus must be reached first on the indicators' overall weighting and then their specific weighting.
3. There must be discussion and agreement regarding the measurement approach to be adopted.

All these stages were completed during January 2002. The measurement strategy had to be reliable regardless of the stage of implementation at which it would be applied. As well, its application needed to be simple to manage, since it was to be repeated at six-month intervals. Further, in order to avoid the pitfalls associated with assessment of the quality of procedures and activities, which would have required a more complex methodology, we were to focus on factors subject to objectification. The method of calculation, which was structured on the basis of the three mechanisms and the three instruments/tools that comprised the group of six components, imposed both an overall and an individual weighting for items, which was based on their relative significance.[1, 2]

Certain aspects of an integrated services network that have to do with professional and management relationships and practices were not taken into account in the monitoring of the degree of implementation, since they were viewed as conditions for the success of an integrated network rather than components of it.

Roles of the components of the integrated services network

In building the assessment gird, it was first necessary to determine what would constitute optimal implementation. Rather than limit ourselves strictly to the presence or absence of a given component, we opted to break down each component into its functions. Thus besides considering whether a certain structure had been put in place where necessary, we took into account the presence, partial presence, or absence of the functional aspects of each component. What follows is a functional description of the components.

Coordination (20 pts.)

Coordination played a strategic role in the implementation of change, because the players involved were so numerous and their professional and organizational affiliations so diverse (they belonged to public-sector home-care organizations, community groups, private enterprise, and the cooperative and collective economic sectors), as well as because of the issues raised around clinical and management practices. In exploring the degree of implementation of coordination, we treated the existence of a structure for coordination and its use by the players involved, with a focus on its role in providing systemic feedback, as the salient aspect. In examining this component, we dealt with factors such as players' representations of coordination, the stability of those representations over time, members' regular attendance at meetings of the coordination committee, information sharing about the integrated network at these meetings, and the adoption of a critical perspective on change in services to the elderly.

We define a critical perspective as a group process that expresses diverse levels of involvement, as illustrated by the decisions made. Coordination committees on services to the elderly had a role in bringing about change in services to the elderly. This role varied from territory to territory, since it had not been formally delimited and the coordination committees were given a degree of latitude in interpreting their mandates. Thus, in order to assess the degree of critical perspective operating within each committee, we relied on a method of modeling involvement levels.[3] These are the levels of involvement:

> Level 1: The committee sponsors activities that meet the needs of the target population (collaborative model).
> Level 2: The committee develops partners' degree of involvement in a common shared cause, which entails partners' taking ownership (mobilization model).
> Level 3: The committee contributes to effecting changes in the structure or functioning of one or more community action sectors, which implies the ability to influence both context and players, as well as partners' involvement in the action (social development model).

Single Entry Point (20 pts.)

The purpose of putting in place a single entry point for the elderly is to promote ease of access to services by enhancing referral of "the right person" to "the right place". The single entry point should also improve the nature of the information about public, community-based, and private services that is disseminated to the elderly, their family, and their caregivers, ensuring that this information is concentrated as opposed to dispersed, and that it is accurate and full as opposed to fragmented. As well, the single entry point should contribute to the process of triaging the vulnerable elderly by creating a point of convergence for all referrals and by the use of screening tools. In some cases, there could be telephone call back. In the performance of these functions, the qualified service providers at the single entry point would contribute to strengthening the links between elderly individuals and the services best suited to them.

Case Management (20 pts.)

To assess the degree of implementation of case management, we identified those aspects that are subject to objectification. The actual number of full-time equivalent (FTE) case managers was compared with the estimates that had been made on this score. (The procedure used may be consulted in Chapter 23 of this book.) When case management is not used as an intervention mechanism, a whole set of other factors will also be affected. A smaller number of elderly than intended will benefit from a comprehensive assessment of their circumstances based on the SMAF, from service coordination, and from individualized service plans (ISPs). The specific weighting assigned to the components of the SMAF and the ISP reflects this concern. The other aspect to be taken into account is the average caseload as compared with the recommended one, namely 45 for the first years of the experiment, gradually tapering to an average of between 40 and 45. Any deviation from this norm, whether by exceeding it or falling below it, incurs penalties, in that an excess of cases risks harming the entrenchment of the role of case management while a low rate reflects poor case-management penetration in the target group.

The ISP: A Specific Coordination Tool (10 pts.)

Case management constitutes a new professional role for which the ISP is the tailored tool for service coordination. This tool is specific to case management because the case manager is formally designated as the person responsible for ISPs and the systematic follow up they entail. For clients followed in case management, the expected norm for ISP fulfillment is 100 %. Regular monitoring in the three experimental territories made it possible to follow how many ISPs figured in the records of new clients registered for case monitoring over periods of six consecutive months. We only took into account whether an ISP was in place and not its precision nor the quality of its contents.

Computerized Clinical Chart (15 pts.)

Following an analysis of software with the potential for functioning within a system such as the health and social services network and for operating with the required kinds of information and degree of power, the Estrie region opted for the computerized clinical chart known as the CCC-SIGG, or just SIGG. (SIGG stands for Système d'information géronto-gériatrique, or gerontogeriatric information system, while CCC stands for Computerized Clinical Chart). This was put into use progressively in the various MRCs beginning in the spring of 2002. The proposal to adopt it had been passed by the executive directors of the Estrie health and social service institutions in December 2001. While implementing the SIGG presents numerous challenges, it nevertheless offers not just case managers but all the partners involved in the network of integrated services to the elderly a level of efficiency that cannot be gainsaid. The factors to be considered in assessing its level of use relate to installation of the software and workstations and the use made of these by the clinicians for whom they are intended.

SMAF and Iso-SMAF Profiles: Shared Instruments (15 pts.)

In contrast to the ISP, which is specific to case management, the objective for use of the assessment and needs-classification instruments known as SMAF and Iso-SMAF is that this use will extend to professionals from a variety of backgrounds working in different institutions and organizations, but serving the same users, who live with reduced independence. Use of these kinds of instruments by diverse partners and caregivers necessarily involves all these individuals in a process in which certain past gains are given up as new modes of operation are adopted. The use of shared instruments represents a key factor in keeping the network updated, since these instruments serve as a vehicle, or a common language, for professionals practicing in different fields to convey essential clinical messages to each other when they must coordinate an adjustment in their work. When vehicles of this kind exist in online form, the messages in question can be conveyed right away to all the professionals working with a given patient. In theory, this will prevent the duplication of assessments and interventions, as well as the numerous requests for patient history that the elderly and their family caregivers tend to encounter. The norm for use of the SMAF for the case-managed target group is 100 %.

Implementation of use of Iso-SMAF, the instrument for classifying and managing resources by profile, entails changing the methods of managing service supply and demand based on the key criterion of functional autonomy. Its primary function consists of drawing up the independence profiles of a given target group and relating these to resources' intake profiles, so that individuals living with disabilities are referred to the resources best suited to meeting their needs. A second function, whose importance should not be minimized, is to serve as a yardstick for funding services. The detailed assessment grid for the degree of implementation of this instrument was published in the first book on PRISMA.[1]

Findings on degree of implementation after three years

Interim findings on implementation were published at mid-point in all three territories, so that the policy makers, managers, and clinicians involved could get some sense of the order of magnitude of the degree of implementation for each component. Following a year-and-a-half of implementation, it was observed that coordination had attained a high degree of implementation in all three territories, that the single entry point was running into delays, and that case management too was lagging. Use of the ISP showed no stability over time: results were sometimes high and sometimes low. Overall, Sherbrooke and Coaticook scored 55.5 %, while Granit scored 63.4 %, mainly because it had been designated the pilot territory for SIGG first implementation, which gave it a head start. These interim findings were published in the first PRISMA book.[4]

The findings for the each territory after three years of monitoring are reported in Table 2.1. The cumulative score is 85.2 % for Sherbrooke, 77.6 % for Granit, and 69.3 % for Coaticook.

Table 2.1
Progress in degree of implementation in the three experimental territories

Monitoring period Sherbrooke	07/2001 %	01/2002 %	07/2002 %	01/2003 %	07/2003 %	01/2004 %	07/2004 %
Coordination (%)	93	93	91	91	76	90.5	90.5
Single entry (%)	0	0	50	80	85	85	90
Case management (%)	0	30.5	53	55	53	58.5	75
Use of the individual-ized service plan (%)	0	81	47	69	62	63	78
Use of shared assess-ment instruments (%)	40.7	88.7	80	88.7	88.7	92.7	93.3
Use of Computerized Clinical Chart (%)	0	0	0	20	76.7	82	82
Total (%) /period	**24.7 %**	**46.1 %**	**55.5 %**	**68.4 %**	**73.8 %**	**79.3 %**	**85.2 %**

Monitoring period Granit	07/2001 %	05/2002 %	11/2002 %	05/2003 %	11/2003 %	05/2004 %	11/2004 %
Coordination (%)	79	82.5	82.5	82.5	72.5	67.5	67.5
Single entry (%)	0	50	70	70	70	70	70
Case management (%)	0	67	67.5	63	76.5	90	89
Use of the individual-ized service plan (%)	0	65	50	50	66	58	57
Use of shared assess-ment instruments(%)	36	80	76.7	77.3	82.7	83.3	86
Use of Computerized Clinical Chart (%)	0	0	80	80	80	91.3	91.3
Total (%) /period	**21.2**	**58.4**	**72.5**	**71.7**	**74.8**	**77.5**	**77.6**

Monitoring period Coaticook	07/2001 %	05/2002 %	11/2002 %	05/2003 %	11/2003 %	05/2004 %	11/2004 %
Coordination(%)	63.9	76.5	86.5	86.5	85	86.5	86.5
Single entry (%)	0	50	70	70	70	70	70
Case management (%)	0	27	54	58.5	62.5	57	52
Use of the individuali-zed service plan (%)	0	62	59	53	13	100	41
Use of shared assess-ment instruments (%)	35.3	77.3	78.7	76	87.3	87.3	83.3
Use of Computerized Clinical Chart (%)	0	0	80	80	80	70.7	73.3
Total (%) /period	**18.1**	**48.5**	**71.8**	**71.7**	**69.9**	**76.4**	**69.3**

The components that emerged as high scorers (over 90 %) were not the same across territories. In Sherbrooke, coordination, single entry, and use of the SMAF and Iso-SMAF instruments scored very high. In Granit, use of the CCC-

SIGG scored highest of all components. In Coaticook, no component scored as high as 90 %.

Components that scored between 70 % and 89 % were case management, use of the ISP, and use of the CCC-SIGG in Sherbrooke; case management, the single entry, and use of SMAF and Iso-SMAF in Granit; and coordination, the single entry point, and use of SMAF and Iso-SMAF in Coaticook.

Sherbrooke did not score low (defined as lower than 70 %) for any component; Granit did for ISP use and coordination; and Coaticook did for case management and ISP use. The overall low rates of implementation for ISP use were drawn to the attention of management right from the earliest data collection (when interim findings were compiled). This contributed to the development of a research project led by Dr. Dominique Somme; its findings appear in Chapter 9 of this book. Initial findings from the study were published in the first volume on PRISMA.[5] These emerged from a review of the literature and enabled a reflection on the concept of the ISP and the use made of it. With the second phase of the research project, it was possible to investigate case managers' perceptions of the true usefulness of this tool and then go on to conceptualize an online tool far more focused on assessing clients' needs as well as being more user friendly and dynamic. This new conception allows for adjusting the ISP to suit changes in client needs or resource capacities. The revised ISP version was not available as of 2006, however, because work was in progress across Quebec to create an online version of it. Case managers are disinclined to use a tool they perceive as being of little use, static, and rigid. These factors may partly account for the poor results for ISP use in two out of the three territories. Another aspect of the situation may be that the workload was especially heavy in these territories, where clients are never placed on waiting lists. This leaves little time for the performance of tasks viewed as being essentially administrative and having no clinical usefulness. The ISP's current form, as integrated into the SIGG, undoubtedly did not help, since it entailed writing/reading many lines and columns of text.

In Granit, coordination scored low mainly because the initial dynamic commitment of members of the territory's coordination committee gradually changed. The committee shifted from being a catalyst and prescribing expected service-quality standards to a remote observer of faster or slower progress in implementing the various components. Setting up an advisory committee responsible for monitoring implementation relieved the coordination committee of some of its responsibilities vis-à-vis the integrated network.

Finally, case management scored low in Coaticook because insufficient human resources were assigned to undertake it and few clients were registered for it during its first years of implementation. Case managers in this territory carried mixed caseloads: elderly with mildly, moderately, and heavily reduced independence; clients with short-term needs alongside clients with long-term needs; palliative-care clients; and handicapped people. It proved very difficult for them to develop a new approach, because they could not really see how case management differed from what they were already doing and the lacked the time and the opportunity to reconsider their practices, especially with respect to services at the regional level.

The Progress of Implementation in the Experimental Zone

After three years, overall, the experimental zone, consisting of these three territories, attained a 77.6 % implementation level. Table 2.2 reveals that there has been a steady progression over the years. After one year of implementation (that is, in July or November 2002, depending on the territory), it reached 66.6 % implementation. This rose to 72.8 % the following year and reached 77.6 % on completion of Year 3.

Table 2.2
Yearly progress in overall degree of implementation in the experimental zone

Monitoring period	Time 0 07/2001	After 1 year 07-11/2002	After 2 years 07-11/2003	After 3 years 07-11/2004
Sherbrooke	24.7 %	55.5 %	73.8 %	85.2 %
Granit	21.2 %	72.5 %	74.8 %	77.6 %
Coaticook	18.1 %	71.8 %	69.9 %	69.3 %
Average for the whole experimental zone	21.3 %	66.6 %	72.8 %	77.6 %

In the more rural territories, the pace of progress slowed following the steep climb of the first year of implementation. In Sherbrooke, on the other hand, the slower pace of progress that marked the first stages remained steady until the end of the monitoring period. This contrast between Coaticook and Granit on one hand and Sherbrooke on the other was to be expected. The components that were easier to implement were put into effect early on, when participants' motivation was high. In Sherbrooke, the network's complexity (owing to the number and diversity of services and the nature of their distribution) entailed a significant degree of restructuring, which required more time. In this regard, less populous settings have an advantage. There are fewer players to be brought together for coordination and change can occur more rapidly. On the other hand, implementing use of the individualized service plan was harder in these settings and ultimately leveled off, largely because case managers, its main users, saw little usefulness in it and because ISP data entered in the SIGG by other caregivers in the network were too rarely consulted.

Discussion

Our observations on the ground and our regular measurement taking lead us to conclude that, considering the difficulties encountered during implementation, all three territories achieved impressive results. In particular, the funding was lacking that would have been required to assign the human and material resources needed to reach the target levels suggested by the research team. The number of FTE personnel necessary for case management and, in the rural setting, for maintaining the reduced caseload level of 45 was not provided. Besides this, home-care services in Quebec remained underfunded in relation to the increasing level of need in the population of the frail elderly, which did not make case managers' task any easier. In a difficult climate, managers and clinicians made significant efforts to reach the implementation objectives set for the integrated services network for the elderly on their territory.

References

1. Veil, A., Hébert, R. Évaluation du degré de mise en œuvre d'un réseau de services intégrés pour les personnes âgées en perte d'autonomie. Dans Hébert, R., Tourigny, A., Gagnon, M. Intégrer les services pour le maintien de l'autonomie des personnes. EDISEM Québec, 2004: 125-134.

2. Hébert, R., Veil, A. Monitoring the degree of implementation of an Integrated Delivery System. International Journal of Integrated Care, 2004; vol. 4 (September): 1-11. ISSN 1568-4156 (www.ijic.org).

3. Lebeau, A., Vermette, G., Viens, C. Bilan de l'action intersectorielle et de ses pratiques en promotion de la santé et en prévention des toxicomanies au Québec. 38 – Collection Études et analyses. Gouvernement du Québec, Ministère de la Santé et des services sociaux, Direction générale de la planification et de l'évaluation. 1997, 102 pages.

4. Veil, A., Hébert, R. Interim process evaluation of the implementation of integration mechanisms and tools for frail older people experiencing functional decline in three eastern townships sub-regions (Québec). In Hébert, R., Tourigny, A., Gagnon, M. Integrated service delivery to ensure persons' functional autonomy. EDISEM, Québec, 2005: 73-116.

5. Somme D., Hébert, R., Bravo, G., Blanchard, F. Individualized service plan (ISP) concept and utilization: a review of experiments on integrated services for the elderly in Québec and elsewhere. In Hébert, R., Tourigny, A., Gagnon, M. Integrated service delivery to ensure persons' functional autonomy. EDISEM, Québec, 2005: 273-290.

Chapter 3
Results of Service Integration: Perceptions of Managers and Service Providers

Anne Veil and Réjean Hébert

Highlights

In order to determine the opinions of key actors involved in implementing the integrated services network for the elderly about how effectively it was put into place, evolved, and functioned, we met with more than 75 people in individual or group interviews focused in the three territories in the experimental area in Estrie.

Synthesizing the analysis of this information revealed that the six components had been implemented, but that certain of them were not functioning optimally. The obstacle that stood out as a predominating factor among those raised by the interviewees as a whole was the inadequacy of resources, both human and financial. The facilitating factors raised relate to aligning the change along three levels of action or authority (decision-making, management, and clinical) as well as the leadership evidenced at the local and regional levels. The managers and practitioners perceive a change in the paradigm occurring on the heels of the integrated networks. In other words, the health and social services network is becoming aware of the importance of its elderly patients and their needs related to frailty and chronic disease, of the predominance of long-term care and services, and the choices that this trend imposes on service organization and professional practices. Services are being increasingly organized within a framework of partnership between public, private, and community providers of a large range of health, rehabilitation, and social services.

This new awareness of the needs of the elderly and their increasing numbers has created room for change in how the providers interact. Indeed, they are now aware that interdependent partner support is necessary to effectively help solve the complex problems of the frail elderly while, at the same time, striving to avoid or postpone their institutionalization.

> Despite the staff shortage, marked by difficulties in accessing basic services, managers and practitioners remain convinced of the value of the integrated network model. Moreover, they tell us that the model could be applied elsewhere, since it is relevant to the problems experienced in the field. While the criticism that the trail hadn't been blazed was occasionally raised, the interviewees felt that they had sufficient time and room to take ownership of the model and for the local territories to make it their own.

Introduction

The study for implementing mechanisms and instruments for integrating services was monitored over three years in the three territories in the experimental area. This process including participation as observer on governing boards, collecting data from information systems (I-CLSC and SIGG) to discover, on one hand, to what extent the six components of the integrated network had been implemented (degree of implementation) and, on the other, to find out if the main functions of the mechanisms and instruments were observable. Consequently, statistics on use of the single entry point and screening for functional decline were inventoried; descriptions of structures and dynamics of participation on the governing board were produced; surveys of interventions and patients under case management made it possible to determine that the professional activities of case managers actually reached the target groups; and SIGG data brought to light the main users of the computerized clinical chart. The results of these follow-up activities on implementation progress were presented in an interim report[1] (formative assessment) drafted especially for policy-makers and the heads of the three territories. It provided them with objective data to guide their decisions about the efforts to be put into deploying or aligning any of the components. Presentations on the interim results as well as the final outcomes after three years of follow-up were given during conferences. This chapter represents the state of things at the end of this process, when the actors looked back on what had been accomplished, what facilitated matters, and what difficulties were encountered.

Methodology

An embedded multiple case study[2] is indicated as an assessment method when: 1. the boundaries between the phenomenon and its context are not clearly identified; 2. the study of the context variables are appropriate for understanding the phenomenon; and 3. the relevant behaviors being studied cannot be manipulated or controlled. We opted for an embedded multiple-case study to examine implementation because all three conditions were met. Based on the nature of the study objectives, we decided on a mixed method. The quantitative aspects were presented in an interim report and in Chapters 5, 6, and 7 of the first

PRISMA book[3]. Other quantitative information is presented in Chapters 2, 4, 6, and 23 herein. In this chapter, our interest lies with qualitative elements.

Interviewees were identified in two ways. The group of policy-makers and managers consisted of key position holders: executive directors of institutions and community organizations, heads of professional services and nursing departments, heads and administrative managers of services for the elderly, and head nurses for specialized services (geriatrics, intensive rehabilitation, day hospital). On the clinical side, group interviews (four in Sherbrooke and one in each rural territory) brought together social-service professionals, nurses, rehabilitation practitioners, and community workers that were identified either by case managers from a list of their main spokespersons or because of their positions in key services, such as the single entry point, long-term services, and specialized services. This sampling was designed to achieve the highest degree of representation possible of the continuum of services for the elderly. The interviews were audiotaped and transcribed verbatim, and analyzed by synthesis. The basic structure of the interviews dealt primarily with their perception of implementation, the operation of the six components of the integrated services network, and the aspects that facilitated or impeded implementation of the integrated network. In addition, they were asked to provide their assessment of whether other regions would benefit from implementing the integrated network model, based on their three years of experience (generalization). The process took a summative perspective, which, in other words, means taking a position on the potential of generalizing integrated services networks for the elderly with respect to the model's efficacy. For the purposes of the implementation study, efficacy basically takes in accessibility, continuity, and integration of services as perceived by the actors. Since each territory had some leeway for taking ownership of or buying into the various components to maximize the chances of sustainability (transfer logic), generalization, in this instance, pertains solely to the components as a whole and their synergy, even if the appropriation process gave rise to initiatives of interest in the three territories.

Results

We present the results by territory so as to not conceal the specificities reported for each of them. We group the statements of policy-makers and upper and middle managers because they are convergent, on one hand, and those of the various practitioners, on the other, because they concern clinical aspects.

Sherbrooke Managers

Although joint action has been undertaken with the public, community, and private institutions subject to an agreement as a whole, they do not all have the same involvement in the problem or direct interests respect to the planned change. Some are therefore actively involved in the process without receiving an immediate, direct benefit from the changes. For example, the Centre de réadaptation de l'Estrie shares a limited number of frail elderly people with its partners. Partners share basic values so that *"the actors work as a single team,"* despite the fact that the efforts during initial years focused on managing interfaces. The integrated services network model in Estrie provided an opportunity to develop a structure. It now remains to fine-tune clinical management, using typical clinical-management models that could be disseminated among partners and in which each would have definite roles, in particular with cognitive problems and other chronic diseases. Implementing the SIGG[a] computerized clinical chart provided an opportunity to gain familiarity with the new confidentiality rules specific to computerized systems for transferring clinical information.

The CHUS[b], a regional institution with a staff of 5000 providing general and specialized care, feels that it has established a closeness in discussions and shared common concerns about the problems experienced by the partners. Yet knowledge about the concept of "integrated network" and about what case management and SIGG can contribute on the short term has remained limited. Many CHUS providers are unaware of how the integrated network can help them in organizing care. SIGG access is restricted to social workers and nurses on the geriatrics team. While emergency-department staff does not consult very often, it was pointed out that slowness in accessing the regional network discouraged certain users from the outset. The CHUS's prime interest in participating in joint action is that community partners would be taking greater charge of the elderly, who were spending too much time in acute-care beds once medical intervention had been completed. The work carried out resulted in a "clear improvement," although work remains to be done. As for case managers (CMs), the CHUS noted their presence in the emergency department and units. CMs are invited to talk about the nature of their contribution and role. CHUS staff shares their concerns and expectations with CMs, which should allow for closer ties based on better mutual understanding. In the case of large organizations such as the CHUS, there should have been more people under case management so that the true impact would have been evident: *"It's like a drop in the ocean."* Indeed, it makes it difficult for the medical staff to see and feel any impact without a significant volume of managed cases. It was also observed that not all CMs had the same perception of their role and that the CHUS social workers remained apprehensive about CMs infringing on their area. Even if each organization were attempting to improve the system, *"without a regional mechanism, the patient is the one who would suffer."* The CHUS made a beginning in case-finding for frailty among emergency-department patients using PRISMA-7. At the outset, the CLSC was apprehensive about being swamped with referrals, but the increase was actually gradual. On the other hand, case-finding for frailty is also

---

a   SIGG: Gerontogeriatric computerized information system
b   CHUS: Centre hospitalier universitaire de Sherbrooke

useful in the institution, since geriatrics nurses will be involved more quickly in the case when an elderly person is screened and hospitalized. This often allows them to suggest management by the geriatrics team. This networking gives rise to apprehensions about increasing the caseload of geriatricians, who are already in short supply. Nevertheless, more organized screening in the emergency department would make it possible to determine whether or not the traffic is due to repeat visits by the same individuals. Other parts of the hospital could also be used to screen for the frail elderly (pre-surgery clinics, ophthalmology, etc.). There is not necessarily a consensus at the CHUS on screening in the emergency department, but mentalities must change. People are impressed when this case-finding reveals that the elderly person is in case management, which authorizes rapid intervention by the CM and increases the chances of the CM having an impact on the length of stay. Despite this proof of CM responsiveness, interviewees wonder about the alleged caseload of case managers, especially when they want to have more people receiving case management. On the interorganizational level, the CHUS and CLSC[c] are working on a shared management instrument. These initiatives will foster confidence and help identify problems, rather than having everyone consulting statistics on their own.

At the SGUI,[d] generally speaking, interviewees feel that they have moved beyond the starting concepts to actual case management. They also stated that certain issues that appear quite difficult initially, such as the SIGG, had finally become realities. The SIGG has been completely implemented and training on Iso-SMAF profiles is moving forward, despite the fact that few people feel completely at ease using them. Long-term care physicians, with some exceptions, are not very familiar with the profiles. After the merger of the CLSC and SGUI, discussions were initiated about sharing information and processing requests, in particular, for temporary placement, and alternative placement. When working as a network, decisions such as closing placement beds must take into consideration the impact on partners: *"(...) our concern isn't just within the institution ... now it's a system."* Managers must therefore adjust their roles and help make their staff more aware of obligations throughout the continuum of services. Based on experience with using Iso-SMAF profiles in order to determine the resource that the individual should be referred to (e.g. profiles 10 and higher to a CHSLD[e] and profiles 6 to 9 to an intermediate resource[f]), it appears that we need to *"look beyond the profile"* and then take into account professional clinical judgment. The majority of practitioners share this viewpoint, decrying the current use of Iso-SMAF profiles as cut-and-dried and categorical. The profile is no longer a decision support tool: it's the decision

---

c   CLSC: Local Community Service Center
d   SGUI: Sherbrooke Geriatric University Institute
e   CHSLD: Residential and long-term care center
f   IR: Intermediate Resources

itself. Given the shortage of home-care resources, people arrive at the CHSLD in a state of distress and exhaustion. Currently, resources come from within the system itself, so we are taking from one hand and giving to the other. If no resources are allocated to development, the network cannot achieve maximum performance. The waiting list for geriatric evaluation, alternative placement, and physiotherapy were brought up. Despite these difficulties, there is much that case managers can do to support families. There were also interesting results for the day hospital and day-care center, which are working together to clarify roles, strive to avoid duplication of assessments, and to better direct the elderly within the respective services. More must be done to make practitioners and clinicians at the hospital more aware of the geriatric approach as well as the constraints under which staff must work in a CHSLD. Each week, the DNC,[g] CHUS, and SGUI nursing departments meet together. A lunch was recently organized with clinicians in order to share common concerns such as managing infections in both institutions. *"I'm just so pleased with that!"* What still lacks visibility is cooperation with physicians in private practice. Other initiatives are described in order to compare how an IFRU[h] works with the SIGG compared to the single entry point (SEP) assessment team and also between the single entry point and case management. This is done in an effort to tie things together more closely, target the most important issues for both teams, and use the same clinical language. An example of this would be the way that the two departments interpret an emergency, high-demand cases, and caregiver exhaustion. At the same time, the bureaucracy was reviewed with a view towards streamlining it. The IFRU had the expectation that the SEP would improve information returns about the management of patients referred to home care—particularly the waiting time for the requested services *"to take that responsibility off of us."* This is important in rehabilitation because maximum recovery occurs in the first three months following a stroke. In this context, any delays must be monitored.

With respect to information systems, there is a desire for all tools and instruments to be computerized for all patients and that hardcopy use be avoided. Yet since members of the clinical teams have different levels of skill in keyboarding and using computers, software user-friendliness is an important consideration. Improving the transfer of the clinical information already available in the SGUI specialized services would be of even greater help in home care. Having less than full coverage with all computer tools means that certain information is not conveyed. When an individual at the day hospital comes under case management, the change in status is more difficult to manage with the SIGG because it involves migrating from the local server to the regional server or from hardcopy to the regional SIGG. Information falls through the cracks during the transition. Moreover, the sharing of offices and computer

---

g   DNC: Director, nursing care
h   IFRU: Intensive Functional Rehabilitation Unit

workstations as well as examination rooms without computers imposes some limitations. It means that information must be transcribed from hardcopy to electronic form, which is an unnecessary duplication. The same kind of bond with CHUS practitioners would be of interest but, for the time being, difficult to carry out due to organizational scope. While the real gain experienced by the day hospital and the IFRU was achieved through the use of common instruments, consultations between partners are very important in terms of joint action *"so that people feel involved in the change."*

The CLSC is the most central organization from the standpoint of putting into place case management and single-entry-point mechanisms, especially because of the positioning of its primary-care mission. Although case managers were first located along the periphery of CLSC facilities in order to clearly show their interorganizational role, this approach was reconsidered after a while. On one hand, the case-management model was revised (unique to mixed). On the other, many of the oldest institutions were merged, which facilitated clinical integration and made the physical location of case managers less critical. Moreover, primary-care providers were hoping to be grouped with the area teams with a view to improved overall functioning. Managers feel, however, that it would be better to maintain a dedicated team of case managers, given the catchment population. Once these arrangements had been completed, CLSC upper management felt that the difficulties had been smoothed out and that case management was being increasingly accepted by the actors as a whole and seen as a major player in the network. *"It's an advantage."*

Work is still needed on the ISP.[i] Indeed, this tool has not been accepted into the culture; some state that it is unwieldy in design and use. The ISP did not receive the required support: the concept lacked clarity and training; the tool still needed some work. The Ministère de la Santé et des Services sociaux and its scientific committee has undertaken to bring this tool to a state that would respond to the needs of CMs and practitioners as a whole. As a result, they will make greater use of it on the SIGG if it is clearer and more representative of the current state of services delivered to patients. Recently, about 15 physicians from a medical clinic requested ISPs for their patients in case management. While the need is clearly present, the instrument does not yet meet expectations. The single entry point is increasingly evolving towards a single-access system, since there is always more than one possibility for accessing services in larger cities. Yet there is now a clear process defining the course through and registration with the network. Joint-action mechanisms were marked by the initial coexistence of several institutions involved in separate missions (one hospital, two CLSCs, and five CHSLDs) and several private and community partners. With the computer and communication system managers in the integrated network have given themselves, *"not a manager in Sherbrooke feels that he or she*

---

i   ISP: Individualized Service Plan

is working in isolation; they are jointly responsible for a network. I'm fairly convinced of that." Private partners were the most difficult to insert into the joint-action structure (physicians, pharmacists, and private homes), but the conditions are not easy for these actors, who are called on to go outside of their prime sphere of activity: serving their clients. In the case of physicians, valuable links were forged with the DRMG[j]. It would have been helpful to sustain the interest of certain physicians by, for example, having a remuneration system with provisions for invoicing a certain number of hours every month for taking part in a network and attending multidisciplinary meetings. The issue for pharmacists revolves mainly around networking the information and the technical capacity of installing the SIGG in community pharmacies outside of the RTSS[k] network. *"We need to break ground on this issue."*

While the SIGG has been set up in all public services, the ideal situation would be to extend it to FMGs (family-medicine groups) and private doctor offices. The SIGG and Iso-SMAF profiles are now currently used for home services: people understand and know what they can get out of it. Since not everyone is entering data in the SIGG, its content is less than optimal. Many clinical contributors (CHUS, day hospital, etc.) perform SMAF and MCAT[l] assessments without entering the results in the SIGG. Case managers, on the other hand, use the SIGG to the utmost and more than 500 patients have been put in the system. The single-entry-point assessment team uses the SIGG on a laptop, which is a major step forward. The concurrent use of hard copy and an electronic instrument is not a winning situation. The existence of another electronic issue (diagnostics and laboratories on Ariane[m]) requires an interface with the SIGG. It would be very formative to put other types of clinical assessments on the SIGG. To illustrate, having protocols for cognitive disorders could support the relationship of trust and cooperation between services, the management framework would be shared, and the convergence of interventions assured. Using such shared instruments for assessing and classifying needs creates a shared clinical language and reference schemes. When used in larger-scale operations, such as assessing the profiles of all the individuals in the placement group, it yields very rich information with a new analysis potential. It brings out the number of profiles with cognitive, physical, or mixed impairments within an institution. It further becomes apparent that the profiles, although used for service financing purposes, fail to take into account the health problems that require intensive medical or nursing management. Managers consider that this represents an initial phase in interpreting longitudinal data about individuals living in an institution. Not all is clear yet, but the results are very interesting.

---

j   DRMG: Regional department of general medicine
k   RTSS: Health and social service telecommunications network
l   MCAT: Multiclientele Assessment Tool
m   Ariane: CHUS computer system

While many partners subscribe to the Ministry guidelines on integrated networks, some professional practices have been changed. Moreover, several managers are skeptical, not about joint action and coordination yielding visible benefits, but about using the MCAT in certain contexts. Clarity seems to be lacking for the managers who would like to implement the integrated network on the basic model alone; guidelines were progressively implemented as work advanced in the territories. Nevertheless, the model is viewed as being quite valuable: 1- the elderly must be taken care of in the community; 2- when the loss of independence is significant, the single entry point detects it and, since it is linked to front-line care in the community, management within the continuum is assured; 3- screening can also be carried out in hospital emergency departments as well as in the vaccination clinics so that the vulnerable elderly can be referred to the CLSC component for an overall assessment of their situation and, if needed, be referred to case management. The simpler the criteria, the easier it is to make the process systematic. This is what was done in Sherbrooke when the access criteria for case management were simplified (Iso-SMAF profiles 4 and greater). The traditional CLSC procedure is that a practitioner responds to a request and then closes the file. Operating from the concept of management within a continuum leads to another way of doing things in which the CM and family physician form a tandem with which caregivers can be associated. We also know that STGU[n] and day-hospital patients must be linked to case management, since the average SMAF values in these services indicate a significant loss of independence. If practitioners make little reference to case management, it's because private homes and families fulfill most of the needs. In reality, however, the individual still has significant disabilities and professionals must assume responsibility for the need for long-term management, since neither private homes nor the family are responsible for continuity. Many network practitioners have gone further than hoped for in terms of avoiding duplication. Nevertheless, the clinical component must continue to move towards harmonization of clinical practices. The model with its six components, which are indissociable from one another, can be exported. The remainder *"takes on the color of the territory."* The only thing that was proposed is to add a 7th component to the model pertaining specifically to family physicians. They have completely different organizational methods that require specific incentives. The advent of specific medical activities should make it easier to deal with complex cases. It is also important for remuneration to be adjusted to the type of medical intake required for the elderly. Two physicians currently serve on the management committee in order to bring the medical perspective to network management.

In Sherbrooke, a number of indicators of interesting results was raised: 1- The service offer is adapted to needs; 2- Resources have been increased, espe-

---

n   STGU: Short-term Geriatric Unit

cially in intermediate resources, where Sherbrooke was experiencing a shortfall (*"This represents a major gain."*) 3- Before putting our mechanisms in place, an average of 60 people were awaiting placement in short-term beds. This number dropped to below 10 people and recently to an average of 4.7 people, while the response for management clearly improved and the waiting time at home before placement did not increase. 4- More people have home-care services. 5- The circulation of information among partners has improved, although it is not yet perfect. 6- Screening is carried out in CHUS emergency departments and at vaccination clinics. 7- The SIGG is being used increasingly and staff members now talk in terms of patient profiles. 8- Joint action and coordination has been maintained. Over the years, access has improved to better, reliable, and current data for discussions between partners. There remains to examine the methods for instituting 24/7 medical services and to promote communication with the emergency departments. Attention is also being given to the possibility of allowing elderly people leaving the hospital to have access to a place of convalescence so that they can take advantage of a setting conducive to recovering their independence, which would prevent potentially precipitous placement in a CHSLD. There is also a desire to form an assessment team based in the emergency department or to establish a linkage between the emergency-department triage and the single-entry-point team. All in all, the return on investment is real: *"I'm convinced, but it still has to be proven, which is not easy ... the real integrated network will come into existence when everyone is connected."*

At the outset, there were two private CHSLDs with public agreement. Since then, one has closed and the public CHSLDs have merged. The road has been rather rough for the private CHSLD with public agreement. When the public network was going through turbulent times, transition beds were opened, which has relieved some of the pressure on the public network. Seeing as how they were involuntarily committed to a subcontracting relationship with the public network, the private CHSLDs subject to an agreement felt that their efforts were not always adequately appreciated. All things considered, they had no power or influence over the situations to which they had to quickly adjust. Their perception is that they provide quite a bit of support to the network without receiving much in return. In addition, they have to constantly hire and fire staff, which is hard on employees. The private CHSLD subject to an agreement lies along the periphery of public institutions, which are the core actors. It sees itself as being small and not having the same problems to solve as the big players. The difficulty of working in concert with smaller actors should give rise to other consultation methods, such as using the multidisciplinary team models with respect to the family, in which information is exchanged before and after team discussions. This would allow representatives of the elderly, private homes, and their practitioners to participate more fully in the decision-making process. Because it enjoys a closeness with its patients and their families, the private CHSLD is sensitive to imposed relocations from one institution to another depending on the bed situation and the public system as well as patient's independence status as represented in the Iso-SMAF profile. Managers questioned the funding guidelines for services based on profiles, while no account is taken, for example, of an individual's difficulty in swallowing or the specific nursing care required. The profile indicates that the individual requires assistance, but not how much resource time is required to fulfill the specific need. Financing on this basis remains a concern, yet it does not prevent them from appreciating the mechanism for accessing local placement, whose functioning based on profiles has the merit of creating categories and refining the lists. They consider that implementing case management would be the ideal approach to accompanying the elderly person through the maze of the network, *"which is not a luxury."* It appears that the elderly living in private homes (some 3000 individuals in Sherbrooke alone) lack supervision. Their caregivers are in no way integrated into the network and the reflex to turn to the emergency department remains. The private CHSLD would have appreciated having the SIGG in their institution for the use of physicians coming in to see their patients (and interface with the CHUS's Ariane system would be worthwhile) and for managers in calculating patient profiles. This return on their investment in the network was never offered to them.

A general practitioner opting for elderly patients reported that case management is a major element for the elderly and their families, claiming that it can make the difference in continuity of services: *"Yes, yes, I'm convinced of that."* Having a dedicated CM provides the means for going beyond the difficulty of CLSC practitioners availability. They are *"people with an extremely high workload who do nothing but respond to an acute demand. ... It's clear to me that the integrated network is a necessity. In no way am I calling that into question."* Administrative mergers do not solve the problem of accompanying the vulnerable elderly through the network. The realignment of the CM model, which transitioned from the single role model to a mixed model was fortunate. It could be applied to other vulnerable target groups such as mental health, physical impairment, and chronic diseases with which there is a significant continuity problem and where *"we continually duplicate."* Awareness of the CHUS's situation with respect to other partners, certain of whom believed (and some still do) that the hospital is like an *"open bar."* While attitudes are changing, the changes in spokespersons, particularly on the management level, is not helping matters.

The single entry point is comprised of a multidisciplinary team of professional practitioners who receive all requests for services for the elderly and who go into the home to carry out MCAT assessments for the purposes of service allocation. Since this is a time of curtailed access to services due to operating difficulties, single-entry-point practitioners often find themselves between a rock and a hard place. Despite these conditions, *"I believe in it. We have to keep moving forward. The change is really big, but it is truly necessary."* Reorganizing the entry point of CLSC requests proved very beneficial, requiring centralized processing of requests. They are sent by telephone, processing, and forwarded to zone teams. Since the entry point also receives requests for patients aged from 0 to 100 years, there are 7 full-time equivalent (FTE) resources and 2 part-time resources to cover the hours. In the case of individuals with profiles 1, 2, or 3 referred to community organizations, certain vulnerability criteria are checked and telephone callback is used to confirm a certain level of safety. Voicemail is supposed to be eliminated but hasn't been so far. The single entry point has become significantly more efficient by centralizing requests, since now it is possible to tell if a person is enrolled in three physiotherapy clinics and what service is really required. While requests are better routed now, it is still difficult to put a figure on the number of bad referrals that the system has been saved from. The single entry point is also well-placed to maximize resources: when this service has a waiting list, the individual is directed to another.

Practitioners in Sherbrooke

According to secondary-care practitioners, the collaborative relationship with case management has not achieved its full potential. Certain CMs have a tendency to be directive, which is not appreciated. Moreover, it was pointed out that a positive effect could be felt when the CMs take on several cases. The pressure, however, has returned now that a waiting list has been set up. From the clinical perspective, there is still no agreement about defining the individual's need and determining which practitioner would be appropriate. *"Unlike what they believe, it's not always up to us to do the work."* Certain practitioners in key positions at the CHUS appear to be targeted by CMs in an effort to get the maximum out of the hospital stay. This tactic is not appreciated. It appears that everybody has their own definition of sharing of responsibilities and which can vary from case to case. It would be better, however, to establish rules on the level of teams or departments. When assessments performed at the secondary-care level arrive at the CLSC, such as a profile 6, and the primary-care assessment was a profile 9, they challenge our assessment and *"that hurts"*, yet the reality is just that: it's a kind of degradation. The picture of a patient described in secondary care is often different from that at home; often, it is necessary to insist before primary-care staff accepts it. Use of Iso-SMAF profiles is now to the point that the geriatricians and nurses on the geriatrics team do so on a regular basis. The geriatrics nurse prints them out and puts them into the patient record. CMs attend multidisciplinary meetings fairly often. If the patient does not go back home, the CM is responsible for filling out the placement request. Sometimes the meetings are held as conference calls. As far as this team is concerned, the process appears to be well established. The perceived gain is that the geriatrician has a portrait of the elderly person's functioning at home and can determine the objective to achieve during hospitalization. After the patient is discharged, the CM is responsible for seeing to subsequent interventions. When the hospital social worker (SW) works hand in glove with the CM, the hospital becomes the SW's purview and the home the CM's; each knows what to do and they work together in the patient's interest. The multidisciplinary model of case management is reported as being a positive element. At the same time, it would be good to standardize CM knowledge to the extent that those trained in social work receive targeted training in health/nursing and vice versa.

At the CRE[o], it is believed that participating in the integrated network by referrals to the CLSC that end up being put on a waiting list could generate disinterest. Nevertheless, the CMs hit the ball back into the court of CRE practitioners such as when the visual impairment of an elderly person appears to have gotten worse, *"that happens. It's even the most important aspect for us, anyway."*

Mental-health problems led to CMs submitting a high number of information requests to the geriatric psychiatry sector, especially in the beginning. It appears that some basic elements had not been learned and that some of the CMs needed training. Such situations make it difficult to establish confidence at the outset. Some secondary-care professionals find it difficult to work with Iso-SMAF profiles: they are familiar with the table, but they haven't integrated its use into geriatric psychiatric practices, such as at the CRE. For others, in particular, in physiotherapy and occupational therapy at the CHUS, having the profile is quite helpful. Moreover, it makes it possible to set realistic objectives with respect to the individual's functional level prior to hospitalization. A computer workstation should be made available so that these professionals can consult the SIGG. Sometimes hospitalized patients have not been referred to geriatrics and it's the physical/occupational therapists that suggest it to the attending physician.

Not everyone uses the SIGG. Physical/occupational therapists would like to have access to it, because it would help resolve cases more quickly. When the patient is managed by a case manager, physical/occupational therapists state that they find printed information in the medical record, but not always systematically. The situation has not improved for patients without case management. CHUS physical therapists have trouble communicating with home-care services: the three lines on the continuity sheet is not enough for them to record certain required specifications. If they knew in advance that it would be impossible to have the required service at the right time, the patient could be directed to other services and alternatives would be sought. The instructions given to the elderly are often too complicated for them to follow. They should not be directed to a resource unable to respond to their needs. Sometimes, during a telephone call with the patient, we learn that it took three months for the bath requested of the CLSC to be given, but no one alerted the referring practitioner. In the case of certain services that involve mobility safety, the referring practitioner experiences a certain level of uneasiness if he or she is unaware if the ser-

o   CRE: Centre de réadaptation de l'Estrie

vice has been provided. Sometimes, patients are discharged rather quickly from a hospital, which means that the equipment they need must be found quickly. A similar situation arises with loaned equipment: you don't know what the patient is going to get. Yet CHUS and CLSC caregivers *"should work as a team ... If we knew how they worked, we would stop bothering so many people."* Physiotherapy and occupational therapy are key professions for the elderly. Significant problems were noted, especially in Sherbrooke, in completing requests for primary care.

The CLSC is in a similar situation, where there are long waiting lists for basic services (assistance with hygiene, psychosocial follow-up). The lack of resources is so flagrant that when CLSC practitioners are unable to ensure the safety of the individual in the home, requests for care get transformed into placement requests, which makes no sense to them. CLSC practitioners observed that the information about patients from the hospital setting too often states that the individual is incapable of returning home, whereas he or she still has a potential to do so with home support. Many undesirable situations are caused by the bottlenecked access to services. As a single-entry-point practitioner stated, however, *"we have a snapshot of the patients that we have never seen before and an idea of who they are."* Even if there is nothing that can really be done for them, we inform and refer them. Priority cases are marked as such. While it is clear that the single entry point goes beyond its assessment role, there is really no other alternative. Despite this unfortunate situation, collaborative relations have developed between case management, the day care center, and the CLSC assessment team. The team of CLSC social workers (SW) or human relations officers (HROs)[p] have stated that CMs evidence a quality and intensity of interventions that few in the network are able to deliver. Being a CM brings greater self-esteem, which is why many HROs are switching to it. CLSC HROs consider that they also provide case management, specifically with mental-health patients, the intellectually impaired and persons with disabilities, but *"we get no recognition for it."* They are of the opinion that the difference lies mainly with the load of lighter cases given to CMs and that the majority of home-care social workers could have become case managers. With respect to CLSC and day-care center primary-care services, short-term care staff are perceived as *"not yet partners,"* because they don't have much interaction with the SIGG and are unaware of what primary-care practitioners do for their patients. According to them, case management is still poorly understood by the various CHUS practitioners. Opinions were divided during discussions to move the case-management team to a location separate from home-care services. Some people thought that the decision was necessary in the beginning to make a distinction and to get the function off the ground. They consider that the financial

p   HRO: Human relations officer

resources were lacking, resulting in all the problems related to access to services.

The collaboration between practitioners could have been more open, especially with certain SGUI and CHUS departments, except for the day hospital and STGU, who are SIGG practitioners. In their opinion, broader SIGG use and entering progress notes would help broaden this collaboration. They would also like to be invited to the last multidisciplinary meeting before the patient is referred to the CLSC and have access to secondary-care expertise in order to take into account any subsequent interventions. Clinical collaboration also means having a CLSC practitioner serve on the services committee in a setting where discussions are "truly patient-centered." It can also involve meetings between the program heads and their clinical effects, such as standardizing SMAF scoring in the MCAT: *"The MCAT, well, you know, it's been a longtime that...you know, when you have confidence in the other, when you read someone else's MCAT and you can say to yourself that you really trust that, well, then, you've come a hell of a way."* The enthusiasm of primary-care practitioners is evidenced by the fact that the integrated services network places greater value on the mission of home care services, an area they know so well but which has often suffered: *"we were at the very bottom of the basement,"* whereas the value of the work is now starting to make itself known.

SGUI staff believes that the components of the integrated network are not functioning optimally and that a certain amount of breaking in is still needed. The SWs primarily believe that the predominating impression left when there is no minimal basket of services is that nothing is working. These shortcomings in service access negative impact on the operation and image of the integrated since the outcomes at the end of three years of effort should have resulted in better communication and tighter links and that *"things would be breezing along."* Instead, services are doled out *"drop by drop."* CMs should have services to manage. Currently, however, it's more a question of seeking compensatory measures. This dynamics in the field does not make it easy to focus on recipients. Despite everything, experience brings out that case-manager involvement in the case is particularly helpful: *"Things went well with the case manager when there was enough money"* to fund services. For a while, the case manager controlled access to certain services, which facilitated interventions. When a case manager is involved, even when the patient is completing a care episode, *"we can close the file with confidence. We separate tasks. Everybody knows what everybody else is doing and that works well. There is no duplication."* Case management therefore provides security that can be felt by both patients and caregivers.

One issue brought up in dismantling the obstacles to collaboration between clinicians is having a meeting between the single-entry-point assessment team and secondary-care practitioners, so that they can share problems and solutions as well as create a corridor to work together more effectively: *"We have to work as a team for service continuity, but we don't know each other and we don't know what the other one is looking for."* While the integrated network model embodies sound principles, certain elements need to be pushed to the maximum, especially service corridors, in order for information to be conveyed. There is also a belief that the Iso-SMAF profiles should not be used alone in making decisions. Development of the SIGG should be continued and more practitioners should be involved. As things now stand, there is a waiting period of eight weeks for assessment when a request for case management arrives at the single entry point, which really isn't good. An elderly person derives a good deal from case management. The case manager is responsible for linkages with the network and the patient enjoys greater security. On the other hand, services are not adequately available and this includes those that come under case management. Too few patients are covered by case management; too many people still wonder where to go and what to do. Thought should also be given to developing information campaigns targeting the general public. Furthermore, it appears that family physicians need to be more integrated and informed.

Community-organization workers feel that they are on the network's periphery, especially since the confidentiality rules observed by CLSC practitioners prevent them from having basic information that would enable them to adapt the service to the patient's actual needs. That is the main issue raised in interviews with them. They decry the difficulty in reaching home-care providers, who are the main people they talk to. Others also have trouble understanding the network's language. Those who attended some joint-action meetings at the outset of the project said that *"it was kind of Greek to me. Jeez, it was just so new that maybe we had a hard time getting our bearings. But after that, the case managers got in touch with us, which was a tremendous help in dealing with those cases. We were just so lucky to have someone like that to talk to. The contacts, information, service complementarity, we have. Since CMs have been around, I swear by them."* Interaction with CMs centers on exchanging information using a "more human approach" and CMs deliver better follow-up. In referring to attempting to get information from the CLSC about one of their patients, community workers say *"it's nearly impossible. Forget about it. We've tried and it doesn't work. - At a certain point, it really bothers us because we want to help, but when the cases go beyond the scope of our roles, we would like to transfer them to the appropriate resource, if there is one. If not, we need to do something else. If we aren't aware of the resource, however, then they fall through the cracks."* In addition to the impact on the elderly person, the disadvantages include lost caregiver time, inappropriate referrals, frustrations, and impaired quality of service.

A number of comments made by community-organization workers lead us to believe that corridors for information exchange must be created between the CLSC and community organizations, mainly to more effectively direct referrals and follow up current cases. These corridors for information exchange have been established between certain community organizations and case management, positively impacting on collaboration. They would like to give further and obtain the ISPs on which they appear as service providers. Things are blocked on that level, too. They still don't have SIGG access, although they think having it would be *"fantastic."* It would provide the means for informing the right caregivers about abandoned services and hospitalizations as well as better informing their volunteers when people are temporarily away from home. Some of them would like to see the CHUS take a greater role in disseminating information and making referrals to community organizations. Despite the shortcomings raised, *"I clearly think that the integrated services network is a great thing. And it shows that we all have a stake in working together. On the other hand, as a community organization, we have to make ourselves be respected. We also have the right to refuse, too. That's a more political aspect."* They also consider that they are competent to identify the nature of certain unanswered (respite, food, heavy work) and the elderly themselves (moving, heavy housework). Sometimes the community network puts in place services relevant for the elderly and would like to make practitioners aware of them, which is not always easily done. They would like to have a formal annual meeting between community organizations and CLSC practitioners. In summary, the community network was informed about the deployment of the integrated services network and practitioners have gained familiarity with the vocabulary (e.g., single entry point, SMAF, integrated network), but that the network was inadequately integrated as a partner in Sherbrooke.

Granit Managers

For management, the experience of implementing the integrated network represented an opportunity to update *"services in place and the service continuum that should exist,"* and identify duplications, gray areas, and how to obtain better coordination mechanisms. Based on the state of affairs in Granit, they feel that they gotten off in the right direction with accessibility and continuity: *"I believe that we must go even further with this model."* The main improvements reported were exchanges between practitioners, the three missions of the institution working better together, and the concentration of information and associated tools, which *"have only have a positive impact on the best ways to work with people"* to ensure that they receive better overall service, given by the right person. It has given us a bit of perspective in how our services are organized and in *"conceptualizing our approaches, which we don't often have time for."*

The first step got underway with the work initiated during administrative merging of the three missions. This represented convergence with the integrated network project, which rapidly yielded benefits. The managers had to adjust to the *"opening of their specific field of activities to a much broader overall perspective of the offer of services."* For their part, practitioners and clinicians were prompted to *"see what the other could bring, making it a two-way street"* and exposed to working with a common language. A number of them worked with partners outside the institution. Management deemed that it wasn't possible to be against the integrated network because, as the population ages, *"the offer of services must be approached from an overall perspective, not one based on missions."* It is important to have a shared understanding of the integrated network; starting off too quickly prevents appropriation. Moreover, the change must be managed by putting the right people in the right positions. This takes time and should not be hurried. Bridges have been built using the joint-action mechanisms and case management. The challenge for us has been to tie in the medical aspect. Many physicians do not necessarily feel concerned for the time being, except for some dedicated to the elderly, who are deeply involved. More work should also be done with the private homes for the elderly in our territory.

For a region as extensive as Granit, where services are spread across three points of service, the challenge is to work on the corridors of services from the medium- and long-term perspectives. One of the tools for working on the corridors effectively involves computerizing work processes, exchanging clinical information, using computerized clinical charts, teleconsulting with specialists, and so on. The desire is to work in real time and not have to put up with the inconvenience of delays because specialized services are located at a distance. Initiating this component allowed us to implement the SIGG, whereas, for the region, it was just scratching the surface of work on the professional practice setting. The institution's executive committee organized training in the use of the SIGG. Now, *"we manage the needs categories."* This tool is a patient record that provides an overview of the services for the individual that *"I see as being kind of symbolic of a change in practice,"* but the medical component of the tool must be improved because it doesn't respond to physician needs. Using the SIGG raises the issue of getting beyond the technological challenge faced by many users who are not computer literate and who can't type. On the other hand, hardcopy is a thing of the past. Home-care, day-center, and long-term services lend themselves to this tool, as does the placement access mechanism. Nursing presents some problems, because nurses do not work with similar tools on a daily basis.

As for the functional assessment, all the ingredients have been brought together, the tools are in place, practitioners have learned how to use the tools, and *"they are happy with that, asking for still more, and even want it expanded to take in other patient groups."* Work remains to be done, more specifically at the gateways to the network, such as the emergency department and short-term care, which still operate according to the silo approach, in spite of positive experiences in collaborating with certain practitioners. Practices require more work and greater networking is needed when caring for the frail or disabled elderly. Case management is committed in this regard, but the model must be disseminated and the practitioner must not feel that he or she has to carry the whole burden. Moreover, CMs have the power to ask questions about their partners' offers of services of partners and to identify the required adjustments, since CMs see the unfulfilled needs.

In adopting the CM model, the advantages and disadvantages of the different models were weighed. Finally, they were very comfortable with the mixed model in which CMs are dedicated to complex cases. The idea is to prevent families from being exposed to too many different practitioners, unless absolutely necessary. To determine if the CM team members were to all be in the same discipline or not, we consulted staff, who thought that there should be more psychosocial workers in this position. CMs repeatedly approached community services to increase their visibility and explain what they did. They intend to do something similar in the near future with the medical clinics in the territory.

This organization has relieved a great deal of pressure on long-term placement. In fact, there has been discussion of closing beds and investing in home care. Profile-5 patients no longer go into placement facilities, which also influences occupational-therapy, physical-therapy and pharmacy practices. When a crisis occurs, the patient is stabilized and returned home, whereas, in the past, they would have been sent directly to a placement facility. The beds that have been freed up are used for transition, so that the elderly do not spend much time in short-term care. The nurse in the short-term geriatrics unit uses PRISMA-7 to identify cases at risk and makes referral to the single entry point. Assessment is carried out and services set up more rapidly. Various irritants have been acknowledged. Home-care practitioners feel that they have difficult cases, too, with palliative care and disability; they believe that case management is needed in such cases, too. Gray areas were identified, especially pertaining to the assessment roles at the single entry point and case management, and assignment of cases to home care or case management. The model must be adapted *"but not abandoned."* Relief for CMs on long-term leave is not always possible, which has slowed the progress of joint action. Application of the ISP is encountering difficulties as in the other territories.

Both for the organization and partners, the single entry point is the hub for requests. Receiving requests requires the most space. Case-finding remains marginal; follow-up lacks the underpinning needed for insertion into the entry point's operation. Requests for home services are assessed by the case managers using PRISMA-7 (four or more risk factors), but the process for assigning cases must be reviewed.

Joint action gets more effective as things advance and people get to know each other better. Granit benefited from having committed leaders: one among management and the other with the home-care team and at the community level. As a manager, what this new vision holds must be seen: *"Well, I believed in it. But it wasn't until I saw that my interest was improving the quality of services to the public, and how implementing the integrated network was going to change the organization ... that was going to give my manager leverage to have a pro-*

active relationship with my staff that I really believed in it and really came on board." Beyond the efforts within the system, work was carried out with the Centre d'action bénévole (volunteer center), which takes an interest in finding cases of frailty or disabilities. Volunteers were met with and they learned about the loss of independence, which *"earned their confidence in us."* The Service d'entretien domestique (home maintenance service) is in the process of modifying its offer of services, within its legal confines, in order to eventually offer personal services such as bathing, meals and hairdressing. This organization with 75 attendants and dispatchers reaches some 600 beneficiaries and has *"become an essential collaborator."* Our visiting homemakers no longer do cleaning. Their roles are shifting to more specific and technical care (safe movement, patient lift, physical mobilization). It came out that management needed to be firm; not necessarily wait for a perfect consensus, which leads to inaction; and identify strong tendencies to create *"a movement and follow the parade,"* with the important consideration being that people believe that they belong to something positive for the general public.

Granit Practitioners

From the outset, the day-care center manifested satisfaction with the dynamics established with the CLSC, who makes more referrals, many with cognitive disorders, *"so we work together more often than before."* The day-care center is located in a separate building so that the SIGG provides a means for communicating about its beneficiaries referred by case managers, which make up three-quarters of its users. Other practitioners in the public network speak enthusiastically about their experience with the SIGG and their meticulousness in entering notes to make them rapidly available for other practitioners: *"I know that the others are going to consult them, so I do it right away. I try to do it quickly because I like it, too, when others do the same ... because fair's fair."* Although network practitioners see the patient's Iso-SMAF profile when they consult the SIGG, access to it is not across the board. One individual who is quite familiar with profiles and serves on the placement access committee deems that profiles should be used during interdisciplinary team meetings to lead people to become familiar with the tool.

A short-term hospital practitioner indicated that since individuals requiring several home services have come under case management, they consult at the hospital less frequently and services are put into place faster. In the past, such heavy home-care cases could not get the attention they required due to an excessive caseload. Hospital units acknowledge SIGG existence but don't use it, primarily because of the challenge in using computers, but also because their job is already quite demanding. They feel that the data could be entered by the medical-records department. This alternative would mean that the physician's notes would be transcribed by someone else and left unsigned, since physicians do not enter their data in the SIGG, either. The issue has not been resolved. Community organizations don't have the SIGG and when case managers are on extended leave (maternity, accident, illness), the community is at a loss.

Little progress has been noted in the emergency department (ED). In response to a request to take part in case-finding among the elderly with PRISMA-7, the team refused mainly because it lacks the resources to perform its own triage tasks. The SIGG hasn't been implemented there and no notes are taken, but the emergency department can call if a case-management patient has visited there. The ED staff can recognize CM patients because it is indicated on the admissions form. ED staff must be won over by making them *"see the impact that it has on all the other departments; we want to work with other disciplines, but the issue is how to make them understand that it's important."* ED staff doesn't see the real gains with case-finding, which doesn't enhance their motivation.

As for the value of the integrated network model, one participant stressed that, even if sometimes things become cumbersome, *"I think that, with time, we've got everything to gain with continuity. That's clear. And I think we're doing it more and more. Anyway, that's what I feel on the job, and I wouldn't limit it to just to case management. That may have gotten things rolling, but it also created a kind of linkage ... I think it's going to be a bigger challenge to work together, to recognize that we all have our own philosophies in each of our settings, because we don't work the same way ... Our challenge is to accept each other's reality."*

As for individualized service plans (ISPs), practitioners are not specifically informed when information is entered on them. It comes either through referral, during an interdisciplinary meeting, or by e-mail. In the case of community workers, meetings are sometimes held to coordinate a sequence of services, but the telephone is also used. They find these methods suitable for initiating services. The community setting would like to know if the service is appreciated, which has not been communicated to them adequately. While emergency services do not fit into these plans, *"we really would like that."* Suggestions have been made to add resources to the emergency department for liaison purposes or to locate case management in the emergency department. Concurrently, it was pointed out that there is a great deal of paperwork and electronic messages, and there were reservations about *"time with the patient"* and the importance of a meaningful relationship with the patient, which can make all the difference.

Inserting the new role of case manager into the home-care team was difficult because *"it caused a split"* and it appears that the roles of case management and psychosocial work carried out in home support were not clarified to the satisfaction of the parties involved. While there are still grey areas, the team has gained maturity through this experience. One of the main issues in the split focused on the designation of "complex cases" requiring case management, whereas palliative care is left up to the regular team, despite the burden that such cases impose and without any reduction in their caseload. The other issue dealt with the transition from regular follow-up in the home-care department towards case management: *"After being with a patient for 2 or 3 years, she gets hit with a stroke and that's all she wrote. I'm not going to be taking care of you anymore; case management is going to take over ... and what's more, it's like I was telling her that I'm not competent to take care of her and that I'm sending her into case management. That really doesn't make me feel good about myself."* Therefore, putting case management into the organization of home care can affect the practitioner-patient relationship and continuity. The argument put forward is that, for the elderly, *"continuity of service means keeping the same practitioner."*

Practitioners in Granit believe that the elderly are being well served and that their needs are being answered, although, if more services were offered, *"it would be much nicer."* People sometimes have specific needs that we cannot fulfill because *"we don't have a panoply of services yet."* This is all the more true in remote municipalities, but users are satisfied.

Professional referrals to occupational therapy and physiotherapy from the SGUI and CHUS are directed to colleagues in the regions for follow-up after a stay in short-term care or rehabilitation. This bypasses the single entry point. This tendency also occurs in nutrition. Basically, this practice points to the concern of limiting response time and ensuring a response to a specific need.

Coaticook Managers

Implementation is operational in Coaticook, since all the components have been put into place but are not functioning optimally. The prime reason for this is the delay in hiring an adequate number of case managers, due to funding shortages, and SIGG implementation (having portable computers for in-home assessments). Joint action on the local level allowed the institution to score some points. Momentum is harder to achieve, however, on the regional level because the area is small and has less weight. In addition, relations with partners on the regional level (CHUS and SGUI) need to be *"more closely knit so things work better. ... You always have to call back (...), it's up and down."* Because of staff turnover, collaborative practices established with one individual are not necessarily maintained by the replacement. The fact that these practices depend on individuals and are not sufficiently supported on the organizational level results in varied performance. The issue of prime importance is that local practitioners know as soon as possible, from the first day of hospitalization, that an elderly person with impaired independence from the Coaticook territory has been admitted to the regional hospital (CHUS) or to a secondary-care department (STGU or IFRU), so that the return can be prepared in an appropriate manner. Efforts are continuing along these lines.

This territory is handicapped by not having short-term hospitalization. It's quite difficult to make an integrated network out of a few beds in an emergency room, *"with us supposed to do miracles with a poor-person's budget."* The limits imposed on using local emergency-room beds (maximum of 8 hours) seems unrealistic for patients with impaired independence, who need more time to recover from an acute episode. The geriatrics unit has only five beds, but it needs about ten in order to function properly. Coaticook managers believe that consolidating this department would yield advantages for patients as well as the CHUS and the local institution.

In this context, providing specialized medical care represents another challenge. Managers felt that services needed to be provided in the territory by consultant geriatricians, who would visit on a regular basis. There is also a desire to have telesupport options that would enable local physicians to make rapid, relevant decisions and that would promote access to specialized clinics for as-needed assessments. Experimentation with this approach for psychiatric care was conclusive: physicians and other practitioners are better able to carry out follow-up, which converges on harmonization of care and valuable multiplier effects. In working with specialists, family physicians gain knowledge about pathologies, work tools and medications. It's a question of doing the same thing in geriatrics.

The integrated-network project was unifying. Actors can be rallied around this kind of project, but *"the partners must feel there is a place on the level of service organization..."* Leadership must be able to overcome resistance from within and mobilize partners to accomplish their work. Management provided support to the leader in working with partners but did not interfere in the leader's work. The Board of Directors monitored the project and obtained statistics.

Work targeting continuity was carried out with pharmacies in which the exchange of information between physicians in the local emergency department and geriatrics unit and community pharmacists, making it possible to offer safer conditions when patients were discharged: *"implementing the integrated network locally yielded real gains. What was set up really produced added value,"* Information is still conveyed over the telephone because the SIGG is not accessible outside of the RTSS network. This is, however, an objective to be reached eventually, which will benefit all of the elderly, not only those under case management. The value of putting into place local partnering strategies has been acknowledged as long as it targets first and foremost the more vulnerable, but also provides a means for improving communication and work processes.

Service continuity was clearly benefited in this small territory by putting into place a geriatrics unit, which has fit right into the range of services that case managers can offer. A link is systematically maintained between this unit, home care, and the emergency room, since a social worker / case manager visits the unit daily to see if home care is aware of the patients there. The emergency room constitutes a valuable setting in order to *"read the situation"* and then direct the case, avoid hospitalization, and prepare for the patient's return home. The geriatrics unit brings together a team of professionals and a physician, who takes charge of interdisciplinary management, which is necessary for these frail individuals who can no longer live at home. Efforts are made to ensure that the patient doesn't fall between the cracks. There is constant concern about returning the patient home, because *"we have to work things out so that the patient becomes independent."* Shortages of certain professionals—in particular, occupational therapists and physical therapists—cause problems of access to the services needed for the elderly with impaired independence to remain in their homes. The problem is generalized. There is a policy under which a family physician is assigned to anyone who does not have one. Each physician goes on house calls during the week that he or she is on duty at the geriatrics unit. The perception of physician joint action is satisfactory, especially as it applies to the different missions of a local institution or coordination is carried out quickly and effectively in order to prevent the states of patients from deteriorating. Coaticook physicians feel that an integrated network benefits the elderly person, the system, and the physician, who will be working less and less alone. That represents genuine progress. It becomes clear that joint action among the different professionals caring for an elderly patient benefits the individual in terms of quality of life, so that he or she can remain in the home for as long as possible with the addition of home care. The system benefits because this postpones placement or long-term hospitalization. In the case of a physician alone with an elderly patient with impaired independence, making progress on all fronts is neither simple nor straightforward. Most physicians are satisfied with the interventions carried out under case management and that relieves them of *"a burden of responsibilities."* More and more, it's not up to the physician to manage all the work, seek out services, and run around after everyone. Now, everyone does their part according to their own field of expertise. No need to go back and work individually; interdisciplinary work is a *"positive value, it's a plus."*

The first rule in making a successful integrated network is working in partnership. There is no getting around establishing local partnerships. This broad openness towards partners makes elderly people in the territory aware of the services offered. The institution supports initiatives (services in English, conferences on health care and services for the elderly, therapeutic leisure activities with community meals, and so on), which ensures a population base. It also enables the institution to adjust services, such as, in working with community organizations or private homes for the elderly, essential services in a territory which has no intermediate resources. If there's a problem somewhere *"someone sounds the alarm."* On the other hand, recent experience indicates that the patients in case management are too demanding to truly benefit from certain local volunteer community services. Meals on Wheels is an important component for serving home-dwelling patients and it is working well. Organizing respite for caregivers, which lends itself less to volunteerism, is a different situation. Work is ongoing to improve access to home-maintenance and paratransit services for all of the municipalities in the territory.

Certain gains in Coaticook have been deemed appreciable: 1) broadening the use of the SIGG to all elderly people receiving home care; 2) patient satisfaction; 3) expanding the single entry point to the entire population from age 0 to 100. Although all the partners are familiar with the single entry point, it is nonetheless difficult to estimate to what degree the elderly population is, despite the articles published in the local media. Because the CLSC and CHSLD missions are located in the old hospital building, some elders might have the impression that they are calling the hospital, whereas they are really reaching the single entry point. The perception may take some time to change. Request triage and linkages with the emergency room are working well. Reminders must often be made about case-finding with PRISMA-7. Practitioners don't immediately take up its use because they feel that they are quite familiar with their patients with impaired independence, since the setting is small. Implementing the single entry point, in contrast to the past intake process, led to the perception that greater focus was being placed on the elderly. When a caregiver calls the single entry point, the practitioners will call back and are more caring. This function could be developed further and carried out systematically.

While all the components are really important in an integrated network, case management is essential because the elderly have *"multiple problems"* and the network is too complex. The elderly get confused, they are worried, they don't know what's going to happen. The case manager therefore has the role of ensuring continuity as they move throughout the various services. Having a small institution with limited resources makes it difficult to avoid opting for the mixed case-management model. This is all the more true since the three psychosocial professionals must be used in the various sectors covered by home care, namely, intellectual impairment, physical impairment, and the elderly, including palliative care. As a result, the mixed model is not so much a choice as the only possibility. In a larger team, there can be a certain amount of maneuvering room in sharing responsibilities and caseloads. As for continuity, however, having a small team means that members are more familiar with the patients, who experience fewer negative impacts when replacements are made. Having the same practitioner is not a given.

The idea of having an interdisciplinary case-management model was also seen as being valuable. There is, however, a shortage of professionals, in particular, nurses, who have a significant volume of service requests to handle. The assignment of a patient to case management is rarely discussed on a team basis. The issue in this regard is perceived as nonexistent since the role of the social worker (or HRO) and the case manager is filled by the same person: *"There is no boundary between the two."* There is no need, either, to preselect patients to be direct to case management because, one way or another, a professional is there to organize services. It was not deemed necessary to distinguish roles with partners. Physicians and community workers, for their part, found it difficult to identify which individuals in the elderly population that they served came under case management. After making the situation known, the physicians began receiving notes identifying which patients were under case management, which was appreciated. This is one advantage of small settings.

Recently, significant progress appears to have been made with the addition of a full-time resource in case management: the number of cases managed increased in the distribution of tasks is better balanced. Each practitioner has administrative tasks, sectoral responsibilities (intellectual disability, physical disability and aging-related loss of independence) and case-management functions with each having a variable caseload. Assignments to case management and entry into the SIGG were done too late in the initial years. Efforts to improve were undertaken, but the results are less than perfect. For example, emphasis was put on the SIGG and SMAF identification sheets, but the ISPs are not all completed. The problem is lack of resources. The delay in SIGG use pointed out by management has resulted in case managers having to use paper forms for longtime when carrying out in-home assessments and then transcribe the information into the SIGG back at the office. This duplication is perceived as impeding their efficacy. Portable computers for in-home visits were relatively latecomers. Physicians do not use the SIGG sufficiently, in spite of their training with it, which accounts for their requests to obtain paper copies of the ISP. The training was carried out at the beginning of implementation, but since they haven't practiced very much, they have forgotten what they learned.

The integration of the case-manager role among home-care nurses was slow and work remains to be done. While the sharing of the pivotal role of nurse with case manager has not been completely mastered, evident progress has been made. It is important to go back over the vision of continuity in the home-care team. Case managers must do a better job of explaining and selling their role to their home-care colleagues, which, until now, was the responsibility primarily of the department manager. Consequently, perception of the roles still causes a few hitches and is moving forward slowly. Eventually, each practitioner must have a clear vision of the roles and they must be distributed more efficiently. Managers pointed out that, since their arrival, the case managers tend to seek out more information that they need at the regional level. Meetings with the CHUS's social-services department and the Institute are planned to improve collaboration: *"We're working on our linkages."* Given the distance and time constraints, case managers would like to be able to count on CHUS and Institute professionals keeping them informed.

Not having a waiting list for home care sometimes requires them to take action to "put out fires." Patient groups other than those under case management have less intensive follow-up: *"clearly, we carry out less interventions."* On the other hand, work within the organization is not carried out using the silo approach. The process is horizontal: home-care staff goes to the emergency room; there's continuity in terms of placement, home care, and the day-care center: *"it's a continuum because that's what we want. We're not interested in silos between sectors."* The perception of the elderly has changed because *"we note that somebody's going to be there and we see them differently."* The day-care center is now used for individuals with a severe loss of independence. *"We are decompartmentalizing all that."* The main theme is to examine the response to patient needs and to see who is the best placed for doing so. Efforts are being made to intervene before the problem gets worse so as to prevent emergency-room visits. *"It wasn't difficult to bring about the changes because the practitioners are patient-centered."* Flexibility has been used in allocating home care in order to better respond to the needs. In addition, there have been opportunities for collaboration with the mental-health team in caring for certain elderly people.

Iso-SMAF profiles provide an indication of the needs for services as well as enabling practitioners to share a common language. The advantages of being familiar with the Iso SMAF profiles of our patients in home care and at the day-care center are undeniable. Deployment for patients as a whole, not just for those under case management, was very important. The sharing of these tools is also a major point because *"we all have the same language and I think that's important for continuity."* Internal practices have changed in that now discussions about cases are only held if a profile has been developed. The profile provides a means for taking the direction that is supported, which *"gives us reasons to head in one direction."* Staff must therefore be familiar with computerized tools. Management must support the use of computers and equip and train staff to use them. In addition, staff must be induced to use computers on a daily basis. Management must be aware that there is a learning curve in computer use. Adequate time must be taken so that staff members who are not very computer literate can learn to use different software programs.

In terms of more overall outcomes, progress has been noted in the perception of the elderly, their needs, and the necessity of responding promptly. Now that practitioners are aware of the problem, they can act quickly, propose things for the home to prevent hospitalizations, better fulfill the needs of patients and their families, and put off institutionalization. It's an impact of interest. The results of continuity and efficiency are relatively obvious to managers and physicians in the territory.

In terms of management within the institution, all programs that affect the elderly were already managed by one person, who is responsible for overall coordination. Tackling this kind of change rests mainly on people who believe in it, work hard, and see the difficulties. While this takes vision, it is based on the experience of people, which accounts for the importance of respecting the course taken and allowing adjustments. There are professional and budgetary issues involved. An overview is needed and change managed to avoid overloading. The manager must be able to grasp the implications of changes before they are implemented. Staff must also clearly see the benefit in implementing any project. While the leader must have relational and communication skills, he or

she must be able to imbue the project with an overall direction in order to atten-
uate the impact of ambiguities and vagueness. Local issues must be understood;
implementation of changes that reflect the locale must be fostered. That takes
people with sound knowledge of the integrated network for the elderly, who
have current knowledge about budgets, who are capable of managing staff as
well as personnel and interprofessional conflicts, and who can rally support in
the anticipated direction. They were lucky enough to have all this. Finally, taking part in research clarified model elements, whereas certain territories in
Estrie experience difficulties in this regard.

Coaticook Practitioners

Practitioners perceive case management as being "very much in vogue." Since
the Ministry wants it, however, it is also an obligation. They believe that the service is for all elderly patient groups since the distinctions between the roles of
case manager and psychosocial worker have barely been touched on. They have
noticed that an increasing number of people have been entered in the SIGG.
Practitioners see duplications with the regional level. Steps already taken on the
local level are redone or patients return to their homes without the transition
being organized. Occasionally, the service plan proposed on the regional level
does not appear logical to local practitioners, who are quite familiar with the
elderly person's situation and the limitations of the local offer of services. To
illustrate, the hospital indicates that in-home physiotherapy should be provided
three times a week, whereas local capacities are limited. Practitioners must
negotiate with patient expectations. Moreover, some patients live some distance
away, which means that caregivers must receive much more instruction and
must be given an exercise program. After that, they are on their own. Certain
improvements have been noted, such as the continuity sheets that arrive at the
single entry point.

The single entry point is not perceived as a new service; since intake was
functioning quite well, it is viewed as continuity. The people at the single entry
point are quite familiar with the network and how the services fit together. Since
the setting is small, partnering is a normal state of affairs and people respond
readily.

Iso-SMAF profiles *"are well-known ... and used to offer services to any
patient requiring them. ... And we need that for access to any kind of service."*
The profile is a good indicator, providing a clear picture of the individual without having to read the entire SMAF. People put considerable effort into completing the profile, which is increasingly becoming a guide for identifying what
must be compensated for and which services are required from outside the institution. Since Iso-SMAF profiles are commonly used, it it easier for the day-care
center to anticipate intake and manage the day, because they will know ahead of
time the level of requirement for the practitioners, making it possible to form
groups. This planning aid was not available before, which is a real help.

One community worker sees that the integrated network has made genuine progress; gains have been made, in particular, in the area of transmitting relevant information. Yet community providers were like to know each other better. It was also emphasized that with no access at all to patient records, even if the organizations signed the protocol for sharing information, it is sometimes difficult to offer the service appropriately. For example, it is important to know if a particular patient has cognitive disorders. If our attendants or volunteers find moldy food in the refrigerator and the individual is no longer eating properly, this information is conveyed to the single entry point. We are unaware of what, if any, action is taken. The type of information that an organization requires mainly depends on the type of services rendered. To illustrate, in the case of transportation, it is important to know if the individual uses a cane. Feedback would therefore be appreciated. There is also the question about how to react to increasingly demanding cases in the home. There are gaps on this level and community organizations could work together to find solutions. When the practitioners do not have the SMAF, Iso SMAF profiles, or the SIGG, it is difficult to know whether the patient is under case management. For them, this information serves as an indicator of the patient's vulnerability and can be used to heighten vigilance. If practitioners are unaware, they have no means for taking an active role in follow-up. Most of the time, organizations are not aware if they are part of a individualized service plan. Even the elderly are unaware of it. When services are requested, practitioners never state that the individual is under case management. Lastly, community organizations wonder if they serve this patient group.

The experience is quite different for practitioners using the SIGG: the information is available, each practitioner makes progress notes, the expected hospital discharge date is provided, it is known if a pacemaker has been installed and if physiotherapy has been requested at the day-care center. *"I've only been entering notes into the SIGG for a week and I really like it!"* Since all cases go into the SIGG now, there's no longer any need to wonder if it's worth the double checking in the SIGG. Shared computerization is a necessity. *"The day-care center has traditionally been the most isolated of caregivers. We were like you guys (community organizations). We were almost partners in the same box, it's true, but we didn't have any ties. We didn't talk to one another ... it was rough ... But case manager, all I need to do is pick up the phone."* The case manager does the rest. The information is circulated. *"We're much less isolated now that we're part of a team."* Where SIGG participation should be requested is at the local emergency room during the evening and night shifts. The length of the notes still presents a problem for physiotherapists. The SIGG would have to include pain and transfer assessment grids, which would be a significant gain for physical therapists, who need 30 minutes to enter notes for a single patient, whereas the paper version can be filled out very quickly. The medical file always requires duplication, which is a problem, for example, for cases that get shifted between geriatrics units. The shortage of computers is another obstacle: currently, for practitioners use the same computer, which isn't practical. If the computer isn't available, the practitioner writes up the notes on paper but then they are not entered into the computer afterwards.

After three years, the result is better patient follow-up and continuity. It is reassuring, for example, when a patient is discharged from a geriatrics unit, has follow-up, and is not left to his or her own devices. On the other hand, things still need tightening up. While organizations have bought into ISPs, something like a service contract, it would be important to clarify the role played by all in this contract at least once a year. If needed, it should be amended. Patients who sign authorizations allowing the sharing of information must renew the decision every year; the parties to the contract should also do so. Liaison between short-term care and home care sometimes fall short of the mark. When the call informing about the discharge is the same day as the hospital discharge itself, there is no time to prepare services or the response time needed to contract for oxygen, provide new prescriptions, get equipment, and no one to explain everything for two or three days. It's a difficult situation.

In summary, in the three territories, all of the interviewees stated there were gaps in access to basic home-care services, inadequate financial resources, and a shortage of professional human resources (nurses, occupational therapists, physiotherapists, and geriatricians) as well as difficulty in planning succession for case managers. The steady rate of service requests from the hospital sector should encourage regional partners to better integrate local providers in their process so that preparations can be made for the discharge, which is not always the case. When the interviews were carried out in 2005, the health and social services network in Estrie was faced with a fairly generalized lack of access to basic services in Sherbrooke (assistance with bathing and hygiene, in particular). Regionally, the issues were transportation problems and partial service in certain remote municipalities in delivering meals and home maintenance. Sherbrooke describes bottlenecking in many services for which the elderly had to be put on waiting lists (day-care center, temporary placement). This reflection of inadequate access to services, however, did not prompt participants to withdraw from or limit their support of the integrated services network. For the most part, they were convinced of the necessity of adopting this approach is so that the system would be able to adequately serve the elderly now and in the years to come.

Presented as a conclusion, Table 3.1 (see below) depicts the elements that participants raised as being satisfactory (we appreciate ...) as well as those that might merit amending or a warning (we suggest ...).

Table 3.1
Satisfactions and Suggestions
Related to Implementation of the Integrated Services Network

Coordination

We appreciate ...	We suggest ...
A clear position from management so that the system shifts towards integrated networks and case management. It allows participants to speak the same language and take converging actions: a framework for managing the interfaces between services. The change in philosophy generated by joint action between partners: exchange of information, tools, and expertise.	Stability in organizations (at least during the phase of instituting the dynamics of joint action). The turnover of clinical and management staff does not support continuity and makes it difficult to transmit values and knowledge related to the network.
Having created a shared vision, done groundwork, and introduced mechanisms for cooperation before having budgets enabled senior executives to use this money differently, since the consensus on priorities had been achieved.	Defusing the fears of partners about having resources or mandates withdrawn. These issues eat up energy unnecessarily.
Consulting with one another is an effort: Everything that is done (for better or for worse) is visible. We have to accept it when our partners for their services into question and we must respond to their questions.	Transparency Use methods that systematically sample information that affects institutional functioning.
Coordination yields a great deal of information about the state of the network and collaboration between partners while giving everyone better knowledge of the other's work. It makes managers more aware of the upstream and downstream repercussions of their decisions.	Encourage initiatives that enable practitioners and managers to grasp the reality of the work and partner constraints. Foster a desire to improve practices and tools. "Why reinvent the wheel?"
The leadership exercised in the three territories: strong, convinced, competent, unifying opinions, in touch with every level of the system. The leadership shared between the Ministry, the Agency, and managements of the integrated networks makes a strong case for legitimacy.	A "must" for any region implementing an integrated network: no one person can bring integration about.
Awareness about avoiding duplication is carried out.	The instances of poor interorganizational functioning must be put before an authority with the power to settle them or submit recommendations (e.g. loaning the home's adaptive equipment).

Single entry point

We appreciate ...	We suggest ...
The single entry point as the referral hub for requests for services.	The public and practitioners should be better informed about how the single entry point functions.
An interdisciplinary in-home assessment team based at the single entry point.	Activities for harmonizing assessments between secondary care and primary care.
The single entry point receives many requests for services from the hospital, which only uses Iso-SMAF profiles for placement requests. In preparing for the patient's return home, the profile indicates the current level of functioning as well as the required services.	Iso-SMAF profiles should be fully deployed throughout the hospital setting, which would clarify the need for services when the patient is discharged.

Iso-SMAF profiles

We appreciate ...	We suggest ...
Implementing local mechanisms for access to placement would provide the means to manage placement dynamics locally.	The use of Iso-SMAF profiles in financing services raises issues (e.g. the profile doesn't take into account the time a practitioner puts into dealing with a handicap, such as the specific care required for gavage and glycemia testing).
Operating with Iso-SMAF profiles makes it possible to rationalize placement access and to distinguish major categories of needs.	Using the profile as a criterion for directing patients towards intermediate resources, family-type resources, and CHSLDs should be completed and validated by a professional advice.

SIGG computerized clinical chart

We appreciate ...	We suggest ...
Use of the same language and implementing common tools: SMAF and Iso-SMAF system, SIGG.	Easier access to computer stations with the SIGG (many stations are shared or too remote); additional stations for hospital units are required (occupational and physical therapy, geriatrics).
Technical support received in taking ownership of computerized tools.	Enriching the SIGG with medical, pharmacology, and rehabilitation tools.
	Improving the ISP (links with SMAF and computerization).
	Personalized assistance clinics for individuals unfamiliar with the computer keyboard and mouse; the software must be user friendly.

Computerizing records is a springboard to operating methods that reduce the impact of time and distance on the quality of service and prevents duplication.	Connecting all service providers to the elderly through computers will make it possible to optimize the integrated network ... but practitioners must have confidence in it, that's a condition.
The SIGG is perceived as a tool that could also be useful with other patient groups.	Community pharmacies should be connected to the SIGG; medication profiles are absolutely necessary for physicians.

Clientele

We appreciate ...	We suggest ...
Have an overall vision of patient's movements. Be able to distinguish situational and occasional needs of patients who require long-term management. Link the degree of loss of independence with the need for services.	When access to basic home-care services is defective, all efforts to organize management are negatively affected. In-home services must be intensified to avoid placement, especially in the case of couples, who would cost more in a placement setting than if they were supported to remain in their own home, when that is what they wish to do.

Case management

We appreciate ...	We suggest ...
The presence of case managers and their roles as translator and guide for caregivers and the elderly. Families greatly appreciate what the case manager does for them. Better understanding case management opens the way to developing collaborative practices. After taking part in a joint intervention with a case manager, it becomes obvious that we need a professional dedicated to elderly patients who isn't constantly changing.	Working on access delays to case management and having more case managers. Giving case managers privileged access to certain buffer resources (respite, temporary placement, bolstered home-support measures). Use of the initial case management team (supervised waiting list) should be avoided when it appears that things are wavering.
Have a simple criterion for access to case management (i.e. Iso-SMAF profile of 4).	Practitioners and clinicians who do not have Iso-SMAF profiles can have a difficult time knowing who is eligible for case management.
The lighter caseload allows the case manager to truly play an interorganizational role.	That more patients should be allowed in the case management. Why not increase the caseload?

Physician who have experienced case management appreciate sharing the burden of cases. When a close working relationship is established between the physician and case manager, the physician is kept well informed when his or her patient is hospitalized, so that subsequent steps can be initiated in a more balanced matter.	The physician-case manager tandem is not yet functioning optimally, but solutions to this proximity problem are not evident. Establish a partnership between the physician and case manager before a patient is enrolled in case management. The medical management of the elderly in private homes should be better structured. Improving case-manager training related to specific aging problems (e.g. geriatric psychiatry).
The role of geriatrics nurses on hospital geriatrics teams and geriatric-psychiatry to link secondary care with primary care and case management.	Geriatricians have been inadequately associated with the overall process and they are essential.
	A solution must be found for patients being hospitalized without their physician's or case manager's knowledge. Does the medical-records department have a role to play?

Resources

We appreciate ...	We suggest ...
Division of the densely populated territories into zones helps improve services, especially because it affords greater familiarity with practitioners, their practices, and local resources.	Transportation is a constant, unsolved problem in rural territories.
While the integrated network project provides adequate structures, tools, and mechanisms ...	... we lack the resources to fully implement them. Transition budgets are indicated because the situation is very hard on managers and practitioners alike: *"Exhaustion is rife throughout the network."*

Discussion

The experimental zone revealed some very hard work that got done despite the context being unfavorable along several lines. On the provincial level, the funding of health and social services is perceived as significantly lower than merited by needs. Moreover, there are professional staffing problems for key positions in home support for the elderly, such as nurse, occupational therapist, physical therapist, family physician, and geriatrician. The health and social services sector is characterized its by complexity and fluid nature. Many people have noted and deplored the incessant changes and staff turnover. Despite the operating difficulties as much for the public as practitioners, this universal access system receives the support of the general public and even more so of the elderly, who lived through a time when health care was beyond their financial means. On the regional level, underfunding is evidenced by significant gaps in the basket of services. This is the context described to us when we explored the topic of implementing integrated services network in the three territories.

From the viewpoint of project success factors, the program implementation theory brings out the following elements:

1. Overall context. Several context levels overlap and converge on the inadequacy of resources in the health and social services field. Yet the Ministry's policy directives have well served the integrated networks project, since the integration of services and the size of the ageing population lined up directly with the principles guiding the Ministry's policy with respect to the elderly.

2. Organizational context. The emergency departments and hospitals have been involved on the policy and managerial levels, but less able to make changes at the level of front-line practitioners, subjected to significant pressure from the demand for care with a nursing shortage. This situation has persisted. The daily pressure in CLSCs is likewise considerable for practitioners when they have a waiting list and few or no basic services to offer.

3. Human and financial resources. An important factor in a project's success or in implementing change concerns the capacity to provide the right level and type of resources. In most cases, the financial and human resources were inadequate. Only a few new resources were invested, which means that the change would have had to be funded from an already inadequate budget. Many actors decried this problem.

4. Physical resources. These resources, required primarily for implementing the SIGG computerized clinical chart, were planned for and assumed by the regional agency. Despite everything, partners considered that the CHUS and hospital care in general have an inadequate number of computer workstations.

5. Target group. The great majority of patients targeted for case management met the access criteria. They did not abandon the care proposed by the case managers, despite the inadequacy of services.

6. Practitioner and clinician training. The initial training for case managers should have required subsequent coaching sessions and discussions about the role, guidelines for interventions, and problems associated with aging. Many of the services involved in the integrated network had presentations about network components that were sometimes extensive with a question period and sometimes briefer. Individual motivation and adherence to the

project depends in part on how the change underway is perceived, which is why extensive information sessions are important.

7. Motivation, adherence. Some actors who were uninterested or slightly interested in the project did not fully adhere to it, although they were not fundamentally against it. An example of this is family physicians who stated it was like jumping between two moving trains. Nevertheless, they supported most of the project's principles. The tandem arrangement expected between case management and family physicians was partially achieved, although the structural conditions for the collaboration were not all pulled together (e.g.: physician remuneration for attending multidisciplinary meetings, allowance for caring for demanding cases of the elderly with impaired independence, excessive caseload, inadequate access to the SIGG). Steps were taken, sometimes after a period of reflection that made it possible to better understand and see the positive impact of the proposed change on the quality of life of their patients and their passage throughout the continuum's services.

8. Perception of the project itself: The model of the integrated services network was well received on the policy-making and management levels of public services. They describe it as a "promising project" and as a focal point for enthusiasm, making it possible to learn, progress, and go beyond traditional structural limitations. Despite this potential, a timeframe of several years could appear inadequate to resolve certain situations, especially those that require a complete reexamination of the problem (e.g. if the hospital is glutted with patients, you should ask yourself if coordination with services offered in the community is working effectively). That is even truer when resources are lacking.

If we sift through this amalgamation of situations to look for the main conditions of success in implementing an integrated services network, we always come back to the same leitmotiv: *"I believe in it."* Undoubtedly the product of perception of coherency between the problems identified in the field and the type of solutions advocated by the integrated network model, the confidence of key actors played a determinant role exactly because of the system's state when all these efforts were being carried out and because all the proof had not yet appeared in the literature.

Here, we underscore four elements of success that are essential.

*   A clear regional stand with clear expectations and a role assumed by the Agency that formalizes a change resulting from clinical concerns. The forums organized by the Agency resulted in a large consensus on the development of home-care services as well as on the action plan and targets to be achieved.

- A firm commitment by the institutions' managements that have directed their resources so that the entire region can follow suit, especially as regards the SIGG computerized clinical chart.
- Sound clinical work carried out by people with a great deal of clinical credibility and recognized researchers applying rigorous methodology to their work—"the project was promising"—the people on the front line couldn't think that it was simply an "administrative fad." Therefore, it is important to have a model with clinical and organizational consistency in order to win over the greatest number of people.
- In a territory such as Sherbrooke with a major pool of services, elderly persons, and case managers, one of the conditions for success was having an integrated-networks coordinator working full-time on its implementation: organizing partner collaboration and implementing tools, case management, and the single entry point. In rural territories, those responsible for implementation were people recognized for their expertise in managing services for the elderly. In all three territories, these managers were able to link the policy, management, and clinical levels as well as having legitimacy of action.

After three years of work, the collected statements do not convey a flawless picture. The actors, however, proved that they now have the keys for understanding the system in which they find themselves and leverage for change that did not exist before this project came to their region. Once the change has been better targeted, its many facets better grasped, and disseminated to a large number of people at every level of action, then hope in progress can come into being. This is what we draw from this privileged encounter with the interviewees.

References

1. Veil, A., and Hébert, R. Évaluation de l'implantation des mécanismes et outils d'intégration des services aux personnes âgées en perte d'autonomie – étude de cas comparative entre trois MRC de l'Estrie, Interim report, Dec. 2002.

2. Yin, R.K. *Case Study Research: Design and methods*, 2nd edition, *Applied Social Research Methods Series*, No. 5, Sage Publications, Beverly Hills, 1994.

3. Hébert, R., Tourigny, A., and Gagnon, M. Integrated service delivery to ensure person's functional autonomy. EDISEM, Québec, 2005.

Chapter 4
Measuring the Integration of Services between Stakeholders in the Continuum of Services for the Elderly in Three Territories

Anne Veil and Réjean Hébert

Highlights

Integrating services is a relatively recent topic in the literature. What has been written on this subject, however, reveals to us that integration is a broad, complex concept comprised of many aspects. The authors have yet to achieve consensus on the organization of these dimensions into a hierarchy. This should give pause to researchers who wish to measure integration, especially with respect to the definitions of the dimensions and variables of the concept to be measured. No instrument is currently capable of measuring all the facets of integration and taking into account its complexity, as demonstrated in the first part of this chapter.

Within the framework of the PRISMA-Estrie implementation study, we wanted to determine and apprise partners in the service continuum of their own perceptions about the state of collaboration they were experiencing three years after implementation of the integrated service network. We have adapted an instrument validated by Gina Browne and her collaborators (Ontario, Canada) that can be used to classify service providers in five levels of knowledge, communication, and collaboration. The results are presented as charts and tables that reveal which services are less well-known and which are perceived as involving interaction in terms of communication, cooperation, or collaboration.

The results show that the three territories had general averages in the upper bracket for communication, just a few tenths under the threshold for cooperation. While their general averages differ only slightly, the scores attributed to the different services identified those that are perceived or that perceived themselves as having a high, moderate, or low level of interaction and collaboration. In this regard, the results, presented as charts and tables, lend themselves quite well to taking stock of the degree of integration between diverse services in the continuum, even if they come under different sectors.

Introduction

When actors work together, they can identify and agree on targets for action. The discussions leading to agreement provide an opportunity for identifying the main values of the moral contract binding them because they subscribe to an overall philosophy of quality of care for the elderly. In particular, they have adopted the PRISMA model, which identifies the means for promoting the integration of services using three mechanisms (co-ordination, single entry point, and case management) and three tools (the SMAF / Iso-SMAF system, the SIGG computerized clinical chart, and the individualized service plan). The integrated-network implementation study focused on these six features with the objectives of monitoring implementation, of identifying the advantages and drawbacks to putting them into place, and of determining what value partners placed on the model. We hoped that this process would yield their perceptions about the state of integration in their networks. To achieve this goal, we used an instrument that has been recently validated to record how network-associated partners perceived their own degree of integration. This chapter reports on the outcomes of this process. Before presenting the results, however, we describe the aspects of integration that the instrument enables us to measure because the concept is broad and complex.

The integrated services network model implemented in Estrie was unique in that it tried to fit into the health and social services network, taking advantage of the opportunities offered by the network and dealing with its limitations. Moreover, the different territorial realities within Québec's regions produce a variety of contexts representing challenges for the integrated network project. Québec has an advantage over many countries in that health and social services issues come under a single Minister. Moreover, a certain amount of spadework was carried out through the merging of the complementary missions of hospital centers, placement services, and CLSCs during the 1990s. That being said, such mergers do not automatically change clinical and management practices. Influencing work habits in isolation means setting up projects that open up new ways of perceiving the system and new ways of working. The PRISMA project aimed, for the most part, at enhancing coordination between structures offering complementary services, although some concurrent services were also involved (private sector). Some had been merged administratively (CH-CLSC-CHSLD public services*), but there were few practices involving joint action and coordination with all of the services pertaining to problems specific to the frail elderly.

An embedded model of autonomous structures such as that proposed in Estrie cannot be achieved without a significant degree of joint action and coor-

---

* CH-CLSC-CHSLD: *Hospital Center – Local Community Service Center – Residential and Long-term Care Center.*

dination. This involves not only the organizations whose operating methods and systemic incentives are geared to "silo" performance, but also calls for an interactive process between many actors operating according to different principles (public, private, community, social economy) and at different levels of action (policy-makers, managers, clinicians, and practitioners). While joint action is not the equivalent of integration, no integration process can be successful without it.

Conceptual Approach

The topic of integrating services can be broached from a number of perspectives. In Quebec, service integration is often associated with an administrative operation (institutional mergers) or expected outcomes (efficiency, quality, continuity of services). Yet a survey of the literature on integration demonstrates that the concept is complex and multifaceted. There is general agreement about the objectives in terms of users: *Integrated services protect the user from inconveniences resulting from compartmentalization within and between levels of government administration (Office de la langue française, 2004) [translation].* *Le Robert* dictionary (1998) refers to integration as being a desire to tighten the bonds between actors or components within a structured whole in order to attain desirable objectives. Certain authors have pointed out the disparities in the meaning of integration from one country or continent to the next, where it may be associated with *managed care (USA), shared care (UK),* or *disease management,* which betrays a lack of conceptual clarity.[9]

The initial attempts at integrated systems in the United States used the definition of a network of organizations that offered a range of services to a target population or negotiated service provision from a service continuum. The organizations comprising the continuum accepted accountability for the results.[15] Integration is often perceived solely from the administrative point of view, which involves a merger of structures. Yet viewed from the viewpoint of improving management of certain groups of vulnerable people, integration stands first and foremost for shifts in clinical and management practices with a view to improving the continuity of services within the context of efficacy and efficiency. This goes fairly far beyond the administrative perspective.

During the last decade, a number of authors from industrialized countries turn their attention to the notion of service integration because they were looking for solutions to the impacts of population aging on their health and social services systems. For example, in France, the term "proximity coordination"[6] is used instead of integration, which is unattainable given the current state of relations between the many actors and payers. In the United States, Shortell[14] talked more about an "organized delivery system," associating it with the concepts of value generated by the care delivery process as well as accountability, since the American system is actively involved in seeking arrangements between actors and program-based dispositions to reduce the cost of care and services. Shortell presents the notions of clinical and functional integration, and the American medical system as means for supporting competencies, outcomes and the actors involved in creating value for patients despite the fact that the system is dominated by the interests of insurance companies.

Kodner and Spreeuwenberg[9] view integration as being at the heart of systems theory. As described by O'Connor and McDermott, cited by Foote and Stanners,[5] "a definition of a system is something that maintains its existence and functions as a whole through the interaction of its parts." Therefore, system boundaries can be entirely virtual, since what rallies system members are the shared goals, network communication, and the fact that each one benefits in some way. The notion becomes pivotal in the development of health-care organizations, which present as separate but interrelated with roles that should be, in theory, complementary. Integration binds the entity together to accomplish the goals shared by the constituent parts. As a result of the complexity of the health and social services system and its tendency towards specialization, the services become fragmented. If integration is not carried out with all the actors and various levels of action, the problems will persist. Family physicians, because of the key role they play with specialists and patient living environments, have often to bridge the gap between the medical system and social services in order to ensure their patients received quality management of care. The need to stop the cost of services from spiraling upward (economic imperative) has made this role increasingly important. In contrast, family physicians no longer have the time to take on everything. Furthermore, they are not certain that the role should fall to them.

Faced with definitions of integration often centered on organizational objectives to be achieved, Kodner et al.[9] proposed their own based on patient needs in which integration is "a coherent set of methods and models on the funding, administrative, organizational, service delivery and clinical levels designed to create connectivity, alignment and collaboration within and between the cure and care sectors. The goal of these methods and models is to enhance quality of care and quality of life, consumer satisfaction and system efficiency for patients with complex, long-term problems cutting across multiple services, providers and settings." Like Leutz,[11] these authors believe that the level, type, and combination of strategies used (whether financial, organizational, administrative, clinical, or related to service delivery) should be matched with patient characteristics and the specific challenges arising from obtaining quality care appropriate to their situation. Consequently, as needs grow in complexity, the integration strategies must be correspondingly tightened.

An initial imperative in our research into new tools and practices related to service integration was to better define its objective. Leutz and other authors raised some interesting principles pertaining primarily to the organizational and relational levels involved in integration. Let's begin by reviewing Leutz's five laws.

1. You can integrate some of the services for all the people, all the services for some of the people, but you can't integrate all the services for all the people. Leutz is referring to the different levels of needs of people and the corresponding intensity of services.
2. Integration costs before it benefits.
3. Your integration is my fragmentation. All systems have boundaries. Integration touches these boundaries and therefore runs the risk of disturbing by provoking changes.
4. You can't integrate a square peg into a round hole. Integration objectives are very difficult to achieve if there are no linkages between financing and system operating methods.
5. The one who integrates calls the tune. Systemic and political phenomena are at play during integration.

The relational dimension involved in any integration process is complex in and of itself. It concerns many levels of strategic and financial action, public policy, management and practitioners/clinicians.[11] In other words, the referent can be established according to micro (target groups), meso (organization), or macro (society, public policy) strategies.[13] Efforts should not focus on a single level and must be convergent since internal barriers, such as areas of conflicts between professions remain, even when the structural, organizational and financial barriers have been attenuated. Sight must not be lost of the importance of establishing and supporting partnerships between and among professions to achieve a shared vision, mutual trust, and interprofessional cooperation in order to move towards integration of services (Wistow cited in Reed[13]). These intermediate targets are required to achieve integration. They all involve interaction with the other professions and services, which implies putting into place and maintaining a business or service relationship on a long-term basis.

An article on follow-up to a process to progressively integrate partners (Project Chain)[17] describes three dimensions of an integration structure: amplitude (number of providers contributing to integration), action levels (policymakers, managers and clinicians/practitioners) and the degree of vertical and horizontal integration that take place within formal and informal communication frameworks. The relational component therefore relates to network extent, expressed as the number of service providers contributing to the service offer. While they all have fields of specialization differentiating them, they must be linked through some kind of bond. In order to mesh and work together, they must communicate, which involves horizontal actions (such as between clinicians) and vertical actions (such as between managers and caregivers), both intraorganizationally and interorganizationally.

Although rarely approached from this angle, it should be emphasized that one of the priorities in involving case managers in the different systems pertains directly to this relational field. Case-manager attributes include promoting quality communication (honest, direct, relevant, timely, ongoing) between all the actors: managers, professionals, and technicians from the various public and community health and social services sectors, the elderly and their families, third-party caregivers, coordinators, and the staff and managers of private services.

That being said, Contandriopoulos et al.[3] define integration as a process to create and maintain over time "a common governance between independent actors in order to coordinate their interdependencies" within a collective project in which all participants find benefits in better coordinating their practices. Integration is a process that takes different shapes but aims at institutionalizing cooperative relationships by coordinating clinical practices with a view towards improving the continuity of care for vulnerable groups of patients. The dimensions of integration have been defined as follows.

- Normative integration aims at ensuring coherency between the actors' systems of value, service-organization methods, and the clinical system. It "makes it possible to plan governance according to the requirements of cooperation."
- Clinical integration pertains to forming multi- or interdisciplinary teams offering overall and ongoing medical and psychosocial care. These are stable, flexible teams that pivot around the network. They use shared tools and protocols. The active participation of physicians on these teams is a condition to make integration of care and services a success.
- Functional integration brings together the informational, organizational and financial dimensions. It aims at creating the conditions resulting in and maintaining clinical teams and in clustering the network's financial, management and information systems around the clinical system. Therefore, this means creating shared governance with full powers over the resources to be mobilized in favor of clinical projects. This includes the introduction of economic incentives to encourage actors to coordinate their practices as well as using an information system that can support decision-makers in their management choices and caregivers in their clinical decisions, thereby enabling the network to adapt to the constantly changing context and needs. It strives to align itself with shared accountability for collective issues related to health and social services. This form of integration can be measured by the degree of coordination in support functions (leadership, governance, management, funding, information systems) between stakeholders and the different care and service units.
- Systemic integration "implies that the complexity and content of the issues occurring locally in the organization of care are reflected in the larger environment." This type of integration provides for coherence between the local, regional, and national levels.

While certain authors worked to elucidate the dimensions of the concept of integration, others started drawing up a hierarchy between these different dimensions. Ahgren and Axelsson[1] put forward that functional integration is a composite dimension comprised of clinical, informational, and financial integration. Even if the basic work on the concepts doesn't appear to have been completed yet, policy-makers and service managers experimenting with new design and management means now need to be able to measure the progress achieved.

For an Operational Definition of Integration

Measuring a concept begins with finding a working definition whose elements cover the concept completely (collectively exhaustive) with no redundancy (mutually exclusive). Therefore, it would be of use to identify the nuances between the definitions of concepts similar to the one to be measured. In our case, integration is quite similar to concepts such as cooperation (or collaboration), coordination, and interdependence.

In order to clarify the potential and limitations of each, we propose the following definitions derived from the work of Contandriopoulos et al.

Interdependence: "Interdependence exists when independent stakeholders (or organizations) must resolve collective problems (Bryson and Crosby, 1993, cited in GRIS[3]), which means that none of the actors involved have all the resources, skills, and legitimacy needed to contribute a legitimate, valid response (in scientific, professional, technical, and social terms) to the problems faced by each actor (or organization). Stakeholder cooperation therefore lies at the core of the integration issue." Operationalization of this concept calls for a network vision of the problems and solutions.

Cooperation: "Cooperation is the type of relationship that interdependent stakeholders (individuals or organizations) tend to prefer instead of competition when they share the same values and agree on a common philosophy for action; when they have a positive assess of the work of other stakeholders; when they are in agreement on sharing their areas of expertise and tasks; and, lastly, when they are in a conducive organizational context (Benson, 1975, cited in GRIS[3]). Cooperation is never absolute; it does not exclude competitiveness between stakeholders (individuals or organizations). Sustained cooperation requires that stakeholders (individuals or organizations) continuously negotiate among themselves and assess the outcomes of their cooperation" (Friedberg, 1993, cited in GRIS[3]). The operationalization of cooperation depends on communication between stakeholders (organizations) and on interdisciplinarity within a formal framework involving relational codes promoting a given philosophy. Cooperation is a spirit and attitude before becoming an action. It exists as a sharing of values and a common philosophy, recognition of the value of the work of others, and openness in sharing their field of competency (interdisciplinarity). It is fostered by a conducive organizational context.

Alter and Hage (1993, cited in GRIS[3]) define three types of coordination on the basis of the clinical complexity required by the state and situation of the patient and by the care and services organization to be put into place.

1. Sequential coordination refers to a linear process in which expertise is accessed through a referral system on a case-by-case basis. This type of coordination is appropriate solely in situations in which uncertainty is low. Sequential coordination, more commonly referred to as liaison, is already the norm in the health system.

2. Reciprocal coordination is indicated when there is interdependency between the actors and when the patient must receive care and services from several organizations or professionals at the same time. The conditions for success are 1) taking into account the interventions of others in making one's own clinical decisions; 2) having adequate information to respond coherently to the patient's needs. A patient often acts as his or her own coordinator. Reciprocal coordination is indicated when the situation is not very complex, the number of caregivers is low, the care episode is well defined, and an effective information system is used. If any of these conditions are missing, collective coordination is called for.

3. Collective coordination is required for patients with multiple health problems of uncertain evolution. Collective coordination requires organized management and formal agreements between organizations to ensure adequate accessibility to the required care and services. Uncertainty increases as does the interdependence between actors, which drives up the need for collective coordination. No single procedure is appropriate for all cases. Each coordination situation must be personalized and adapted to the context for which is required.

As explained by Kralewski,[10] the involvement of many actors in a continuum requires a definite effort. In order to facilitate their efforts to strengthen coordination, continuum members must absolutely have a reliable information system that can provide information that is current, accurate and comprehensive in terms of use of services, the work loads of clinicians and caregivers, the outcomes, their costs, the quality of care, and the level of satisfaction of the patients. One might believe that the greater the perception that caregivers and service providers have of information-system functionality, the greater the chances that the information required for proper management will be available when needed and the greater the perception that there is coherency between services when more complex cases present themselves.

Measuring Integration

The concept of integration is rather broad in view. Moreover, it is also important to take a position with respect to other work that has been done when attempting to measure it. The concept's complexity makes taking a position mandatory because there is no single measurement that can simultaneously assess all facets of integration. To illustrate the different ways of measuring service integration, we present three articles that take different approaches. We used one of them for the Estrie implementation study.

Compared Measurements of Integration

Shortell[14] states that integration is supported by key organizational functions: human resources, strategic and financial planning, information systems, and quality assessment. From his perspective, measuring integration means determining the degree to which these functions and activities are coordinated all along a continuum of services so as to add the best possible value to the system. While the definition is of interest, its current formulation doesn't provide the means for delimiting the exact dimensions of the object to be measured.

Other authors have made valuable contributions in measuring certain aspects of integration. An article by Ahgren and Axelsson,[1] based on Swedish experience, only looks at the degree of integration between the various providers of health-care services. Social services were not included. The authors basically consider that integration can be more or less developed, consisting of a continuum from full segregation (distinct, independent entities) to full integration (merger, resources pooled within a single unit). The intermediate levels are linkage, coordination and cooperation. They make a distinction between coordination and cooperation. Coordination aims at smoothing operations between various health-care units without the need of a network manager. In contrast, cooperation requires network managers to improve contacts between the units, who retain their distinct independent characters. Ahgren and Axelsson also state that most existing models of measurement of integration services deal with structural integration. They use notions contributed by Lasker and colleagues (2001) to place certain concepts with respect to others. Ahgren and Axelsson do not refer to organizational integration, which, as mentioned above, predominates in Contandriopoulos et al.[3] They pay scant attention to the structural aspects of integration, which appears to be seen as the presence of structures supporting integration or as the merger of structures. Rather, they report on Lawrence's and Lorsch's idea, stipulating that the highest degree of integration between certain units is not necessarily the maximum and that, in fact, a lesser degree could be acceptable. In other words, the optimal level of desirable integration would be linked to the central role played by certain actors in the continuum being assessed. The idea has a great deal of merit.

The concepts discussed by Ahgren and Axelsson[1] lie at what they deem to be the heart of the integration process. Their instrument is called the scale of functional clinical integration. Its conceptual organization is depicted in Figure 4.1.

Each degree of functional clinical integration is linked to indicators that help identify towards what level integration is heading towards. Consequently, the separation of organizations translates into a referral mode in which patients must navigate the system on their own. Linkage implies having guidelines to follow and people who are responsible for different types of services. Coordination between networks is associated with chains of care; cooperation involves network managers; and full integration is evidenced by resources being pooled

Figure 4.1
Conceptual organization of integration (Ahgren and Axelsson, 2005)

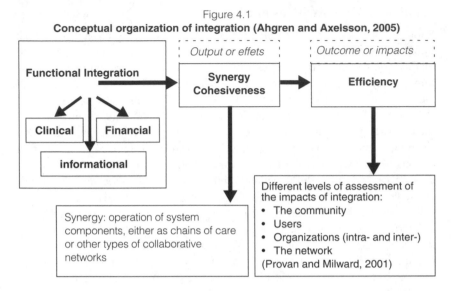

under a single administration. This yields therefore the four main forms of interaction between care and service units: linkage, coordination, cooperation, and integration.

Organizing the integration dimensions enables us to bring out the potential and limitations of the scale at the same time. The primarily medical context in which measuring integration occurs deserves consideration among the scale's limitations. Its end purpose does not focus specifically on patients with complex needs but rather strives to maintain the flow of annual consultations. Moreover, it is interesting to note that the authors view synergy and cohesiveness as the expression or outcome of functional and clinical integration. Their method involves each assessment being reached by consensus in each care unit and that it identifies the current and optimal levels of integration of the unit with respect to the other units, some of which may be outside the organization. In contrast, this type of scale cannot show if the different types of patients were put on a care and services path appropriate for their needs. Furthermore, the network to be measured is not involved solely in the health sector. The social-services sector, which takes in several types of organizations required to respond to the needs of vulnerable patients, is not taken into account. Doing so would have made the exercise more complex. Lastly, there was no assessment of interactions on a network basis.

The second measurement was carried out by a consortium of researchers from 11 European countries under the direction of J.-C. Henrard.[8] From the outset, the authors define integration as a means for improving the quality of health care and social services. This article, centered on home care, proposes an index of items taken from a questionnaire jointly designed by the 11 people in charge of the programs in the countries evaluated. The purpose is to determine the existence of certain basic characteristics in home-care programs for the elderly there. The questionnaire is the *European-Home Care Service* (EU-HCS). The items serving as the basis for formulating the questionnaire were taken from the AdHoc study. Based on Donabedian's concept of quality, which identifies structure, process, and results as the three major dimensions of quality, Henrard and colleagues hold that the literature on integration targets structure and process as the two central dimensions. Structure refers to available resources, service providers, and the organization, whereas process considers the approach used in service delivery. A structured questionnaire was developed based on certain characteristics of services for people age 65 or older. These characteristics could be, for example, the existence of eligibility criteria, referral systems, validated instruments, staff–patient ratios, average length of services, and so on.

On the conceptual level, the authors refer to the structural organizational approach, which involves bringing together staff and resources (social services, primary and secondary health care) under a unified hierarchal structure. Process-centered integration takes in care activities as well as collaborative actions or activities undertaken between health and social services organizations and practitioners brought together under working arrangements between services. For example, comprehensive clinical assessment, hospital discharge management, the participation of a general practitioner at a team meeting, or a case manager were considered as working arrangements of an integrative nature. A total of 29 items cover all of the activities of organizations providing home-care services for people age 65 or older. A score of 1 was given when the item was present. No weighting was assigned since all items were deemed to have the same value. Validation assessment made it possible to break down the services in the study cities into three categories. The first model of services consists of the cities offering several social services with very little process integration (few integrative arrangements) and a certain number of health services associated with social services. The second model consists of the cities offering health services with integrative working arrangements but with few or no social services, except for one city, which has certain working agreements for health care or social services. The third model is represented by two cities offering few services with few or no integrative arrangements.

Reviewing the instrument items reveals that only 2 of the 29 items are related to the hospital or medical system: a general practitioner attending a team meeting and preparation for hospital discharge. The health care identified in the questionnaire is nursing care; no mention is made of medical consultations. Although the objective refers to measuring the integration of health and social services, the scope is limited by the fact that the assessment questionnaire does not deal with hospital emergency departments, rehabilitation, or medical services. As the authors indicated themselves, the organizational dimension and practitioner attitude was not broached; neither was the experience of patients along the path services. Despite its limitations, this work is of interest for raising the notion of working arrangements as a central functional feature of the integration process. This made it possible to compare a number of countries with structures and service organizations that are inevitably different.

The third measure of integration we present is the one we used for the implementation study for PRISMA-Estrie. Developed by Gina Browne,[2] in Ontario, within the framework of integration of perinatal services, this scale makes it possible to display the results of interaction between a number of partners on a single chart. The concept of integration is defined according to types of collaboration, partnership, or networks in which different autonomous organizations work together in order to improve health care and social services. Browne's operational concept includes collaboration, partnership synergy, and network efficacy. It provides a basis for discussing the notion of continuity of care and services. Partnership synergy (i.e. to what degree a partnership functions well) is related to effective leadership, greater efficiency, effective management and administration, and sufficiency of resources. Synergy as studied by Weiss et al.[18] in relationship to functional partnership is the prime characteristic of a winning collaborative process. Weiss's study on synergy made it possible to describe how well a partnership was functioning, but didn't reveal the degree of integration achieved or with which actors. Browne's contribution aimed at identifying the level of collaboration partners achieved with the network. She proposed a three-dimensional model that quantifies the extent, scope, and depth of the integration effort.

Since Browne's measurement makes it possible to distinguish levels of collaboration, the focus is on the dimension of functional integration, which, in other words, is how well service providers are collaborating with each other. While the results of this kind of measurement are more difficult to communicate to interested parties (since they are provided in chart form, which may appear abstruse at first glance), measuring the function is of undeniable value because it represents the system's capacity to mobilize itself.

Measuring Integration in Estrie

We adapted and applied the measurement of services integration developed by Browne[2] to services for the elderly. The definition of integration within the framework of this measurement covers the different types of collaboration, partnerships, and networks in which autonomous organizations work to improve health care and social services for a target population. While the literature often makes no distinction between collaboration, synergic partnerships, and network, Browne considers that these terms describe the concept of integration. She uses the notion of continuity in the sense of the continuation of services at different points in time to prevent, screen, identify, and then treat the disease or problem. This precision sets the guidelines for identifying the partners in a continuum of services.

Browne describes a three-dimensional model of service integration that quantifies the extent, scope, and depth of the integration effort. The model identifies which sectors, services, or agencies collaborate in an integrative manner with the others and which network sectors could improve their collaboration efforts.

According to Provan and Milward, as cited by Browne, the success of a network should be assessed from several perspectives: that of the administrators, service providers, users, and community members. Yet a single set of instruments is not appropriate for every group of actors because they have different interests depending on their position in the system. Browne's measurement can be applied to service providers in a continuum but not to clients or the general public.

Adapting Integration Measurement

Browne's three-dimensional model can be adapted and used in any sector of activity related to human services with overall intervention goals. This is particularly true in the case of vulnerable clients requiring services that fall within a number of spheres.

Composition of the Integration Structure

The three axes of Browne's integration model are described below.
A. The vertical axis comprises the major sectors of activity** involved that refer to the mission or objective. They belong to the cross-sectoral area of integration, making it possible to offer services covering different aspects of the lives of individuals (e.g. health, education, recreation).
B. The horizontal axis identifies the types of services that together provide a continuum of services. They form the intersectoral area of integration in which coordination is required between services and programs in a given sector, such as when prevention is linked to screening and, when necessary, to clinical services.
C. The third axis comprises the main sources of funding (public, private, non-profit). Funding integration would be the pooling of human or material resources between organizations that do not belong to the same sector. Examples of this would be a home respite program organized jointly by community organizations and a CSSS or a convalescence program organized by a hospital with private homes.

** The sector is a segment of health care and social services generally grouped together in the community for budgetary control or historical reasons.

The integrated services network for the elderly, by definition, belongs to the local level. The other levels (regional, supraregional, and national) are ways of describing services from the view of territorial access. The typology that we have adopted in measuring integration in the integrated services network for the elderly (primary, secondary, and tertiary care or services) reflects instead service organization. It often refers to the nature and intensity of patient needs, providing a conceptual connection to patient evolution, which mirrors the continuum of services. A recent document by the Ministère de la santé et des services sociaux (MSSS) du Québec[12] states that a number of different nomenclatures have been used over the years to designate services. In an effort to harmonize them, MSSS authorities arrived at a consensus on this terminology, namely, primary, secondary and tertiary care or services. This choice was motivated by the fact that the "classification refers to the organization of health care and social services from the perspective of accessibility, continuity, and availability, regardless of the location of service delivery" [translation]. The definitions below, which have been used to categorize the services in the integrated network for the elderly, were derived from this document.***

Primary-care services: They respond to common and varied health and social problems affecting the entire population (1st level: general services) and vulnerable or specific target groups (2nd level: specific services). Case management for the frail elderly falls under specific services. On this level, the individual's situation is transient; the problems are temporary or acute, but reversible; or the condition comes under an intervention plan (IP) or individualized service plan (ISP) extending over the medium or long term. Primary-care practitioners often provide ongoing management of the patient. These services require easy and foreseeable conditions of access, continuity of information (caregiver access to relevant information about the person), and relational continuity (sustained ongoing and quality relationship).

Secondary-care services: They respond to complex health and social issues for individuals that have been referred (excluding exceptions) to experts or specialists. These services are for specific groups or the entire population under the mandate of health-related promotion, prevention, protection, and surveillance. Such services are generally of limited duration. While the secondary-care practitioners may take charge of management, the patient is returned to primary care for the overall interventions required. Secondary-care practitioners keep primary-care practitioners apprised of the secondary-care episode (or the event that caused it).

*** The type of service corresponds to an intervention momentum in the development of a problem or issue. In the health and social services community, this typology follows the following categories: prevention and screening, primary-care services, secondary-care services, tertiary-care services.

Tertiary services: They respond to very complex health or social problems of very low incidence and are for individuals referred for problems requiring very specialized skills or highly specialized or costly equipment. Management is only provided by tertiary-care practitioners in exceptional cases. Such services are generally of limited duration. Tertiary-care practitioners keep primary- and secondary-care practitioners apprised of the tertiary-care episode (or the event that caused it). Since tertiary care and services are rarer and do not take in management, they were not broached in forming an integrated network for elderly.

We used this structural base to identify two major sectors major for the frail elderly (health and social), both involving primary-care and secondary-care services. In the health-care sector, we identified 14 primary-care programs (including prevention programs) and 13 secondary-care programs. In the social-services sector, we also identified 14 primary-care programs (including prevention programs) and 9 secondary-care programs. Each sector had programs with public, private, and nonprofit funding as well as blended funding.

Method

Ideally, practitioners, representatives or service coordinators from each sector identified in the list of services are asked to rank the perceived level of integration between their service and all the others. During the implementation study, the governing boards were not able to bring together all the types of services, which limited the breadth of respondent representation. The scale used was developed by Narayan and Shier, as cited in Vanderwoerd,[16] which has 5 steps within an increasing integration continuum scored between 0 and 4.

Ordinal Scale

0 points: *Unawareness:* Programs or services are not aware of other programs or services.

1 point: *Awareness:* Discrete programs or services in the community are aware of other programs or services, but they organize their own activities solely on the basis of their own program or service mission, and make no effort to do otherwise.

2 points: *Communication:* Programs and services actively share information and communicate on a formal basis.

3 points: *Cooperation:* Programs or services modify their own service planning to avoid service duplication or to improve links among services, using their knowledge of other services or programs.

4 points: *Collaboration:* Programs or services jointly plan offered services and modify their own services as a result of mutual consultations and advice.

Questionnaire Administration

The ratings can be gathered in a number of ways, such as by telephone interview, web forms, in person, or during workshops. Each response is entered in the box aligned with the name of the service being rated. In the case of Estrie, the questionnaire was filled out immediately after an interview (either individual or group).

In terms of extent of services in Estrie (active or potential members of the continuum for the elderly), the services were grouped into 22 categories. While these categories are usually distinct from one another, certain services, such as fall prevention (public-health program), operate interorganizationally and are therefore spread across more than one category. We did not measure respondent perception of the extent but only the scope (number of service providers aware of other continuum providers with a result > 0) and depth of service integration (type of linkage between providers) among the integrated network's active partners and not all the organizations belonging to the service continuum. Our results therefore reflect the perception of members who took part in implementing the integrated services network and not that of the entire membership of the continuum. The rate of response, moreover, was calculated using this breakdown of respondents.

Our prime interest consists in identifying the intensity or degree of collaboration perceived by the various providers in the service continuum for the elderly once the integrated service network had been implemented. Since many health-care and social services are accessible locally and, moreover, the localities carried out the process for implementing the integrated services network, the results should be delivered on a local territory basis. The questionnaire used appears in the appendix.

Scoring

Since the set of services available in the continuum were grouped according to similarity, we adopted the same approach with the respondents, who were grouped according to their home institution. As a result, respondents do not rank their own services (blacked out), which prevents any bias related to self-reporting.

The scoring system therefore takes the shape of a table. Results for each group of services fall between 0 and 4. Reading across a row indicates how each service provider is perceived by the other groups of respondents in addition to giving its overall average (with standard deviation). The last two lines are particularly useful in determining how each of the groups of respondents perceives the continuum as a whole, expressed as averages and standard deviations. Reading down the columns gives how each group of respondents perceives each group of services in the continuum and the overall average (last two columns on the right), representing the level of interaction (or depth of integration) experienced by respondents, expressed as averages and standard deviations.

In order to facilitate comparison of the results and interpretation of the overall averages, we used a group of five levels of integration as a reference instead of the eight categories used by Browne. We also compare the overall average obtained in Estrie with that in Browne's study, in which case, we use the same indicators. Figure 4.2 gives the indicators used.

Figure 4.2
Indicators for Interpreting Results

Browne's Study		Prisma-Estrie Implementation
Clinical Indicator*	*Score*	*Group according to Level*
Very little integration	*0.0 to 0.49* ⟶	Unawareness
Little integration	*0.5 to 0.99* ⎫	
Mild integration	*1.0 to 1.49* ⎬⟶	Awareness
Moderate integration	*1.5 to 1.99* ⎫	
Good integration	*2.0 to 2.49* ⎬⟶	Communication
Very good integration	*2.5 to 2.99* ⎫	
Excellent integration	*3.0 to 3.49* ⎬⟶	Cooperation
Perfect integration	*3.5 to 4.00* ⟶	Collaboration

* Browne et al. (2004) Table 2, p. 9

Results of Integration Perception in Three Estrie Territories

The rate of participation in the integration measurement was high. Nearly all of the individuals (97.5 %) that we invited to an interview (individual or group) subsequently completed the questionnaire about the integration of services for the elderly available in their locale.

Description of Participants

Each of the individuals who took part in the assessment interviews on the implementation of the integrated services network completed a sheet requesting sociodemographic and professional information. It was filled out at the same time as the questionnaire on integration after the interview. A total of 77 respondents provided sociodemographic information: 23 case managers, 15 executives or managers, and 39 practitioners or clinicians. One individual completed the service integration measurement without providing a sociodemographic-information sheet (Granit), which resulted in a total of 78 responses to the integration measurement. Tables 4.1 to 4.3 provide the characteristics of respondents based on professional affiliation and territory.

Table 4.1
Sociodemographic Characteristics of Respondents
Profession: case manager (n = 23)

Variables	Sherbrooke (n = 15)	Granit (n = 4)	Coaticook (n = 4)	TOTAL (n = 23)
Sex (F)	86.7 %	100 %	75 %	86.9 %
Age gr.: under 40 (%)	53 %	100 %	aucun	52.2 %
Same duties for (years)	2.0	2.3	2.2	2.1
Same employer for (years)	4.7	5.3	12.1	6.1
Undergraduate training (%)	14 (93.3 %)	2 (50 %)	4 (100 %)	20 (87 %)
Graduate training (master's degree and diploma) (%)	4 (26.7 %)	2 (50 %)	1 (25 %)	7 (30 %)
Exper. with elderly (years)	10.3	3.5	11.6	9.3
% of clients 65 years or over	99 %	98 %	85 %	97 %

As shown in Table 4.1, most case managers are women. They are younger than 40 in Granit and older than 40 in Coaticook, while the age groups in Sherbrooke are mixed. Coaticook has the case managers who have worked the longest for the same employer (average of 12 years). The average number of years of experience with the elderly is from 10 to 11 years, except in Granit, where the average is 3.5 years. The most common level of training is an undergraduate degree in the humanities, particularly social work. A third of them have training at the master's degree level.

Table 4.2
Sociodemographic Characteristics of Respondents
Profession: Executives, Managers, Leaders (n = 15)

Variables	Sherbrooke (n = 9)	Granit (n = 3)	Coaticook (n = 3)	TOTAL (n = 15)
Sex (F)	7 (77.8 %)	1 (33.3 %)	1 (33.3 %)	9 (60 %)
Age gr.: 40 years or older (%)	9 (100 %)	3 (100 %)	3 (100 %)	15 (100 %)
Same duties for (years)	8.8	4.7	15.7	9.3
Same employer for (years)	11.7	9.3	22	13.3
Training certificates and microprograms (%)	4 (44.4 %)	2 (66.7 %)	–	6 (40 %)
Undergraduate training (%)	3 (33.3 %)	–	1 (33.3 %)	4 (26.7 %)
Master's degree training (%)	7 (77.8 %)	2 (66.7 %)	1 (33.3 %)	10 (66.7 %)
Graduate training (diploma) (%)	3 (33.3 %)	–	1 (33.3 %)	4 (26.7 %)
Doctoral training (%)	1 (11.1 %)	–	1 (33.3 %)	2 (13.3 %)
Exper. with elderly (years)	20.3	17	18.3	18.5
% of clients 65 years or over	83 %	80 %	66.7 %	75.9 %

Table 4.2 shows that executives and managers are most often women in urban areas (rather than from rural settings) and are all older than 40 years. They have held the same position for several years in Coaticook (especially) and Sherbrooke; they have worked for the same employer for at least 10 years on average. Training at higher levels (master's degree, diploma, doctorate) occurs more frequently in urban areas. They also have extensive experience in the different services for the elderly, averaging at least 17 years. Experience with both the elderly and other patients with impaired independence is more visible in the smallest territory (Coaticook).

Table 4.3
Sociodemographic Characteristics of Respondents
Profession: practitioners and clinicians (n = 39)

Variables	Sherbrooke (n = 22)	Granit (n = 9)	Coaticook (n = 8)	TOTAL (n = 39)
Sex (F)	16 (72.7 %)	9 (100 %)	8 (100 %)	33 (84.6 %)
Age gr.: 40 years or older (%)	17 (77.3 %)	6 (66.7 %)	5 (62.5 %)	28 (71.8 %)
Same duties for (years)	7.8	10.2	13.3	11.4
Same employer for (years)	17.3	14.9	12.7	14.2
DEC, DEP training... (%)	6 (27.3 %)	3 (33.3 %)	4 (50 %)	13 (33.3 %)
Training certificates and microprograms (%)	3 (13.6 %)	2 (22.2 %)	2 (25 %)	7 (17.9 %)
Undergraduate training (%)	17 (77.3 %)	2 (22.2 %)	3 (37.5 %)	22 (56.4 %)
Master's degree training (%)	2 (9.1 %)	-	1 (12.5 %)	3 (7.7 %)
Exper. with elderly (years)	15.4	13.8	14.3	14.4
% of clients 65 years or over	78 %	76 %	81 %	79 %

Lastly, women accounted for the greater percentage (85 %) of practitioners and clinicians (Table 4.3) and more women fall into the age groups over 40. Respondents have held their positions for more than 10 years on average, except in Sherbrooke where the length of employment is 7.8 years. In contrast, they have worked an average of 17 years for the same employer in Sherbrooke. In Granit and Coaticook, respondents have worked 13 to 15 years on average for the same employer. While their training is varied, most has been at the undergraduate level. Practitioners in the three zones have an average of nearly 15 years of involvement with the elderly. Their patients are mixed but predominantly seniors (80 %).

Results from the Three Territories

Horizontal Axis (depth)

In the context of the integrated network implementation study, depth of integration stood out as the most important of the three dimensions that the instrument can measure, since we were interested in the level of effective collaboration as perceived by the service providers. Our results are derived from calculating averages along the horizontal axis, that is, using the average scores attributed to each of the different service groups by the respondents as a whole, who are themselves connected to continuum organizations for the most part. The scores along the horizontal axis were either attributed by a single respondent connected to a service group or an average of responses from a number of people in the same group of services. The lower and upper limits of the scores for each of the five levels of integration are 0 to 0.49 (unawareness), 0.5 to 1.49 (awareness), 1.5 to 2.49 (communication), 2.5 to 3.49 (cooperation), and 3.5 to 4 (collaboration). This presentation of results will enable us to discern patterns from one territory to the next.

The chart provides access to data of high interactive value where respondents along the horizontal axis intersect the assessed services along the vertical axis. If an actor wishes to verify with which specific partners collaboration actually exists, looking at the set of services rated provides information that the actor can use to adjust his or her mode of interaction with some of them, if necessary. If a respondent or group of respondents wants to get an idea of how their perception of the continuum as a whole fits in, they can compare it to the perception of the other partners. Tables 4.4, 4.5, and 4.6 provide these charts.

For the depth of integration between services, Sherbrooke had an overall average of 2.47 (SD ± 0.49). Since results between 1.5 and 2.49 fall within the communication bracket, Sherbrooke has an overall result at the dividing line between communication and cooperation. This is the highest average among the three territories. The overall average in Granit is 2.29 (SD ± 0.66). This falls within the communication bracket, as does the average for Coaticook, which was 2.39 (SD ± 0.69). These three results are comparable, since the deviations are only several tenths of a point.

Comparison of Browne's and the Estrie Results

Although the overall results from Estrie cannot be directly compared to Browne's, which concern perinatality services, the use of a reference chart (see Figure 4.2) enables us to situate the results on a progressive scale. The overall result in Ontario was 1.75 (SD = 0.77), which is considered moderate integration. The three territories in Estrie turned in results ranging from 2.0 to 2.49, meaning that they all fall within the good-integration bracket.

Table 4.4

Results on Interaction between Continuum Services: Sherbrooke Table

MEASURE OF SERVICE INTEGRATION (SHERBROOKE)	n=3 #2	n=1 #5	n=4 #6	n=2 #7	n=1 #8	n=4 #10	n=1 #12	n=1 #13	n=1 #14	r=1 #15	n=1 #16	n=14 #17	n=1 #18	n=3 #19	n=6 #20	n=2 autres	Integration Aver. (0-4)	SD (N=46)
Rate of Response 15 gr./22 equals 68.2%																	Depth↓	
1. Info-Santé	1.67	4.00	1.00	1.50	2.00	1.25	1.00	1.00	1.00	2.00	1.00	1.93	2.00	1.00	1.33	1.50	1.57	0.76
2. Single entry point	■	4.00	3.00	2.00	3.00	1.25	3.00	4.00	4.00	1.00	3.00	3.29	4.00	1.33	1.17	2.75	2.72	1.11
3. CLSC MDs and nurses	2.67	4.00	2.25	2.00	1.00	1.75	4.00	4.00	3.00	3.00	3.00	2.86	4.00	1.33	1.33	3.25	2.59	0.97
4. FMGs* and medical clinics	3.00	2.00	1.50	1.50	1.00	0.75	1.00	2.00	2.00	1.00	2.00	2.29	2.00	1.00	1.17	1.75	1.62	0.61
5. Home support	4.00	■	3.25	2.00	4.00	1.50	3.00	4.00	4.00	2.00	4.00	3.71	2.00	2.00	2.33	3.00	2.99	0.94
6. Day care center	3.67	4.00	■	2.00	1.00	2.00	3.00	4.00	4.00	3.00	3.00	3.64	2.00	1.67	2.50	1.75	2.62	0.93
7. Centre de réadaptation Estrie	2.00	2.00	2.33	■	1.00	2.00	3.00	2.00	1.00	2.00	1.00	2.07	4.00	1.00	2.00	2.00	2.03	0.85
8. Hospital emergency department	1.67	2.00	1.25	1.00	■	1.50	3.00	2.00	1.00	2.00	4.00	2.43	2.00	2.33	0.83	1.75	1.92	0.83
9. Ambulance services	1.33	1.00	1.25	1.00	4.00	1.00	1.00	1.00	1.00	2.00	1.00	1.36	2.00	3.00	0.83	1.25	1.56	0.87
10. Geriatrics (hospital)	2.67	3.00	2.50	1.00	1.00	■	4.00	3.00	2.00	3.00	4.00	2.71	2.00	3.67	1.17	3.75	2.68	1.05
11. Public health (prevention)	3.33	2.00	1.75	1.50	3.00	2.00	1.00	1.00	2.00	2.00	2.00	2.07	2.00	2.00	2.17	1.75	1.97	0.59
12. Day hospital	3.33	3.00	3.00	1.50	2.00	2.50	■	4.00	4.00	4.00	4.00	2.86	3.00	2.00	2.00	2.75	2.85	0.80
13. Short-Term Geriatric Unit	2.67	4.00	3.00	1.50	4.00	3.50	4.00	■	4.00	4.00	4.00	2.79	3.00	2.00	1.00	3.75	3.15	1.00
14. SGUI* outpatient clinics	2.00	4.00	2.50	1.00	2.00	2.00	4.00	3.00	■	4.00	4.00	2.57	3.00	2.00	0.83	2.00	2.46	0.99
15. Geriatric-psychiatry	2.33	4.00	1.25	1.00	2.00	1.75	4.00	3.00	4.00	■	4.00	2.79	3.00	4.00	0.33	2.25	2.65	1.22
16. SGUI IFRU*	2.33	2.00	1.00	1.00	4.00	3.50	4.00	1.00	3.00	4.00	■	2.53	3.00	2.33	1.17	3.75	2.60	1.16
17. Case management	3.33	4.00	4.00	2.50	4.00	2.75	4.00	4.00	2.00	2.00	4.00	■	4.00	2.33	2.33	3.75	3.27	0.78
18. Temporary placement	3.00	4.00	2.75	1.00	2.00	2.25	2.00	2.00	3.00	3.00	4.00	3.57	■	2.00	1.33	3.75	2.58	0.95
19. Permanent public placement	2.33	4.00	2.50	2.00	2.00	2.75	3.00	3.00	3.00	3.00	4.00	3.29	2.00	■	1.67	3.50	2.87	0.78
20. Community organizations and HMS*	4.00	4.00	2.00	2.00	2.00	2.00	1.00	4.00	2.00	2.00	3.00	2.93	2.00	1.67	■	2.50	2.47	0.92
21. Paratransit	2.33	4.00	3.50	1.50	4.00	2.00	2.00	2.00	2.00	2.00	4.00	1.71	2.00	3.67	2.00	3.25	2.50	0.86
22. Private homes	3.67	4.00	2.75	1.50	2.00	2.25	4.00	2.00	2.00	3.00	3.00	2.79	2.00	3.40	3.40	3.25	2.66	0.89
Average/respondent services	2.73	3.10	2.30	1.52	2.65	2.01	2.48	2.71	2.52	2.52	3.10	2.69	2.62	2.11	1.61	2.68	2.47	
Standard deviation	0.78	1.04	0.86	0.46	1.14	0.72	1.21	1.15	1.12	0.93	1.12	0.63	0.80	0.86	0.86	0.81		0.49

* Acronyms:
FMG: Family-medicine group
SGUI: Sherbrooke Geriatrics University Institute
SGUI IFRU: Intensive Functional Rehabilitation Unit at the SGUI
HMS: Home maintenance services

Table 4.5
Results on Interaction between Continuum Services: Granit Table

MEASURE OF SERVICE INTEGRATION (GRANIT)										Integration	N = 17
Rate of response 8gr./22 equals 36.4 %	n=3	n=1	n=1	n=1	n=5	n=1	n=2	n=1	n=2	Depth ↓	
GRANIT (n = 17)	#5	#6	#8	#10	#17	#18-19	#20	#21	autres	Aver. (0-4)	SD
1. Info-Santé	3.00	1.00	2.00	4.00	2.00	3.00	1.50	2.00	1.50	2.22	0.94
2. Single entry point	3.33	4.00	1.00	4.00	3.80	4.00	3.00	2.00	3.50	3.18	1.04
3. CLSC MDs and nurses	3.67	1.00	1.00	4.00	3.60	3.00	2.00	2.00	4.00	2.70	1.22
4. FMGs* and medical clinics	2.00	4.00	0.00	2.00	2.00	2.00	1.00	1.00	4.00	2.00	1.32
5. Home support		4.00	1.00	4.00	4.00	4.00	2.50	2.00	4.00	3.19	1.19
6. Day care center	3.67		1.00	3.00	3.60	3.00	2.50	4.00	3.50	3.03	0.95
7. Centre de réadaptation Estrie	3.00	0.00	1.00	4.00	2.40	1.00	1.00	1.00	1.50	1.66	1.24
8. Hospital emergency department	2.67	2.00		2.00	2.40	2.00	1.00	1.00	3.00	2.01	0.72
9. Ambulance services	2.00	1.00	1.00	1.00	1.80	1.00	1.00	1.00	3.00	1.42	0.71
10. Geriatrics (hospital)	2.67	1.00	1.00		4.00	2.00	1.50	1.00	4.00	2.15	1.28
11. Public health (prevention)	2.67	4.00	1.00	4.00	2.80	2.00	3.00	2.00	3.00	2.72	0.96
12. Day hospital	2.00	1.00	1.00	3.00	2.00	1.00	1.00	1.00	1.00	1.44	0.73
13. Short-Term Geriatric Unit	2.33	1.00	1.00	3.00	2.00	1.00	1.00	1.00	1.00	1.48	0.77
14. SGUI* outpatient clinics	1.67	4.00	0.00	3.00	2.20		1.00	0.00	1.00	1.61	1.41
15. Geriatric-psychiatry	2.00	1.00	0.00	4.00	2.20	1.00	0.00	0.00	1.50	1.30	1.32
16. SGUI IFRU*	2.33	4.00	0.00	3.00	2.40	1.00	0.00	0.00	1.00	1.53	1.47
17. Case management	4.00	4.00	1.00	4.00		3.00	4.00	2.00	4.00	3.25	1.16
18. Temporary placement	3.33	1.00	1.00	4.00	3.80		1.00	2.00	4.00	2.52	1.41
19. Permanent public placement	3.67	1.00	1.00	4.00	3.40		1.00	2.00	4.00	2.51	1.40
20. Community organizations and HMS*	3.67	1.00	1.00	1.00	3.80	3.00		2.00	4.00	2.43	1.34
21. Paratransit	3.33	4.00	2.00	1.00	3.40	3.00	3.00		4.00	2.97	1.02
22. Private homes	3.33	4.00	1.00	1.00	3.20	4.00	2.50	4.00	4.0	3.00	1.25
Average/respondent services	2.87	2.29	0.90	3.00	2.90	2.32	1.64	1.57	2.93	2.29	0.66
Standard deviation	0.70	1.55	0.54	1.18	0.79	1.11	1.06	1.08	1.26		

* Acronyms:
FMG : Family-medicine group
SGUI : Sherbrooke Geriatrics University Institute
SGUI IFRU : Intensive Functional Rehabilitation Unit at the SGUI
HMS : Home maintenance services

Perceptions of Service Integration by Territory

The presentation of the results obtained along the horizontal axis in decreasing order (Graphs 4.1, 4.2, and 4.3) highlights which fields of service in each territory returned high, moderate, and low results. That makes it possible to analyze the overall portrait and to look for discernible patterns from one territory to the next.

Service Integration in Sherbrooke

The 46 respondents from Sherbrooke break down into 9 executives and managers, 15 case managers, and 22 practitioners and clinicians. This group has the largest number of respondents since the zone is the region's largest and it brings together all of the specialized services in the territory, while offering many community services. Since Sherbrooke houses specialized services for the entire region, they must be treated as part of the territory, even though they are intended for all of Estrie's territories. The respondents represent 15 service groups out of 22 for a response rate of 68.2 %.

Table 4.6
Results on Interaction between Continuum Services: Coaticook Table

MEASURE OF SERVICE INTEGRATION (COATICOOK)										Integration	N = 15
Rate of response 8gr./22 equals 36.4 %	n=1	n=1	n=1	n=2	n=4	n=1	n=3	n=1	n=1	Depth ↓	
COATICOOK (n = 15)	#3	#4	#5	#6	#17	#18-19	#20	#21	#56	Aver. (0-4)	SD
1. Info-Santé	1.00	3.00	1.00	1.00	1.00	3.00	1.00	1.00	3.00	1.67	1.00
2. Single entry point	4.00	3.00	2.00	3.00	2.25	4.00	1.00	1.00	3.00	2.58	1.12
3. CLSC MDs and nurses		4.00	4.00	3.00	3.25	4.00	0.67	1.00	4.00	2.99	1.39
4. FMGs* and medical clinics	1.00		4.00	1.00	2.25	3.00	0.67	1.00	4.00	2.11	1.40
5. Home support	4.00	3.00		4.00	3.75		1.00	2.00	3.00	2.96	1.12
6. Day care center	4.00	3.00	4.00		3.50	4.00	1.67	4.00	4.00	3.52	0.83
7. Centre de réadaptation Estrie	1.00	1.00	4.00	1.00	1.75	2.00	0.67	2.00	2.00	1.71	1.01
8. Hospital emergency department	4.00	4.00	4.00	1.50	2.00	4.00	1.00	3.00	4.00	3.06	1.24
9. Ambulance services	4.00	3.00	1.00	1.00	1.75	2.00	1.00	1.00	2.00	1.86	1.05
10. Geriatrics (hospital)	4.00	4.00	4.00	1.50	2.75	4.00	0.67	2.00	4.00	2.99	1.31
11. Public health (prevention)	4.00	2.00	2.00	1.50	1.50	4.00	1.33	2.00	3.00	2.37	1.04
12. Day hospital	1.00	1.00	1.00	1.50	1.75	2.00	0.33	1.00	2.00	1.29	0.56
13. Short-Term Geriatric Unit	3.00	1.00	2.00	1.50	1.75	2.00	0.00	1.00	2.00	1.58	0.85
14. SGUI* outpatient clinics	1.00	2.00	1.00	0.50	1.75	2.00	0.00	1.00	2.00	1.25	0.73
15. Geriatric-psychiatry	1.00	2.00	1.00	1.50	1.75	2.00	0.00	1.00	2.00	1.36	0.67
16. SGUI IFRU*	4.00	2.00	2.00	1.50	2.00	2.00	0.67	1.00	3.00	2.02	1.00
17. Case management	4.00	3.00	4.00	3.00			0.67	3.00	4.00	3.10	1.18
18. Temporary placement	4.00	4.00	4.00	2.00	3.00		0.67	3.00	4.00	3.08	1.22
19. Permanent public placement	4.00	3.00	4.00	0.50	3.25		1.00		4.00	2.82	1.48
20. Community organizations and HMS*	4.00	3.00	1.00	2.00	3.00	3.00		2.00	3.00	2.63	0.92
21. Paratransit	3.00	3.00	4.00	2.50	3.00	3.00	1.67		3.00	2.90	0.65
22. Private homes	4.00	4.00	2.00	2.00	2.75	3.00	2.33	3.00	2.00	2.70	0.80
Average/respondent services	3.05	2.76	2.87	1.76	2.37	2.94	0.86	1.80	3.05	2.39	0.69
Standard deviation	1.36	1.00	1.35	0.90	0.76	0.87	0.57	0.95	0.84		

* Acronyms :
FMG : Family-medicine group
SGUI : Sherbrooke Geriatrics University Institute
SGUI IFRU : Intensive Functional Rehabilitation Unit at the SGUI
HMS : Home maintenance services

Graph 4.1 illustrates the results for each category of service, presented in descending order, so that those further to the right have lower integration scores. Out of the 14 services that fall within the cooperation bracket (from 2.5 to 3.49), the 5 with the highest scores are case management, Short-Term Geriatric Unit, CLSC home-support services, permanent public placement, and day hospital. The 5 services with the lowest scores in the communication bracket (from 1.5 to 2.49) are public health (prevention), hospital emergency department, medical clinics and family-medicine groups, Info-Santé, and ambulance services. It should be pointed out that the services perceived as falling within the communication bracket are all health-care services.

Service Integration in Granit

In Granit, the 15 respondents fell into 8 different services out of 22, which translates into a rate of response of 36.4 %. The 14 services with the highest scores are case management, home-care services, single entry point, private homes, daycare center, and paratransit. The lowest scores go primarily to regional spe-

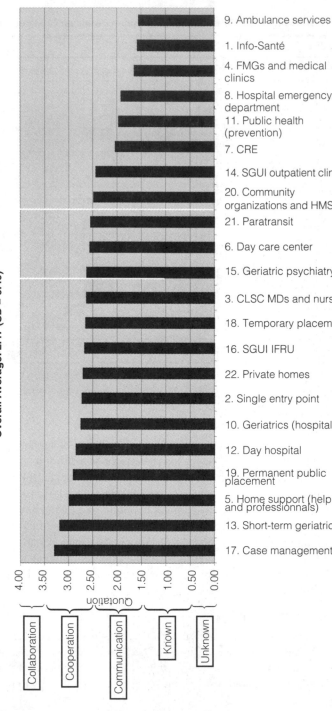

Graph 4.1
Results of integration measurement for Sherbrooke

Integration Measurement for Sherbrooke (n = 46)
Overall Average: 2.47 (SD = 0.49)

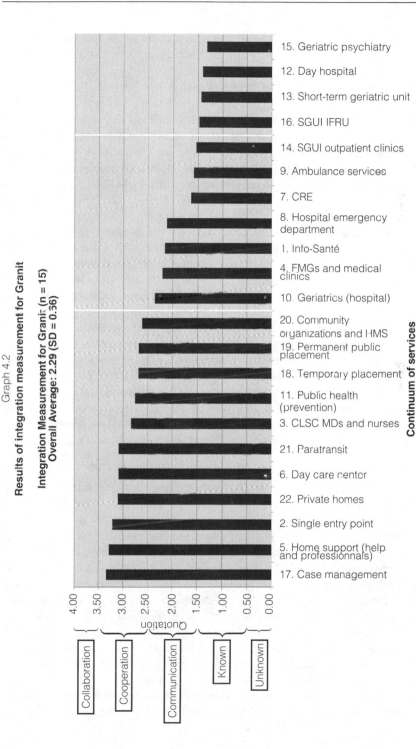

Graph 4.2
Results of integration measurement for Granit

Integration Measurement for Granit (n = 15)
Overall Average: 2.29 (SD = 0.36)

Continuum of services

15. Geriatric psychiatry
12. Day hospital
13. Short-term geriatric unit
16. SGUI IFRU
14. SGUI outpatient clinics
9. Ambulance services
7. CRE
8. Hospital emergency department
1. Info-Santé
4. FMGs and medical clinics
10. Geriatrics (hospital)
20. Community organizations and HMS
19. Permanent public placement
18. Temporary placement
11. Public health (prevention)
3. CLSC MDs and nurses
21. Paratransit
6. Day care center
22. Private homes
2. Single entry point
5. Home support (help and professionnals)
17. Case management

Quotation

4.00 3.50 3.00 2.50 2.00 1.50 1.00 0.50 0.00

Collaboration
Cooperation
Communication
Known
Unknown

cialized services, which means all services provided by the Sherbrooke Geriatric University Institute as well as ambulance services and Centre de réadaptation de l'Estrie (rehabilitation center).

Looking at the overall results for Granit reveals that half of the services are ranked in the cooperation bracket (2.49 to 3.5 points). Nearly all are offered locally, in particular psychosocial services. The moderate category, which corresponds to the communication bracket (1.5 to 2.49 points) includes health-care and rehabilitation services, many of which are offered on a regional basis. Lastly, the "awareness" bracket, with whom perceptions of interactions are less clear, comprises four specialized services provided by SGUI.

Service Integration in Coaticook

Fifteen respondents from Coaticook filled out the questionnaire. When taken together, they comprise 8 service groups out of 22, with a rate of response of 36.4 %. Unlike the other two regions in which case management ranked first, the daycare center ranks first in Coaticook, representing the only partner achieving the collaboration level, followed by many services with similar results. All of the 12 services that received high overall integration ratings (cooperation level: 2.5 to 3.49 points) are local services. In decreasing order, they are daycare center, case management, temporary placement, local emergency department, local geriatric unit, and CLSC physicians and nurses. The intermediate zone, which refers to the communication level, comprises secondary-care specialized services for health or rehabilitation. Seven services out of 22 are present. The services receiving the highest overall scores (awareness level without interaction) include three secondary-care specialized services, namely psychogeriatrics, day hospital, and SGUI outpatient clinics.

Comparison of Results according to Professional Status

We opted for presenting the results according to territory. Nevertheless, it could be of interest to see what the results would be from viewing the data from the perspective of professional status. Since there are many fewer managers and policy-makers in our sample than clinicians and practitioners, rural regions would have had a very low representation of management. We therefore opted to consolidate the data of the three territories in the experimental area according to professional status and the head of community organizations were considered managers. The criterion for inclusion as a clinician or practitioner is to have direct contact with patients as part of their normal duties. The average integration scores for each of the professional groups are similar: 2.38 (SD = 0.51) for clinicians and 2.39 (SD = 0.47) for managers. No significant deviations were noted when the 22 service categories were examined individually.

Based on the information collected until now, the results comparing the three territories are more revealing than those based on professional status. This conclusion strengthens our initial position of considering integration first and

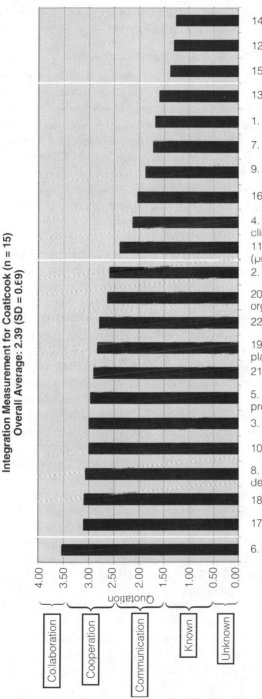

Graph 4.3
Results of integration measurement for Coaticook

Integration Measurement for Coaticook (n = 15)
Overall Average: 2.39 (SD = 0.69)

foremost as a local phenomenon of interaction between services moving towards the regional level and not the opposite.

Patterns Emerging from Analysis of the Horizontal Axis

The secondary health-care and rehabilitation services in both rural territories, delivered by institutions in the central city to all of Estrie's territories, fall among the services with the lowest integration scores. Some were rated as in the "awareness" category and report no interaction; the remainder come under "communication." Most of the psychosocial services received a rating in the "cooperation" category. Interactions in the central city of Sherbrooke appear rather mixed, making it impossible to differentiate the levels of integration in the same way as for the rural territories. Consequently, Sherbrooke has as many health-care services as psychosocial services with high ratings, while primary-care and secondary-care services cannot be separated according to a defined pattern.

Another important observation—the same in the three territories—concerns family physicians. Institutional affiliation appears to determine the level of collaboration that partners can achieve in interacting with family physicians. CLSC physicians and nurses are perceived as belonging to the cooperation category, whereas FMG physicians were rated in the communication category. It must be noted that FMGs were not widespread when the questionnaire was administered. Furthermore, those being formed were set up in the center city, which means that the scores were biased towards private clinics.

Private homes represent the incursion of the private sector into public services. Private homes in the three territories ranked in the cooperation category. Despite efforts to recruit active members for the governing board in Sherbrooke, private homes for the elderly have had no real representation because they have not had a representative or advocacy association. Indeed, such homes tend to view each other as competitors instead of partners. Despite this, private homes were ranked 8th in Sherbrooke. In Granit, there were several representatives of private homes for the elderly asserting on the issue table, but their membership was on an individual basis. Granit partners view private homes as very good collaborators based on their overall score, which puts them in 4th place out of 22 services. Lastly, Coaticook is the only territory of the three in which private homes belonging to an association and have formal representation on the governing board. There, private homes were ranked in 10th place. These results reflect the recognition of this actor as an important member of the continuum of services for the elderly, despite their difficulty in forming a group to have access to governing boards.

Lastly, a look at the overall results makes it possible to target continuum training needs. For example, specialized services at the Sherbrooke Geriatric University Institute, which are offered for the entire Estrie region, would benefit from greater visibility, especially in outlying areas.

Results for the Vertical Axis

Up to now, we have focused on results pertaining to the depth of integration, which are provided along the horizontal axis of the tables. Nevertheless, it would be interesting to see how results along the vertical access could be useful. Taken alone, vertical-axis results enable each of the respondent services to position their perception with respect to all of the service providers. Accordingly, each actor gets an overall view of his or her perception of the integrated network as well as the perceptions of all the other actors in the same network. Consequently, when Granit's geriatric hospital places its perception of the network's integration at 3 out of 4 (high) and the emergency department in the same institution places it at 0.9 out of 4 (low), it can be deduced that certain services or groups of services need to be informed, trained, or better organized in order to communicate with certain key partners, including case managers, who are at the hub of interactions between professionals.

The vertical axis can be used in another way, namely looking at the intersection of the two axes for a single actor. This makes it possible to compare the results of a service assessed by the others (horizontal), how the service assesses the interaction of its partners as a whole (vertical), and to measure the deviation. For example, in Coaticook, the respondents from Group 3 (CLSC physicians and nurses) hold a high overall perception of collaboration between continuum partners, with an overall average of 3.05 (vertical axis). On the other hand, the daycare center, community organizations, home maintenance service, and paratransit have an overall perception of the continuum that falls below the communication category. Yet these same services are perceived by the others as displaying interaction at the cooperation level (>2.5). Case management was a critical component in the arrangements for bringing about the integrated services network, which accounts for the importance of checking the results where the axes intersect. In Coaticook, most of the partners have rated case-management services at 3 (cooperation) or 4 (collaboration), for an overall assessment rating of 3.1 (horizontal axis). Looking along the vertical access—which means the way that case managers perceive interactions with their partners—turns up a score of 2.37. This discrepancy could be explained by the fact that case managers in Coaticook are generally perceived as being more accommodating by their partners than vice versa. The same phenomenon occurs in the case of the daycare center, community organizations, the home maintenance service, and paratransit in Coaticook. This refers us directly back to the question of mutuality of relations between actors. It cannot be considered an isolated phenomenon because case management exhibits the same tendency in Sherbrooke and Granit.

The form of interaction between community organizations and home maintenance services, as perceived by their partners, has received average scores across the three territories at the cutoff point between communication and cooperation, which is a good rating. Comparing these results with those that express how community organizations perceive continuum services as a whole reveals low results (between 0.86 and 1.8) in all three territories; the scores fail to achieve the communication level. This discrepancy could mean that community organizations are perceived by their partners as good collaborators, but that the feeling is not mutual. Community organizations do not have access SIGG computerized clinical chart information, which would give them timely, relevant information. This would avoid the need to telephone around for information and dealing with the hassle of voice mail. Information is a critical element that triggers a sequence of actions to adequately respond to client needs. This is all the more important when the partner is not housed in an institution, as is the case with most community organizations. Access to information therefore allows them to feel more like full partners in the continuum.

In fact, it was observed that, in all three territories, community organizations perceive the level of integration between the various services as being lower overall. Furthermore, rural areas appear to be largely unfamiliar with the regional specialized services provided by the geriatrics institute, as evidenced by a predominance of 0 scores.

Discussion

The general interpretation of the results for the average scores for each continuum services indicates that the three Estrie territories have achieved a good level of integration in the upper third of the communication category. Sherbrooke, on the other hand, nearly attained the threshold of the cooperation level. It would have been interesting to have carried out the measurement before and after the implementation of the integrated network. The instrument, however, was not yet available at the outset of the PRISMA-Estrie project. Nevertheless, our objective of revealing to the partners their own level of integration at the end of the implementation period of the integrated service network has been achieved.

Among the limitations and interpreting the results of this measure, we raised the issue of the hierarchical structuring of services (primary, secondary, and tertiary care). The result is that the more specialized services are often concentrated in urban centers. This could tend to lead residents, users, and caregivers in these settings to place them in the category of nearby services. This would not be the case for rural or more outlying areas, if only because the geographic distance represents an impediment to access and could consequently have an impact on the use of such services. This is often the case with specialized health-care services, which are offered on a regional basis. The results indicate that local services, especially psychosocial services, appear better integrated in rural areas than regional services. One interpretation could be that the integration efforts between the health and social services sectors did not produce the impact hoped for. This interpretation, however, is not supported by the data from Sherbrooke, where health-care and psychosocial services exist side by side with no evident pattern of dichotomy. Another research program would be needed to determine if the proximity of regional services allows collaborative interaction or if there are different forms of interaction between the services and the seven territories served in Estrie.

Lastly, at the end of this exercise, we believe that it is neither possible nor even desirable for all these services to strive to achieve a level of integration that could be termed collaboration. Indeed, the work of Ahgren and Axelsson[1] encourages us to better discern and understand the variations in interaction between the services, which are founded on functional necessities and goals to be achieved. Other work could help us identify a core of services that must be brought to the level of collaboration with others positioned in a surrounding constellation depending on the importance of the role that they play in the con- tinuum. In the case of these peripheral services, achieving the communication or cooperation level with their partners could be completely appropriate. Given the relative novelty of using service integration measurements, we are unable to accurately determine the relative positions between the various continuum part- ners. Subsequent work could examine the positioning of actors with respect to one another with the goal of determining the level of interaction between each of the services that would yield optimal functioning. It would then be possible to measure the discrepancy between what is desirable and the reality experi- enced by care providers, which could open the door to new interpretations.

APPENDIX 4.I

Measuring integration of services for the elderly
2004–2005 PRISMA-Estrie research project

Measurement instrument translated and adapted from the Human Services Integration Measure (2004), validated in Canada (Ontario) by Browne et al.

The service integration measure is an instrument for measuring the extent of integration of services for the elderly (number of services recognized as belonging to the integrated network), the scope of integration (number of services linked to others), and the depth of integration among network partners, assessed on a scale from 0 to 4. The measure of depth comprises an average score for each of the services as assessed by caregivers and managers working in the service network for the elderly.

You have been identified as a respondent. We therefore would like to have your personal assessment of the integration of services for the elderly as well as, overall, the assessment that your service would give. Given the small sampling of respondents, your participation is essential for us to be able to measure service integration in your territory. Follow-up will be carried out, if necessary, to retrieve the completed grid.

The process is straightforward, requiring only several minutes insofar as you only have to transpose your experience (and that of your service) by checking off a box for each of 22 service groups on the enclosed checklist. You have the following choice of responses to assess each service or group of services:

Unawareness:	Programs or services are not aware of other programs or services.
Awareness:	Discrete programs or services in the community are aware of other programs or services, but they organize their own activities solely on the basis of their own program or service mission, and make no effort to do otherwise.
Communication:	Programs and services actively share information and communicate on a formal basis.
Cooperation:	Programs or services modify their own service planning to avoid service duplication or to improve links among services, using their knowledge of other services or programs.
Collaboration:	Programs or services jointly plan offered services and modify their own services as a result of mutual consultations and advice.

Identification of Services in the Integrated Services Network for the Elderly (Estrie)

Unawareness: Programs or services are not aware of other programs or services.

Awareness: Discrete programs or services in the community are aware of other programs or services, but they organize their own activities solely on the basis of their own program or service mission, and make no effort to do otherwise.

Communication: Programs and services actively share information and communicate on a formal basis.

Cooperation: Programs or services modify their own service planning to avoid service duplication or to improve links among services, using their knowledge of other services or programs.

Collaboration: Programs or services jointly plan offered services and modify their own services as a result of mutual consultations and advice.

Service	Unawareness	Awareness	Communications	Cooperation	Collaboration
1. **CLSC Info-santé** and **Urgence détresse** (24/7 on-duty psychosocial assistance) at a CLSC					
2. **CLSC single entry point** (intake, information, assessment, orientation, referral)					
3. **CLSC medical and nursing services** • CLSC basic services • 24/7 on duty (for registered people) • Health-care services offer in the home (by physicians and nurses)					
4. **Family-medicine groups (FMG)** and **Medical clinics** (private practices of family physicians and specialists)					
5. **CLSC home services (social and paramedical)** • Home help (by visiting homemakers and social-services assistants) • Psychosocial services • Occupational therapy, physiotherapy, nutrition, and respiratory therapy • Assistance programs to enable the elderly to remain in their homes (direct allocations, Chèque-Emploi-Service, SIMAD, equipment loans, support to caregivers, etc.)					

Identification of Services in the Integrated Services Network for the Elderly (Estrie)

Unawareness: Programs or services are not aware of other programs or services.
Awareness: Discrete programs or services in the community are aware of other programs or services, but they organize their own activities solely on the basis of their own program or service mission, and make no effort to do otherwise.
Communication: Programs and services actively share information and communicate on a formal basis.
Cooperation: Programs or services modify their own service planning to avoid service duplication or to improve links among services, using their knowledge of other services or programs.
Collaboration: Programs or services jointly plan offered services and modify their own services as a result of mutual consultations and advice.

	Your Assessment: Check a Response				
	Unawareness	Awareness	Communications	Cooperation	Collaboration
6. **Day center (CLSC)** (respite and support programs for caregivers, fall prevention, maintenance, nursing care and physiotherapy, etc.)					
7. **Rehabilitation center** (programs used by the elderly) • Auditive aids • Visual aids • Mobility aids (including maintenance service for orthoses, prostheses, wheeled equipment)					
8. **Emergency department (of your territory's hospital)**					
9. **Ambulance services**					
10. **Geriatrics team or unit** (consultations with geriatrician, geriatrics nurse, physiotherapy, occupational therapy for the elderly in a hospital setting)					
11. **Public health, prevention** for the elderly (such as programs to prevent falls and violence, vaccination programs, and other public-health programs for the elderly)					
12. **SGUI day hospital***					
13. **SGUI Short-Term Geriatric Unit (STGU)***					
14. **SGUI Specialized outpatient clinics*** (memory, incontinence, geriatrics, deafness-vertigo, dermatology, nutrition)					

Identification of Services in the Integrated Services Network for the Elderly (Estrie)

Unawareness: Programs or services are not aware of other programs or services.

Awareness: Discrete programs or services in the community are aware of other programs or services, but they organize their own activities solely on the basis of their own program or service mission, and make no effort to do otherwise.

Communication: Programs and services actively share information and communicate on a formal basis.

Cooperation: Programs or services modify their own service planning to avoid service duplication or to improve links among services, using their knowledge of other services or programs.

Collaboration: Programs or services jointly plan offered services and modify their own services as a result of mutual consultations and advice.

Identification of Services	Unawareness	Awareness	Communications	Cooperation	Collaboration
15. SGUI geriatric psychiatry*					
16. SGUI Intensive Functional Rehabilitation Unit* (IFRU)					
17. Case management (CLSC)					
18. Temporary placement programs (Temporary accommodation, alternative placement, transition, convalescence, etc.)**					
19. Public placement programs (IR-FTR-RLTCC)					
20. Community organizations and home maintenance firms (social economy) offering home-care services: • Meals on wheels • Home maintenance • Escorts for medical and legal appointments • Help with errands • Socialization (community meals, calls to and visits by friends, etc.) • Participation in fall-prevention programs • Support for natural caregivers (respite, mutual help, sitting, information, conferences, etc.)					
21. Paratransit (programs for the elderly)					
22. Private homes for the elderly					

Please get in touch with us if you have a question, comment, or simply want to express your assessment of this instrument for measuring service integration.

_____

_____

_____

_____

_____

_____

_____

_____

_____

_____

_____

_____

_____

_____

_____

Your cooperation is greatly appreciated.

**Anne Veil and the
PRISMA-Estrie Research Project Team**

References

1. Ahgren, B. and Axelsson, R. Evaluating integrated health care: a model for measurement. International Journal of Integrated Care, 2005; 1-14. Site: http://www.ijic.org/

2. Browne, G., Roberts, J., Gafni, A., Byrne, C., Kertyzia, J., and Loney, P. Conceptualizinig and validating the Human Services Integration Measure. International Journal of Integrated Care, 2004; 4: 1-12. Site: http://www.ijic.org/

3. Contandriopoulos, A.-P., Denis, J.-L., and Touati, N. Intégration des soins: concepts et mise en œuvre. Université de Montréal, Groupe de recherche

interdisciplinaire en santé (GRIS), 2001. Site: www.santemontreal.qc.ca/fr/observatoire/

4. Denis, J.-L, Beaulieu, M.-D., Hébert, Y, Langley, A., Lozeau, D., Pineault, R., and Trottier, L-H. L'innovation clinico-organisationnelle dans les organisations de santé. Rapport au FCRSS, 2001, 22 p.

5. Foote, C. and Stanners, C. (2002). Integrating Care for Older People – New Care for Old – a systems approach. Jessica Kingsley publishers, Athenacum Press, United Kingdom.

6. Frossard, M. and Boitard A. Évaluation des réseaux de coordination gérontologique: une approche socio-économique. Revue Épidémiologie et Santé publique, Paris, juin 1997; (45): 429-437

7. Hébert, R. and le groupe PRISMA. L'intégration des services aux personnes âgées: une solution prometteuse aux problèmes de continuité. Vieillissement et santé II – Hors série, 2003; 67-75.

8. Henrard, J.-C., Ankri, J., Frijters, D., Carpenter, I., Topinkova, E., Garms-Homolova, V., Finne-Soveri, H., sorbye, L. W., Jonsson, P. V., Ljunggren, G., Schroll, M., Wagner, C., and Bernabei, R. Proposal of a service delivery integration index of home care for older persons: application in several European cities. International Journal of Integrated Care, 2006: 1-8.

9. Kodner, D.L. and Spreeuwenberg, C. Integrated care: meaning, logic, applications, and implications – a discussion paper. International Journal of Integrated Care, Nov. 2002: 1-11. Web site: http://www.ijic.org/publish/articles/000089/article_print.html

10. Kralewski, J.E., de Vries, A., Dowd, B., and Potthoff, S. The development of integrated service networks in Minnesota. Health Care Management Review, 1995; 20 (4): 42-56.

11. Leutz, W. Five laws for integrating medical and social services: lessons from the United Sates and the United Kingdom. The Milbank Quarterly, 1999; 77 (1): 77-110.

12. Ministère de la santé et des services sociaux du Québec, Direction générale des services sociaux et Direction des services généraux). Les services généraux offerts par les centres de santé et de services sociaux. Sept. 2004

13. Reed, J., Cook, G., Childs, S., and McCormack, B. (2005). A literature review to explore integrated care for older people. International Journal of Integrated Care, 2005; 5: 1-10. Web site: http://www.ijic.org/

14. Shortell, S.M., Gillis, R.R., Anderson, D.S., Erickson, D.M., Mitchell, J.B. et al. (2000) Remaking Health Care in America – the Evolution of Organized Delivery Systems, Jossey-Bass, 2nd edition, 2000. San Francisco, USA

15. Shortell, S.M., Gillies, R.R., Anderson, D.A., and Morgan, K.L. Creating organized delivery systems: the barriers and facilitators. Hospital & Health Services Administration. 1993; 38 (4): 447- 466.

16. Vanderwoerd, J. Better beginnings, better futures. Finding Report, project 1990-1993 – Chapter 11. Partnerships and programs: service provider involvement in better beginnings, better futures, by Narayan et Shier, BBBF Research Coordination Unit: Queen's University, 1996. Ontario, Canada.

17. Warner, M. and Gould, N. (2003). Integrated care networks and quality of life: linking research and practice. International Journal of Integrated Care, 2003; 3: 1-9. Web site: http://www.ijic.org/

18. Weiss, E., Anderson, R., and Lasker, R. Findings from the National Study of Partnership Functioning: Report to the Partnerships that Participated. Center for the advancement of collaborative strategies in health. 2001. Web site: www.cacsh.org

Chapter 5
Local Ownership of Case Management and Its Lessons for Implementing Case Management in Other Settings

Yves Couturier, Sébastien Carrier, Dominique Gagnon, and Isabelle Chouinard

---

Highlights

Without doubt, case management is among the innovations that can enable better continuity of service. An innovation takes on its true form and value when local actors take ownership of it and adapt it to the local setting. There are certain requirements for a successful adaptation:
1. Review the situation prior to implementing case management in a way that takes account of effective continuity practices, real working conditions, and the various parties' expectations.
2. Frame the innovation plan in explicit terms, especially as regards the needs to be met.
3. Analyze how the innovation is to be translated into practice and actually adapted by the parties involved.
4. Modify any working conditions that hinder innovation and, in a second stage, adjust the model in light of information obtained by analyzing the adaptation.

This is a report on our main findings from qualitative research conducted since 2002 during the implementation of integrated services networks for the frail elderly. The main objective of our studies was to better understand how professional actors involved in the implementation took ownership of one of the most centrally operationally elements of integrated services networks for frail elders, namely case management. Beyond being an operational element, case management is the device that embodies the integrated services model presented to local actors and by means of which they experience the model. Examining of the local conditions at work during the process of taking ownership will make it possible to adjust the conceptual model to reality following initial implementation and allows for transferring valuable lessons to other settings, thereby contributing to successful initial implementation.

Some Theoretical and Methodological Considerations

We took the theoretical underpinnings of our research from cognitive ergonomics.[1] Classical ergonomics studies work from a Taylorian perspective, measuring the human factor. The cognitivist trend in ergonomics tries to understand work from the perspective of the professional actor, and more precisely that actor's activity, i.e., the concrete way an actor in a real-life work situation accomplishes the task assigned. Cognitive ergonomics is based on the observation that there are relatively significant divergences between what workers are intended to do, i.e., the expected task; what they actually do, i.e., the task accomplished; and what they say about it. This observation can be viewed as common sense, since everyone has experienced divergences of this kind, often as something to be deplored and with the view that the human factor, as represented by the worker, is responsible for the gaps. The strength and originality of cognitive ergonomics resides precisely in asking what the value of these divergences is, so that the actual conditions of a worker's ownership of a task can be understood. From this viewpoint, the divergence represents not so much a shortfall as practical intelligence at work. In short, cognitive ergonomics views these divergences less as shortfalls than as valuable empirical indicators of local actors' ownership of the task.[2] From our perspective, an attentive examination of this ownership makes it possible to adjust theoretical models to the actual conditions of implementation, and thus to examine the conditions for implementation success. The field of assessing innovations widely recognizes that local adoption represents a privileged moment for examining implementation conditions in order to support those who will be consolidating the implementation at a second stage.[3] Evaluation of this kind also allows for identifying conditions across various contexts, so that local lessons can be put to use in other institutions or further the actors' ownership process.[4]

Qualitative research must be conducted to reach these objectives. The reasons are epistemological and twofold. First, to the extent possible, it is important to be close to the actual context of work in order to document conditions specific to each context and then infer lessons that can be transposed to other settings. Second, it is necessary to access the meaning actors give the expected task, since local adoption of an innovation represents both an adaptive process carried out by actors in the field in a specific setting[3] and the means by which prescribed approaches are retranslated via the interplay of the various actors.[5] For this reason, it is important for the study to pay attention to how actors recount their work experience.

The fact that our study was based in cognitive ergonomics meant that methodologically we had to develop so called comprehensive data-gathering strategies, i.e., strategies attentive to the meaning actors gave to their activities, and that we had to put effort into observing actual practices.[6] We therefore mainly conducted interviews (n = 76) with the various professional actors involved in case management, using an interview method known as the explicitation interview,[7] which allows for getting as close as possible to the action performed by inducing interviewees to access what cognitivists call concrete memory. We also conducted 15 days of ethnographic observation in order to grasp the effective and practical dimensions of case management. Numerous analytical operations were performed on the interviews, mainly content analyses[8] and structural discourse analyses,[9] prior to preparing various models of case manager practices.

A model is a theoretical construct that presents a synthesis of the dispersal and articulation of the conceptual parameters of activities as carried out by individual actors. In what follows, we will present three models reflecting three unique, situated styles of ownership of case management, focused mainly on the role's key function, coordination.

Modeling Coordination as an Activity in Case Management

The main purpose of case management as a device is to support services integration by promoting better coordination of professional actions. It is an interface device positioned between the client- system, consisting of the user, family caregivers, members of the user's close circle, and the community, and the care-system, consisting of all professional and institutional resources.[10] Thus, in the various theoretical models for services integration, the case manager is a cross-institutional and cross-professional coordinator whose mandate is to put coordination mechanisms in operation between the services offered by different health and social services workers, whatever institution they may belong to. Thus, the case manager's actions must accommodate the traditional *clinical* role, oriented wholly towards the professional-client relationship, and an *institutional* role, focused on service and the rules of service delivery. To do this, the case manager assesses needs, plans services, ensures these services are coordinated over time, and provides a degree of clinical follow-up. The case manager is also the human embodiment of services integration, the face of this management approach as seen by the user, seeing to it the user receives the right service at the right time and in the right place. Hébert has said that case managers are the true "blue helmets" of gerontological care,[11] because they have to defend user's rights within the huge health-and-social-services apparatus represented by a program for age-related frailty. Case-manager activities are thus bivalent,[12] in that the object of their actions is both the client system and the intervention system. As will be seen throughout this paper, that bivalency stands for the full complexity of the job and yields a whole series of lessons learned from the successful implementation of case management.

In the PRISMA study, local innovations generated three case-management models. These models are differentiated on one hand by the clientele served by case management and on the other by the nature of the case-management roles.

In the first model, which we call the "exclusive" model, the case manager's role is limited to brokerage and service-coordination tasks, and excludes any clinical tasks emerging from the case manager's own disciplinary background. In this model, the case manager specializes in brokering services, and her or his caseload consists exclusively of users accepted for case management under set criteria, such as age or the number or intensity of the services required. The skills needed for this job are more methodological (ability to negotiate, competency with instruments and tools, networking, mobilizing, etc.) than clinical, precisely because the brokering role predominates.

Under the second model, which we call "hybrid", the case manager plays the role of broker and service coordinator in equal measures and has a homogeneous case-managed caseload, but she or he also preserves a minor clinical role based on professional background. In this model, case managers may provide care to their case-managed clients, so long as their clinical work does not hinder their primary role of service coordinator. For example, a case manager trained in social work could do brief psychosocial therapy with clients. If, however, this requires too much time, she or he will have to refer the individual to another, primary social worker, who will take on the job of psychosocial intervention. Under this model, the case-management team needs not only to have methodological skills, but also to deploy the various clinical skills required by the state of the frail elderly.

The third model, which we called "mixed," is characterized by case-manager caseloads consisting equally of case-managed elders and elders at the onset of frailty, who do not satisfy the criteria for case management. Under this model, case managers are principally health or social services workers within their own fields; and they have an additional role, that of service coordinator, added to their responsibilities to certain clients whose circumstances require more complex and intense services. Thus, this model makes the brokerage function secondary to clinical continuity. It ensures that, when a user who is not case managed but is already being followed by a specific health and social services worker, experiences increased frailty, that same professional continues providing clinical follow-up but also picks up the responsibilities associated with managing the case. Accordingly, while the status of the case changes, there is no change in the client's professional caregiver.

Naturally, these three models for case management took diverse forms over the course of the implementation process. We therefore examined their local appropriation by professional actors specifically with respect to what appeared to us to be case management's foundational function, i.e., service coordination. In order to describe and then model effective coordination as carried out by case managers, we worked with two main conceptual focuses, namely, the kinds of norms actors bring into play in putting together their interventions and their functional relationship with these norms. In the diagram below, what **is prescribed** indicates formal norms that prescribe the actions to be taken. These may take the form of various intervention protocols, administrative rules that govern access to resources, assessment and information instruments and tools, and so on. The concept of the **practice convention** refers to the set of unwritten norms on which practitioners base a significant portion of their clinical judgments. The various clinical judgments framed within an institution gradually come to form a shared history, a practical jurisprudence. This jurisprudence makes it possible to empirically define concepts that are difficult to objectivize, such as a psychosocial emergency, social isolation, compliance with treatment, the capacity for self-management, the degree of protection needed, etc. These conventions constitute a valuable form of collective intelligence, which cognitive ergonomics seeks to understand.[2] They form the shared, informal, normative code that practitioners use to decipher the complex clinical cases before them without having to constantly reinvent the wheel. These practice conventions provide practitioners with significant cognitive gains, because they pool a major portion of the knowledge needed to exercise good clinical judgment, and thereby ensure the effectiveness of services. It goes without saying these various norms are not as automatic as they purport to be; they are the object of constant negotiation and feedback-based adjustment.

Besides identifying the kinds of norms mobilized, it is possible to discern two main ways of relating to these norms, a **formal** one, which complies with prescribed institutional procedures, and an **informal** one, which is open to any of the numerous modes of transacting that elude categorization under professional prescriptions.

When the two conceptual parameters retained for analyzing coordination practices are combined, four categories emerge for the coordination acts performed professionally by case managers. Where prescribed norms meet the formal normative relationship, we find a series of acts that we term **standardized requests**. These consist of coordinating actions in line with various protocols that prescribe the stages of intervention, rules of access to resources, and so on. Viewed in the light of service brokerage, the job the case manager is expected to do fits mostly into this space and takes visible shape in assessment and planning activities. Seen from this angle, coordination is like liaison as presented by Leutz.[13]

More detailed analysis, however, reveals other, sometimes more complex dimensions of coordination. Relying on these same formal norms and yet in some cases acting in contradiction to them, the case manager's effective job is to put **pressure on the apparatus,** for example, on protocols for assigning resources, in his or her client's interests and by virtue of the client's clinical characteristics. Here, coordination is similar to the "blue helmet" role described by Hébert as cited above.[12] That is, it is a role of advocacy *for* the client and *against* the logic of the system, even though the system is key to the service-brokerage role. As we stated above, this reflects the great complexity of the true work done by case managers; but it also mirrors the system's intelligence in

Figure 5.1
Area of Dispersal of Coordination Activities

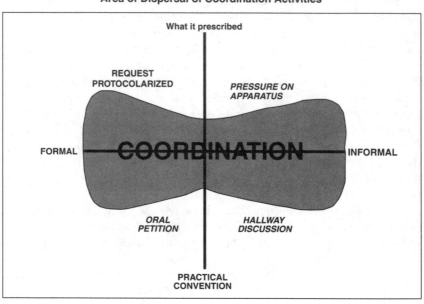

having installed at its heart, by formal means, methods for institutional feedback. This would lead one to hope that case management as here observed will not devolve towards a mechanistic, not to say technocratic, model.

In the space formed by practice conventions, we observed that **oral requests** made by clients or case managers' colleagues, i.e., requests that assessment instruments could allow to slip through the cracks because they are unique or unusual, are formally pulled back into the case-management space and become subject to a translation process by which they are channeled along protocols capable of giving them formal legitimacy. Requests of this kind legitimize the clinical act, because their recognition is a reminder that what matters above all is satisfying demands that come from an actual client and not a system of classification. This translation process that is at the heart of case managers' actual job emerges not just from the presence of clients but also from imperatives inherent in professionalism. What we see here is that case managers cannot confine themselves strictly to brokerage as prescribed by protocol. A significant part of their legitimacy, indeed their relevance, resides in their ability to transform the *clinical* into *service*. Viewed in this light, coordination consists of that articulation of the formal and the informal worlds that is inherent in any clinical relationship.

It is clear that case managers must constantly discuss, negotiate, and retranslate intervention norms with a very broad variety of professional partners, whether medical, paramedical, or social; whether part of the public system or not; indeed, whether professional or volunteer. **Hallway conversations** make it possible for the important meaning-making activity represented by translation to be shared. The most significant result of hallway conversations is assuredly ongoing updates and the adaptive framing of new practice conventions specific to the integrated services network for frail elderly. They are simultaneously both the means and the indicator of the innovation's local adoption.[4] Diversity of modes of action is thus inherent in the task's complexity; and it is also the condition that allows for new ententes to be negotiated, developed, and entrenched among the networks of professional actors mobilizing around the frail elder. On account of this task's complexity, an interdisciplinary ethos emerges little by little;[14][15] i.e., a system of norms and representations of the world that constitutes the culture of a group of actors.

This initial analysis yields several general observations about coordination as the central activity of case management. Coordination emerges as a complex, mobile entity that adjusts to the practical requirements of each clinical situation and each practice context. Thus its form is irreducibly unstable and its necessary adaptability, that is, its unending movement between the formal and the informal, the prescribed and the practical entente, accounts to a significant extent for the divergence between case management as expected and as enacted. Actual case management partly resists prescription, not because the model is not understood, but in order to adapt to local reality. One of the fundamental conditions for this necessary adaptability is the clinical nature of any case-management practice. Clinical action has an ad hoc and here-and-now dimension that cannot be done away with and that is inherent in any professional relationship. No one who promotes case management in any form can cut back on the case manager's negotiating activities with all the actors in the integrated services network, including clients themselves and their close circle.

Three Functional Models of Coordination in Case Management

So far, our discussion of coordination has been based on professional practices; we have sought to identify commonalities across contexts. In what follows, we present three models emerging from three collective local adaptations of coordination by case managers and their partners. These models are referred to as functional, because they allow for reflection on the operational dimension of case management within each context. They were built inductively, with an eye on the three major objects of coordination along which, empirically speaking, the essence of case-management activities are aligned:
- Home-support services for the elderly
- Respite and support services for family caregivers
- Physical and cognitive health services

The diagrams present the way case management is articulated with each of these three broad kinds of service.

Our research made it possible to reconstruct the concept of *service* based on two dimensions that constitute its two conceptual aspects. The first aspect, called *institutional*, relates to access to resources, assessment protocols, and administrative regulations. These foundational materials of the case manager's task shape his or her action as institutional role, i.e., the management dimension of the job. In other words, case management exists as of the moment when institutional complexity is such that it becomes necessary to implement a device for systematizing certain key practices, including coordination. The second aspect, the *clinical* one, relates to all the professional acts performed by a clinician as an actor for the benefit of a single client. This clinical dimension of the job is what is signified by the term "case," which invokes the idea of a broader concreteness, more firmly implanted in a life situation than a problem needing solution or a given pathology would be. We use the term "aspect" to characterize the relationship, simultaneously one of connectedness and differentiation, that links *management* to *case*, the institutional to the clinical. These two dimensions are closely intertwined under the heading of *service,* which designates in a single word both the clinical and the institutional dimensions. Nevertheless, each aspect preserves its distinctive tendencies, its specific logic, which tends to distance it from the other aspect but never wholly severs them. While it is risky to separate the two aspects in empirical practice, we believe it is useful to distinguish them here conceptually, at least for the moment, in order to see how each local adaptation articulates the clinical with the institutional dimension in its own way. We will now present three models, keeping in view the three forms of continuity (relational, informational, and management continuity) defined by Reid et al.[16]

1. Intermediate Functional Model

In the intermediate model, the case manager coordinates the three general functions. While partly intertwined with each of these, the worker's case-management activity does not completely meld with it, remaining to some extent independent of the clinical work. Nevertheless, the clinical and institutional aspects do share territory, territory that allows for a functional encounter between the management world and the clinical world, as is indicated by the word "intermediate." Although it has a clinical component, this model would appear to be closer to the theoretical model of exclusive case management, that is, the model of an agent working to coordinate cross-professional and cross-institutional services, whose caseload consists exclusively of case-managed individuals. For case managers to be able to act this way, their role of cross-institutional coordination must be acknowledged by actors in the whole integrated services network. Under this model, brokering and planning activities constitute the essence of the case manager's work; clinical activities are left to actors present on the daily scene, for example, family and social aides and nurses. The role of the clinical portion of the case manager's work is thus to enable health and social services workers to have an inter-subjective awareness of the incorporation of brokering activities into the clinical plan. This model provides effective support to informational and management continuity but is less effective as regards relational continuity, sometimes even giving rise to ruptures and reduplication. This is accounted for by the lesser place assigned to the clinical dimension, in favor of allowing for an independent professional function focused on service brokerage, which requires that other professionals, whose work is dedicated to clinical practice, be present on the scene. We call this model intermediate because the case manager mediates between available services and the professional actors involved in them and is not wholly submerged within the professional group. The case manager's position must be intermediate to preserve the neutrality of mediation and keep it above the clinical fray.

2. Peripheral Functional Model

Under the peripheral coordination model, the case manager occupies a position peripheral to the three services; and her or his action is focused on acting as liaison or interface among them. Actors in the integrated services network view the case manager as filling a role consisting essentially of transferring information between institutions and professional actors. Here, it is not so much a question of shared territory as of a boundary, an interface, between the two aspects discussed above. Thus, this form of case management mainly supports continuity of information about regarding services, which results in the case manager's

Figure 5.2
Intermediate Model

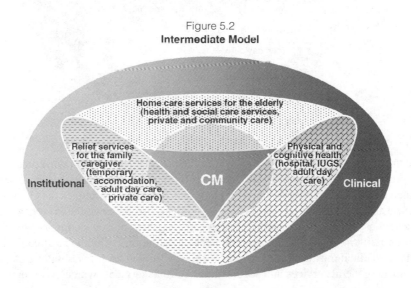

acting on behalf of institutional concerns (access to services, protocols for action, and so on). The focus on information has an important effect on management continuity. For example, it emphasizes planning access to resources and a protocol-based approach to intervention. This model's institutional coloring can have the effect of marginalizing the case manager as member of a team whose main guiding value for action is specifically professional, that is, based on clinical skill.

This approach to case management emerges as less effective when it comes to relational continuity, because of the extremely narrow clinical space the case manager occupies. As with the preceding case, clinical activity is left to those involved on a daily basis; and the case manager retains very few immediate clinical concerns. Outside the case manager's sphere of action, internal cross-professional micro-coordination continues to occur and unfolds following an essentially clinical logic. Altogether, this model does not take coordination as far as the previous one; instead, it allows informal approaches to continuity to develop in various clinical spaces alongside case management.

Figure 5.3
Peripheral Model

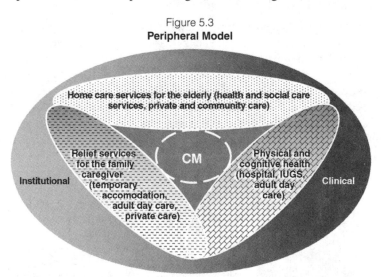

3.   Model of Coordination from within the Practice Role

In the model of coordination from within the practice role, case management is more or less integrated into case managers' clinical acts, because it is incorporated into their disciplinary practice. Here, shared territory occupies the clinical space almost in its entirety and what is specific to case management is less than clear. Case management constitutes an innovation of narrow scope and takes essentially the form of a role supplementary to the tasks that were already in place. While it may appear to have exceedingly limited usefulness with respect to local, general services and second-line regional services, which go on operating just as they did before case management was implemented, it does take on innovative value when it comes to relations between the local integrated services network and specialized tertiary services. And, after all, this does represent an important integrated-services role when it comes to complex clinical situations requiring specialized services.

Under this model, the case manager is a practitioner like any other, but with a supplementary administrative mandate that takes second place to clinical practice. Since case managers are fully recognized by their professional colleagues as practitioners, they are viewed less as enacting a role favorable to systematic institutional coordination than as clinicians who can rely on the emergent practice conventions favoring case management to take coordination a little farther than was done under former non-systematic practices. This model of case management, framed as it is as an extension of modes of action that existed prior to case management's implementation, facilitates informational, management, and relational continuity. It is a model of case management that derives its effectiveness from being closely aligned to informal practices and its weaknesses from its limited ability to transform them.

These three models of local adaptations of case management are easy to plot on a conceptual continuum with case management as brokerage at one end and clinical case management at the other. Their distribution along this continuum is a reflection as much of local choices as of the conditions specific to implementation. Given that this diversity can be observed empirically, it can serve as an object of reflection before the factors to be taken into account in developing the innovation are implemented.

Figure 5.4
Coordination from within the Practice Role

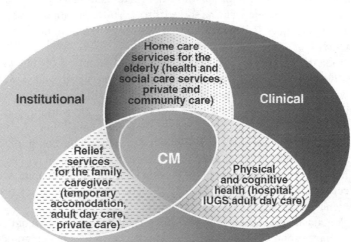

Figure 5.5
Conceptual Continuum of Case-Management Management

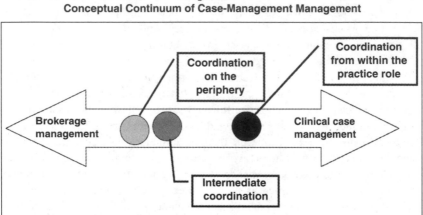

Some Lessons for the Adjustment or Implementation of Case Management in Other Settings

In our view, the way the empirical models of case management are distributed along the conceptual continuum above sheds light on the main object of reflection that case management's promoters must consider in developing their project, namely, in a given setting, what role is to be preserved for discipline-based clinical intervention in relation to the case-management brokerage dimension. The dilemma represented by making a choice between a model of case management with a pronounced brokerage component and a more clinical model, which relies on informal clinical structures in place prior to case-management implementation, can be solved through in-depth analysis of the state of affairs that is especially attentive to tangible forms of continuity prior to implementation.

Both theories about the dissemination and adoption of innovations and definitive research findings on this subject are so numerous and so well-known that we will not attempt to present them here. We will say only that such major conditions as the quality of the leadership available, the working conditions of those targeted by the innovation, the meaning that change holds for the parties involved, the direction taken by resistance—in short all the conditions that play the most important roles in adopting an innovation—have naturally played a role here, just as they do elsewhere. In what remains of this chapter, we emphasize certain conditions with a special bearing on our purpose, which fostered the emergence of a given model over the others.

We consider it self-evident that generally it is essential to monitor the distribution of resources in the setting for which a new services-integration system is intended. This must be done even before the concept of the new system is developed. For example, the relationships of local actors with tertiary services, relationships with primary-care physicians, informal collaborative practices with the hospital, and, still more important, the informal or pragmatic approaches to continuity taken by the various institutional actors before the advent of the innovation, as well as the degree of complexity of services supply, are all factors contributing to the choice of model. It is important to document them because a new system that is founded on positive pre-existing methods of operation has better chances of success. The role of the resulting continuity between the past and the future is not just to contribute to the efficiency of change; it also ensures a degree of continuity in the meaning that the various parties involved give to their work.

Furthermore, implementers of a new case-management device must state their clinical objectives, in particular as regards the relationship they want to set up between clinical intervention and the administrative or institutional role involved in case management. The issue here is a consideration of case managers' professional identities. A clear statement of the innovation's objectives is essential. Will existing coordination practices be made systematic; will new practices be introduced; or will existing practices be gently and gradually transformed? Thus the model chosen must establish early on the depth of innovation to be introduced. A model that targets an in-depth transformation of practices is bound by a different set of requirements than a model that relies on informal continuity practices. In other words, implementers of a project of this kind must make clear the empirical relevance of case management in relation to local coordination needs.

Naturally, both active and passive forms of resistance to the implementation of case management must be anticipated, not in order to suppress them, but rather in order to understand their meaning. While resistance is sometimes a tacit form of conservatism, we view it primarily as a message addressed to innovation promoters about the meaning that change holds and the conditions needed for actors to mobilize vis-à-vis such change. Messages of this kind are conducive to examining the working circumstances underlying resistance. While such resistance is inherent in any innovation, good planning should enable all those involved in an integrated services network for frail elders to better understand the value added conferred by case management, which is too readily deemed to be strictly administrative. This applies in particular to those who view themselves as playing a formal or informal role in coordination, e.g., pivotal providers, liaison officers, and so on. Any perceived duplication could be targeted by specific intervention by innovation implementers.

One of the prime occurrences of perceived duplication is with regular in-home services provided outside the context of case management. When tension does arise, it tends to be observed when a client passes from pre-case management to case management. In our opinion, case management that focuses excessively on such clients leads to a fundamental break with the client group that is at serious risk of increased frailty over time. Good continuity between groups with low-care demands and high-care demands preserves basic continuity between a case manager's formal continuity approaches and the informal continuity approaches that emerge from the clinical links among the professionals situated close to the action. The local way of conceiving case management should take this necessity into account and partition the two target groups who, after all, have more similarities than differences.

While we did observe some resistance, we were also able to document the degree to which care providers were counting on the case-management project. In particular, they expressed the hope that case management and, more broadly, service integration would foster a more collective approach in their work. Too often, work is experienced as an individual responsibility fulfilled in reaction to the system. Case-management promoters must take participant hopes into account in order to support long-term participant commitment. Otherwise, disappointment could set in, causing actors to lose faith in the project,[17] especially among those whose informal clinical continuity roles are under-recognized.

Conclusion: Implementation in Successive Waves

Certainly, the local conditions that play a part in the success of implementation, as well as in the adoption and local adaptation of an innovation, are numerous. On this score, our chapter could be considered incomplete. We would nevertheless ask the reader to retain from it a few key ideas. The most important of these is this: innovation resides not so much in the promoters' capacity to conceptualize a project, even if this capacity if far-seeing, than in how local actors translate the project into practice. An informed and enlightened promoter will view these translations, not as a form of resistance, but as a source of valuable information in adjusting the model to the conditions that await it. The methodological sequence for implementing innovation is:

1) Overview of pre-existing conditions, taking into account effective continuity practices, actual working conditions, and the various actors' expectations.
2) Formulation of the innovation project with an emphasis on needs to be met.
3) Analysis of how innovation is being translated into practice and of its actual adaptation by the actors involved.
4) Alterations in any working conditions that are hindering innovation and adjustment of the model during a second stage.

As may be seen, successful implementation derives less from a thoroughly mastered, efficient prior design of the innovation than from an iterative process of design that remains open to the lessons derived from the way the main parties translate the innovation into practice. From our research, it is possible to infer principles that will serve as a basis for inspiration. Furthermore, it yields information about, and indicators of, successful implementation to guide promoters.

The models we have put forward, however, are to be viewed less as discrete prescribed paradigms that could be transferred to other settings than as design parameters to be taken into consideration before implementation. We believe our contribution consists of breaking ground for a reflective methodology for implementing complex devices of this kind. In our view, that is where the most valuable lessons are to be found.

We have not discussed the role of elders themselves and their family caregivers in implementing case management. No one would disagree that case management is primarily an institutional innovation. Nevertheless, it is equally clear that this innovation only has meaning when it is perceived as useful by the primary individuals involved, the elderly themselves. Their own perception of enhanced continuity must be the primary indicator of the effectiveness of the successful implementation of case management.

References

1. Falzon, P. (2004), Ergonomie. Paris: Presse universitaire de France.

2. De Montmollin, M. (1984). L'intelligence de la tâche: essai d'ergonomie cognitive. Berne: Peter Lang.

3. Greenhalhg, T., Robert, G., MacFarlane, F., Bate, P. & Kyriakidou O. (2004). Diffusion of Innovations in Service Organizations: Systematic Review and Recommendations, The Milbank Quarterly, Vol. 82, No. 4: 581-629.

4. Oldenburg, B. F., Sallis, J. F., French, M. L. & Owen, N. (1999). Health promotion research and the diffusion and institutionalization of interventions. Health Education Research, 14, 121- 130.

5. Callon, M. (1986). Éléments pour une sociologie de la traduction. La domestication des coquilles St-Jacques et des marins-pêcheurs dans la baie de St-Brieuc. L'année sociologique, No. 36, p.169-208.

6. Yin, K. (1994). Case study research: Design and methods, 2nd ed. Sage Publications.

7. Vermersch, P. (2000). L'entretien d'explicitation. Paris: ESF.

8. Patton, M.Q. (2002). Qualitative research and evaluation methods, 3rd ed. Sage publication, 598 p.

9. Demazière, D. & Dubar, C. (1997). Analyser les entretiens biographiques. L'exemple de récits d'insertion. Paris: Nathan.

10. Zuniga, R. (1994). L'évaluation dans l'action. Montreal: Presses universitaires de Montréal.

11. Hébert, R., Tourigny, A. & Gagnon M (2005). Integrated service delivery to ensure person's functional autonomy, Quebec City: Edisem.

12. Couturier, Y. (2006). La collaboration entre travailleuses sociales et infirmières. Éléments d'une théorie de l'intervention interdisciplinaire. Paris: L'Harmattan.

13. Leutz, W. (1999). Five laws for integrating medical and social services: Lessons from the United States and the United Kingdom. The Milbank Quarterly, Vol. 77, No. 1, 1999, p. 77-110.

14. Klein, J. (1996). Crossing boundaries: Knowledge, disciplinarities, and interdisciplinarities. Charlottesville: University Press of Virginia.

15. Couturier, Y. (2003). L'interdisciplinarité pratique entre travailleuses sociales et infirmières: De la nécessité de produire un récit-client commun. Revue canadienne de service social, 19 (2): 245-251.

16. Reid, R. Haggerty, J. & R. Mckendry (2002). Defusing the confusion: Concepts and measures of continuity of healthcare. Canadian Health Services Foundation.

17. Chouinard, I. (2006). Transformation des formes identitaires en contexte d'émergence du modèle de gestion de cas et enjeux pour le travail social. Master's thesis, University of Sherbrooke, Sherbrooke, QC.

Acknowledgements

The study was funded by the Fonds québécois de recherche sur la société et la culture, the PRISMA research program, the Social Sciences and Humanities Research Council of Canada, and the Réseau québécois de recherche sur le vieillissement.

Chapter 6
Perceived Self-Efficacy of Case Managers

Anne Veil and Réjean Hébert

Highlights

Three years after implementation of the new function of case management in services for the elderly with functional decline, we wanted to determine how well case managers have mastered their role, if they felt able to adequately meet the needs of their clients, and if the other network partners accepted them as case managers.

A review of the literature on certain determinants governing the work efficacy of case managers emphasizes the importance of putting into perspective the case-management model and the means for organizational integration of the case manager role that we wish to measure. We adopted a hybrid approach to exploring the specific factors related to the work of case managers with the elderly with functional decline: a standardized questionnaire and triangulation of the results from analyzing group interviews.

The results bring out a perception of efficacy of 79.4 % in Sherbrooke, 85.9 % in Granit, and 67.7 % in Coaticook. Triangulation identified that the perception of efficacy is based on four categories: case-management services, the case-manager role, relations, and resources. We explore the linkages between these results and the methods used to integrate the case-manager role into an organization, including caseload, teamwork, and intervention intensity.

At the end of the process, we are convinced of the importance of environmental determinants with respect to intrinsic determinants of the perception of efficacy of case managers and the pronounced influence of the service network's state on their efficacy, especially with respect to service availability, access to a given level of service intensity, and partner collaboration with case managers.

The literature contains very little information about the practices of case managers (CMs). A review of the literature pertaining to case-management models and caseloads indicates that the boundaries of the profession are rather vague. Moreover, case management is carried out in very different contexts (hospitals, home care, community services) and by individuals with varied professional backgrounds, such as social work, nursing, psychology, and rehabilitation. The clients themselves are quite different. Case management targets fairly vulnerable clients and follows a path that is conditioned by the case manager's organizational affiliation and the targeted goal when the service was put into place. Generally speaking, clinical case management applies primarily to individuals with mental illness and the elderly with functional decline.

While understanding of the professional background of case managers and their practice conditions is growing, we still do not know how their experience differs depending on client type. Consequently, even if there is a significant amount of literature on case management in the mental-health sector because it is older (about 30 years), the published information about caseloads, in particular, cannot be applied directly to the elderly. This is due to the fact that while similar goals are targeted (such as preventing institutionalization), the role is performed differently and the problems to be dealt with are not the same.

Nevertheless, we wanted to determine, at the end of the three-year implementation process, to what degree case managers felt that they were fulfilling their roles, were in a position to act to respond to the needs of their clients, and if they were acknowledged by the people they deal with. We also wanted to determine the status of the lower caseload under the model implemented in Estrie. Accordingly, we used two methods: one quantitative, with a validated efficacy questionnaire; the other qualitative, taking the form of group interviews. Plans for the second series of focus group interviews in the three territories after three years of follow-up were made with case managers; the first series was conducted at midpoint. Since we knew that none of the territories had achieved the optimal number of full-time equivalent (FTE) case managers, we wanted to determine if case managers perceived that they could be efficacious in their working conditions. The practice conditions were not ideal or identical from one territory to the next, particularly with respect to the case-management models put into place and caseloads. Given these facts, it was of interest to determine in which territory and with respect to which aspects the feeling of efficacy seemed higher or lower. Comparing the results from the three territories and exploring certain determinants related to exercising the case-manager role were our two main objectives.

Determinants Cited in the Literature about Case-Management Efficacy

King et al.,[6] in particular, identified seven factors that impinge on case-manager performance linked to caseload: 1) contact frequency; 2) response difficulty (since certain cases are complex); 3) intervention type, since some require more time and energy than others (clinical interventions may require higher workload demand); 4) case-manager competence (experience with the problems of clients care for); 5) caseload maturity meaning the number of new cases over the total cases (time elapsed between initial contact and present time, greater burden of work earlier than later in the process); 6) distance to cover – geographical distribution of clients; 7) other roles played by the case manager within the organization. These factors do not all have the same importance, depending on the targeted goal. For example, if a territory puts case management into place basically to enhance liaison between clients and service providers, then the caseload and turnover will be high, but exposure to clients will be lower, which responds to the objectives set. On the other hand, if the focus is on proactive intervention to prevent unnecessary hospitalizations, the distance to travel to serve clients takes on the importance, since it directly influences the frequency of face-to-face contact as well as creating and maintaining a relationship of trust, which is essential in responding to the needs of the frail elderly.

Diwan[2] places more weight on the time passed on core case-management functions and brings out the determinants related to time use (time-consuming), which go beyond the physical needs of the elderly. These determinants are: 1) client behavioral disorders; 2) problems within the informal support network; and 3) new clients. An assessment of case-manager intervention priorities reveals that case managers give preference to direct interventions with clients. Indirect interventions over the telephone or in the office tend to bring out administrative regulations and processes that are often counterproductive and particularly time-consuming for case managers[1].

We use field data to determine to what degree these determinants are present and if other factors emerge from analysis.

Efficacy and Organizational-integration models in Estrie

We have juxtaposed certain data from the three territories to determine if a link could be established between the overall scores on the efficacy questionnaire and certain practice conditions. The table below provides the descriptive elements for implementing case management. It shows that the territories implemented different case-management models and that the resources and clients reached differed from the initial expectations.

Table 6.1
Case Management: Caseloads and Organizational Integration after Three Years

Description	Sherbrooke	Granit	Coaticook
Case-management model	Outset: exclusive model* Afterwards: hybrid model**	Hybrid model**	Mixed model***
Current CM professional background	Multidisciplinary (social workers, nurse, psy.)	Open single discipline (social workers, psy.)	Single discipline (social workers)
FTE CMs after 3 years	**15/19 FTEs** (79 % of expectations)	**2.8/3.5 FTEs** (80 % of expectations)	**1.2/2.4 FTEs** (48 % of expectations)
Caseload (average)**	**37.9** (± 8.5)	**34.3** (± 4.6)	**56.8** (± 10.6)
No. clients reached	**646**	**234**	**104**
Expectations: No. CM clients/ 10 % 65 years or older, not in institutions	646/1774 = 36.4 % of expectations	234/315 = 74.3 % of expectations	104/218 = 47.7 % of expectations

*   **Exclusive model:** Role limited to coordination of case-management clients.

**   **Hybrid model:** Coordination role in addition to a minor clinical role based on professional background (social worker, nurse, etc.). Homogeneous client group eligible for case management.

*** **Mixed model:** Roles under hybrid model but with a heterogeneous range of clients (regular home-care clients + case-management clients).

**** **Caseloads** are those declared by case managers when responding to the perceived self-efficacy questionnaire.

The elements in this table provide the basis for the exploring the determinants of manager perceived self-efficacy and in the discussion.

Methodology

CMPES Questionnaire

The instrument used was the French-language version of the Case Manager Personal Efficacy Scale (CMPES)[5] developed by King et al. This self-administered questionnaire was validated with 278 Australian case managers working in the area of mental health in a variety of settings. The respondents came from different professions, including psychology, social services, nursing, rehabilitation, and medicine. They all completed the questionnaire after taking part in a focus group.

Our research team produced the French-language version of the questionnaire (see Table 6.4) with professional translators using the back-translation method. The French-language version of the questionnaire (Échelle d'efficacité personnelle des gestionnaires de cas or ÉEPGC) has 17 items rated according to a 5-point Likert scale ranging from "rarely or never" (1 point) to "nearly always" (5 points). The maximum score is 85. It was built around the concept of self-efficacy as described by Bandura (1993) cited in King[5] as the personal belief about one's ability to perform a given activity. A high score is a good predictor of work performance.

The number of participants (n = 25) was inadequate for carrying out more extensive statistical tests on the data. We used triangulation of results therefore to attempt to confirm questionnaire results with focus-group interviews with a view to finding ideas to explore about the case-manager role and how caseload fits into the other elements that affect personal efficacy.

Focus Groups

In an effort to determine if the case-management role had been kept current and if the resources and tools available to case managers enabled them to perform satisfactorily, we conducted group interviews (focus groups) with case managers on two different occasions. The first time occurred 18 months into implementation of the integrated network as part of a formative assessment. Its findings were published in the first PRISMA book.[3] The second occasion took place at the three-year mark to take stock of case-manager experience and progress in the work context.

We held four focus groups: two in the central city and one in each of the rural territories. We went to each site in order to limit the travel and time required by case managers as well as to achieve a high level of participation. The discussion themes were announced prior to each meeting. The two Sherbrooke groups were divided according to year of hiring in order to better grasp the situation of the more experienced case managers (on the job since 2001–

2002) and how their role and context had changed. The more recently hired case managers hadn't gone through the initial period when the local co-ordination committee (Comité local de concertation in French) employed the case managers. As a result, their experience could have been fundamentally different. This distinction did not apply to the rural territories.

We invited all case managers to 90-minute interviews, the last part of which was set aside for them to individually respond to the perceived self-efficacy questionnaire. All the case managers who took part in the group interviews agreed to fill out the perceived self-efficacy questionnaire. The audio of all of the interviews were recorded and transcribed verbatim by an independent third party.

The contents of the interviews were analyzed based on an objective of triangulation of results. Verification with the author revealed that the King scale had not been developed from subscales of the efficacy concept. The items were constructed based on the 13 case-management activities described by Kanter[4] and completed with the role prescriptions from the Australian case-management mental-health program. We analyzed an interview and, through an inductive process, brought out four major dimensions of efficacy:

1) Case-management services (items 1, 2, 3, 5, 11, and 12)
2) Case-manager role (items 6, 8, 13, and 16)
3) Relations (items 4 and 10)
4) Resources (items 7, 9, 14, 15, and 17)

At the same time, the frequency of the connections between what the case managers said and the questionnaire items were observed. This test was conclusive. The matching was then carried out for the three other interviews.

Results

Respondent Characteristics

The rate of response was high at 92 % (n = 23) of the 25 case managers who were working at the time of the focus-group interviews, which took place in the first quarter of 2005. As shown in Table 6.2, most of the positions are held by women with an average of 4 to 5 years of experience with the same employer, except in Coaticook, where they have an average of 12 years with the same employer. Those in Sherbrooke and Coaticook have significant experience with the elderly (on average, 10.3 years and 11.6 years, respectively), whereas their younger counterparts in Granit have an average of 3.5 years of experience with the elderly. The case managers in Coaticook have mixed caseloads, with 85 % made up of the elderly.

Table 6.2
Characteristics of CMPES Respondents

Characteristics	Sherbrooke	Granit	Coaticook	Total
	n = 15	n = 4	n = 4	n = 23
Female (%)	13 (86.6 %)	4 (100 %)	3 (75 %)	20 (87 %)
Age (40 years or more)	7 (46.6 %)	None	4 (100 %)	11 (47.8 %)
CM exp. (years)	2	2.3	2.2	2.1
Same employer (years)	4.7	5.3	12.1	6.1
Exp. with elderly (years)	10.3	3.5	11.6	9.3
Clients > 65 years	99 %	98 %	85 %	97 %

Since caseload is a major variable affecting efficacy, we asked case managers to fill out a sheet about socioprofessional information, in particular, their caseloads at the time of the group interviews. As shown in the table below, Coaticook had the highest average caseload.

Table 6.3
Manager Caseload by Territory

Caseload	Sherbrooke	Granit	Coaticook
Median	36 cases	35 cases	55.5 cases
Average (sd)	37.9 (± 8.5)	34.25 (± 4.6)	56.8 (± 10.6)
Average (sd) FTE* adjusted	37.9 (± 8.5)*	36 (± 2.2)*	60 (± 7.8)*
	↓ moderate to high load		↓ very high load

* The caseload was adjusted on an individual basis to full-time equivalents (FTEs). For example, if the CM normally worked a 4-day week, the caseload was multiplied by 0.8 to establish a consistent, comparable average.

Depending on King's categorization,[5] responsibility for 34 to 46 people is a moderate to high load; 47 to 80 cases is a very high load. In the Australian study, caseloads were weighted according to work status (e.g.: part-time) and the time actually spent on case-management duties. In Estrie, we weighted caseload function according to full-time equivalents (FTEs) and not the time actually spent on long case-management duties, because we did not have the real hours spent on interventions broken down separately from the hours spent on administrative activities, training, and absences.

The results accumulated for each of the items for case managers are presented by territory, since practices are similar within one territory, but not necessarily across territories. Policy-makers chose CM organizational-integration models based on local contexts and available resources, which accounts for the variations.

Perception of Efficacy: Overall Results

The overall average of the perception of CM self-efficacy in the three territories was 77.7 %. That is comparable to the original findings of King et al., who arrived at an average of 75.1 % for a moderate to heavy caseload (34 to 46 cases). Table 6.4 below provides the results for each of the items, making it possible to observe which have achieved the highest and lowest values as well as the differences between the territories.

The items with the highest results (4 out of 5) for all of the regions are 1 (knowledge of needs), 2 (able to respond to client's acute needs), 3 (contact with hospitalized clients, 7 (who I can turn to), 8 (clear idea of my role), 12 (familiar with home environments of my clients), and 16 (effectively advocate for my clients). The items with the lowest scores (< 3.5 points) are 9 (availability of support services when clients are in crises) and 14 (enough time to respond to client needs).

The item dealing with too many different roles (13) returned mixed results. It appears in Table 6.4 with its value inversed since it is the only item expressed as a negative. Therefore, in this table, the higher the score, the easier it is for CMs to accumulate roles. Since hybrid case-management models provide for a service-coordination role with a secondary role (< 20 %) in the CM's background profession (e.g. nursing or social work), the item was important. Granit appear the most comfortable with all CM roles (3.75 points), followed by Sherbrooke (3.36 points). Coaticook, which opted for a mixed model has an average of 3 points. These figures suggest that the CMs from the three regions experience a certain amount of difficulty in assuming the roles expected of them, regardless of the organizational-integration model (hybrid or mixed), but particularly under the mixed model.

Table 6.4
**Results of Perceived Self-Efficacy
in the Three Experimental Territories in Estrie**

Item	Sherbrooke N = 15 Score/5 pts.	Granit N = 4 Score/5 pts.	Coaticook N = 4 Score/5 pts.	All N = 23 Score/5 pts.
1. I have an adequate knowledge of the current state and needs of my clients.	3.87	4.50	4.25	4.04
2. I am able to respond to the acute needs of my clients.	4.20	4.50	**4.00**	4.22
3. I am keeping in contact with my clients when they are in the hospital.	4.50	**5.00**	2.75	4.28
4. I am confident my clients will tell me if they need me urgently.	3.67	4.00	3.25	3.65
5. I feel that I am providing a good service to my clients.	3.60	**5.00**	3.50	3.83
6. I am keeping up with paperwork and record keeping in relation to my clients.	3.93	4.50	2.75	3.82
7. If I am worried about one of my clients, I know who I can turn to for help or support.	**4.67**	4.50	3.50	**4.43**
8. I have a clear idea as to what my role is as case manager with my clients.	**4.60**	4.50	3.50	4.39
9. Support services (such as crisis teams and acute admission beds) are available when my clients are in crisis.	**3.36**	4.25	**2.25**	**3.32**
10. I maintain a close liaison with other professionals who are involved with my clients.	4.13	4.00	3.25	3.96
11. Family and caregivers of my clients contact me if they have concerns.	3.90	4.25	3.50	3.89
12. I am familiar with the home environment of my clients.	3.73	4.75	**4.50**	4.04
13. I have too many different roles to be properly effective as a case manager (*inversed).	3.36	3.75	3.00	3.36
14. I have enough time to respond to the needs of my clients.	3.53	3.75	3.00	3.48
15. I am able to help my clients access services in the community.	3.86	4.50	3.75	3.95
16. I am able to effectively advocate for my clients when they are having difficulties with people or agencies.	4.33	4.50	**4.00**	4.30
17. I receive sufficient regular supervision to support me in my role as case manager.	4.27	**2.75**	2.75	3.74
TOTAL (%)	**79.4 %**	**85.9 %**	**67.7 %**	**77.7 %**
Average by item (standard deviation)	**3.97 (0.41)**	**4.29 (0.34)**	**3.38 (0.60)**	**3.92 (0.34)**

* The values for this item are given as inverses for compatibility with the other items, due to its expression as a negative.

Results by Territory

When looked at on a territorial basis, Sherbrooke obtained 79.4 %, with a per-item average of 3.97. Granit scored 85.9 % with a per-item average of 4.29, whereas the total in Coaticook was 67.7 % with a per-item average of 3.38.

Case managers in Sherbrooke experience problems obtaining assistance services for their clients and do not have enough time to respond to client needs. On the other hand, CMs know to whom they can turn when worried about a client's situation and state that they are quite familiar with their case-management role. Granit case managers feel that they particularly lack coaching (2.75) to support them in their role and that they do not have enough time to respond to client needs. Case managers in this region rated most of the items highly, including 2 that received an average of 5 points (unanimity): item 3 (contact with hospitalized clients) and item 5 (feeling of providing good service). In Coaticook, the coaching problem was raised like in Granit (2.75), but many other items received low ratings: item 3 (contact with hospitalized clients), item 6 (up-to-date on record keeping and paper work), item 9 (availability of support services), item 14 (CM availability), in addition to the item on the multiplicity of roles discussed above.

Comparative Results

Beyond the item dealing with roles, there are disparities between the territories on five items, especially for Coaticook, which shows the lowest results. This territory also evidences a major discrepancy in CMs following up their hospitalized clients since it has no hospital, so that clients must be referred to an urban facility about 45 minutes away. This item appears satisfactory in both Sherbrooke and Granit. Coaticook CMs also gave items 14 (CM availability) and 6 (record keeping and office work) the lowest ratings. As for the availability of services during crises, Coaticook CMs (even more than Sherbrooke) expressed a low level of efficacy. Lastly, the two rural territories indicated a very poor feeling of efficacy in terms of coaching resources to support them in their role. The urban setting turned in a higher rating. It is interesting to note that the number of CMs in Sherbrooke justified the hiring of a coordinator, who provided coaching to CMs. The item related to not having enough time to respond to their clients' needs is among the lowest in all three territories (3.48 points out of 5), similarly to a territory-by-territory interpretation when compared to the other items. Lastly, CMs working in a rural setting rate higher on familiarity with their clients' home environments than their urban counterparts.

Table 6.5 presents results according to subscale (case-management services, CM role, relations, and resources). The table reveals that the relations and resources subscales have slightly lower ratings than services and CM role. Relations with clients and other professionals as well as the resources available to CMs to accomplish their work are the two categories in which case-manager feelings efficacy are lowest. Two kinds of resources support the CM role: the services that their clients need (access at the right time, required intensity, quality) and the conditions to which CMs are subject within their organizations (degree of collaboration with multidisciplinary team members, caseload, training, coaching, etc.).

Table 6.5
Breakdown of Results on Efficacy into Four Categories

Territory	CM Services	CM Role	Relations	Resources	Average per Territory (sd)
Sherbrooke	3.97	4.07	3.90	3.95	3.97 (0.41)
Granit	4.67	4.31	4.00	3.95	4.29 (0.54)
Coaticook	3.75	3.31	3.25	3.05	3.38 (0.60)
Average per Subscale (sd)	4.05 (0.86)	3.98 (0.96)	3.80 (0.62)	3.79 (1.0)	

Exploration of Determinants of CM Perceived self-efficacy

With a view to more fully grasping the meanings underlying questionnaire results, the contents of the group interviews conducted with the case managers immediately before they responded to the questionnaire were analyzed. This made it possible to match questionnaire results to overall and subscale scores. The main themes are provided below according to territory.

Sherbrooke

In general, CM perceived self-efficacy appears approximately the same in four major subscales. It should be remembered that the items that rated low in Sherbrooke regard the availability of support services during crises (item 9: 3.36 points) and enough time to respond to client needs (item 14: 3.53 points). The highest scores were given to contact with hospitalized clients (item 3: 4.5 points), access to assistance for cases that worry them (item 7: 4.67 points), and clear idea of the case-manager role (item 8: 4.6 points).

Generally, the analysis brought out that CMs encounter a major difficulty in terms of availability of resources required for their clients—in particular, home help—but across the board. Furthermore, CMs claim they have a problem with accessing the required intensity of services. For example, one bath a week rather than two, or having a single day at the day-care center instead of the two days required. This information is consistent with the outcome of 3.36 out of 5, the lowest value given in Sherbrooke. Moreover, this lack of resources for clients was also raised as an issue that CMs cannot resolve: *"… we just don't have the authority to decide which services are going to be delivered … we don't have the means to help them."* Another type of resource needed to carry out the work is having the time required for clients. Sherbrooke's rating of 3.53 points indicates a mixed position. Analysis brings out that new CMs—most of whom were human relations officers (HROs) recruited from the CLSC—expressed satisfaction with a caseload that was smaller than what they had known in the past. " ... *It helps to have a smaller caseload; it means that you can be more thorough in your interventions.*" Case managers with more seniority, familiar with the exclusive model under which they did not have to act as a CLSC pivot caregiver, indicate that the caseload is excessive. " ... *as for managing time in our pivot-caregiver roles, that takes a lot of time. It's true, too, that I've neglected files ... I just don't feel constable with that and that's not how it was before. It wasn't like that at all. I'm really uncomfortable with that ....*" Lastly, Sherbrooke CMs highly appreciate professional coaching, which they view as a support resource. " ... *well, our case discussions ... I think they really help ... they standardize our practices and that's very helpful.*"

As for the category of items related to services, CMs can talk positively or negatively about their professional experience, as attested to by the rating of 3.97. To illustrate, when the client is hospitalized, certain CMs are aware of and uncomfortable with the constraints imposed by the hospital setting: " ... *I often get the feeling that I'm imposing when I go to the hospital ... [their attitude says] not that darned CM again. Always taking up time that we don't have.*" Another CM brought out the clinical advantages of follow-up during hospitalization: " ... *Let's say my client is in the hospital. I know him. When I talk to the physician, I really feel that what I say is accepted ... I think it has an impact, that gives credibility to interventions.*"

A specific aspect of the CM role is advocating client rights. Both positive and negative comments came up on this item as well. The category boasts the highest average at 4.07 points. Some feel that the smaller caseload enables them to better serve clients because it allows them to better perform the case-management role. Others believe that being integrated into the CLSC (making CMs de facto pivot caregivers) limits their capacity for independent action with the latitude that some of them had when an interorganizational joint-action authority was the CM employer. The second cohort of CMs did not experience this situation. Since integration into the CLSC " ... *we are like blue helmets tied hand and foot ... but at least we aren't gagged. ... I think we're losing some of our identity as case managers ... losing a bit of specificity ... sometimes I get the impression I'm a CLSC–practitioner like under the service allocation committee.*" In an urban context that provides many services in physically separate facilities, the organizational integration of the CM role in the CLSC has surfaced as a factor determining CM leeway and legitimacy of action in other departments and organizations where the CM accompanies the client on his or her journey throughout the continuum's services. The specificity of the CM's interorganizational role is what distinguished case managers from social workers. Case managers who had experienced the phenomenon feel that repatriation to the CLSC has diminished the role's interorganizational specificity and has restricted the legitimacy of intervention that was perceived as being broader from the outset of case-management implementation in Sherbrooke. Therefore, this repatriation has impacted on CM tasks, including certain additional administrative roles, which, in turn, had repercussions on how CM time was organized.

The items in the relations category were rated fairly high with an average of 3.95 points. To illustrate, in the case of relations with clients with whom the CMs have more contact: *"We have a special relationship in case management ... we have 35 cases. Before, [when I was] a social worker, I wouldn't have had the time to put so much energy into it because I had 100 cases."* Similarly, CMs appreciated improvements in relations with certain practitioners, including physicians: *" ... when you say that you're a case manager, it's true, they (family physicians) take the call right away."*

In conclusion, it appears that CM feeling of self-efficacy is not influenced solely by individual performance of functions and tasks. Indeed, it seems to be linked to high degree to the network's capacity to respond to client needs. This element, raised rather vigorously by case managers, is without doubt due to the fact that the primary resource of case managers is access to the required services without unreasonable delays. It must be remembered that case managers are by definition accountable to their clients for continuity of service, which necessarily involves several public, private, and community services over which CMs have no direct control.

Granit

Overall, Granit returned higher results and kept the lead in each of the categories. The elements scoring lowest in this territory related to shortcomings in professional coaching to support CMs in their new role. As mentioned above, the issue of the many different roles to be played returned an average (inversed) of 3.75 points, which stands out as the second lowest result for the territory. Ex aequo et bono, the item about time available to respond to client needs (3.75 points) also reveals a lower view of perceived performance. Otherwise, the overall results are high, since 14 out of the 17 items were rated at 4 points or more out of 5. The three items with the highest scores are maintaining contact with a hospitalized client (item 3: 5 points), offering good service as a case manager (item 5: 5 points), and being quite familiar with client home environment (item 12: 4.75 points).

The use of triangulation brought out more interview extracts demonstrating a feeling of efficacy than in the other territories, which is consistent with the questionnaire results. In the service category, which presents the highest average at 4.67 points out of 5, the items involving collaboration with hospitals in various regions positively attract attention. *"Well, I call [the hospital] to let them know what's really happening out here because that's going to have an impact on what happens at the CHUS. So, I want to talk to somebody down there and I'm going to ask to keep me in the loop, but I'm the one who's going to make the first move, it's not up to them to check if … "* In this interaction, it appears that the case manager must take the communication initiative and insist on receiving information. In contrast, another CM perceived improvement in system reactivity since implementation of the integrated network, especially with regards to hospital discharge: *"Well, I would tend to say yes, I think that that happens rapidly, not even a week before services are in place, as soon as we get the fax from the CHUS or the Centre hospitalier Beauce-Etchemin, it takes a day or two and then it's in place …."*

The issue of relations with clients emerges fairly positively, with an average of 4 points: *"That's reassuring for them. If something comes up, I call my case manager or the CLSC; they have her name …."* Relations with other practitioners are mostly good; the limited availability of certain services is the primary constraint on CM action: *"Things are improving both within and outside the institution, I find it's going well with other professionals, you know, they are making progress."* Interaction with hospitals, however, can still be difficult to establish: *" … I call to let them know that, uh, I am managing his (patient) case and I say to them "give me a call if something new comes up." I never get a call-back. The next day and the day after day, and the day after that, I have to make the effort to call … "* This is followed by the comment that it would be highly appreciated if the family physician had greater access to the computerized clinical chart to consult the record from his or her clinic. This would be another way to maintain relations between professionals working on the same case.

On items pertaining to the CM role, in second position with an average of 4.31 out of 5 points, Granit CMs feel that other providers and clients should be aware of what makes case managers different from other practitioners. This could quell the argument still persisting after three years: *" … what is our role, what distinguishes us from the other practitioners, even from our partners sometimes, it's not always clear. We often get into a debate … and not everybody is always in agreement all the time."* Even though Granit CMs gave high overall ratings, except for the large number of roles to be played, the interview brought out that the role issue remains a topic of concern and that it affects a group of practitioners, giving rise to confusion, which negatively impacts on the quality of interaction.

Lastly, the overall result for resources accessible to the CM is 3.95 points, making it the category with the lowest rating in Granit. The CMs emphasize, on the one hand, that clients expressed their satisfaction with the services received and that a caseload set at 35 is more appropriate than 40, since travel distances in rural areas is often an obstacle, both for clients and for CMs, who must put more effort into mapping out their itinerary in their territory. The time available to respond to client needs is reduced by the time needed to travel to visit individuals who are geographically distant. *" … that's just the reality out here, but I think it applies across the board, when we were talking about case-management eligibility criteria, when a lady is a 50-minute drive away … it's difficult to put services into place, anyway, that's just the reality, I think, which is how things are for us. ... So, you can allow you to sell follow-up every two weeks if the person lives so far away and, when you do, that's 100 km round trip. [...] That's what we end up doing it regularly. -we try to make the most out of our days ... when we're out, by putting two or three in the same village on the same day to avoid losing time on the road ... but that's not always possible."* Consequently, even though full-time CMs work the same amount of time regardless of territory, the intensity of services provided to the client in-person by the CM could be lower for CMs serving clients who live in remote rural areas.

Moreover, despite the support that CMs receive from their superiors in dealing with complex cases, professional guidance on the role's specificity and CM interventions is deemed lacking: *"Well, in my own role as case manager, what I would've liked was having more supervision in doing my job. Having more guidance, for me, that's somewhat of a restrictive factor. Having it would have made things easier."* Weighing in on the negative side with a mere 2.75 points, the fact that new and replacement CMs do not have access to specific training on the CM role is a contributing factor in the category's low rating. *"Uh, I'm scheduled for training next week ... that I should've had two years ago ... that's a shortcoming."*

Coaticook

The Coaticook results to the questionnaire about perceived self-efficacy were the lowest in the three territories. An overall examination reveals that the lowest ratings fall into four categories. Nevertheless, the resources category contains the largest number of low-scoring items. The 4 items on which case managers perceive the greatest efficacy in Coaticook (4 or more) relate to adequate client current needs (item 1: 4.25 points) and client home environment (item 12: 4.50 points), CM capacity to respond to clients' acute needs (item 2: 4.00 points), and effective advocacy of client interests (item 16: 4 points).

As for the CM role, it appears that CM efforts to ensure that the intervention takes place at the right time do not appear adequately reflected, which impedes expression of the role: *" ... I tell myself, well, the case-manager role, that means following them up [our clients], we should know them. You know, I tell myself, all kinds of things [falls] have been happening to that man for three months now and he needs to be assessed. That was the time, the time to transfer him [from a hospital] to the institute. ... Yet everywhere I turned, I got a no."* It also appears that even the multidisciplinary team is divided over the issue of lack of recognition case-management added value, which impacts greatly on case managers and even the clients experience repercussions: *"... I never told my clients that I was a case manager. ... if we don't have the respect here of our peers ... (-Exactly.) ... [what do] you think that could mean to our clients, that we are case managers, that changes nothing."*

Certain results for CM services are lower, especially those pertaining to interactions with hospital departments. It's not merely a desire on the part of CMs to stay in touch with hospitalized clients; it's imperative for the other party to respond to the call: *"They [hospital practitioners] don't know who we are, where our client is; we have to look for him or her."* Moreover, respondents added that the liaison mechanisms were not effective enough. Despite these difficulties, it was apparent that the families of individuals with impaired independents know who to seek out in problem situations? *" ... when the lady ... got to the CHUS, a family member said: 'My mother has a case manager. Her name is (CM's name). She is in Coaticook. Call her if anything happens.' Although she (the mother) went to the hospital, she came back home without me knowing anything about it. It was a family member who told me: 'What do we do? My mother is home and she needs [a number of services]' ... But, in this case, it was the family who informed the hospital."*

The relations category turned in one of the lowest scores, with an average of 3.25 points. There was a time when CMs had a better perception of their relations with other professionals: *" ... yes, well, I think there was a time when input was easier when you identified yourself as a case manager. It doesn't seem like it's like that anymore ...."* When case management was first being implanted, this momentum promoted certain interventions but, it appears, that it is no longer working after three years. *" ... it's that, all that [the effect of initial momentum], it looks like it's gotten watered down some, our collaborations are less evident. Even on the team, we were obliged to ... now, there is a big controversy about clarifying our roles."* These problems in operations and understanding the role, both within the institution and with partners, can affect relations and collaboration efficacy. What the CMs expressed reflects the necessity of working harder to improve mutual confidence, the recognition of roles, and the value of interdisciplinarity in efficaciously fulfilling the needs of vulnerable clients.

Nevertheless, CMs state that they often hear expressions of confidence and perceived competence in their relations with clients and their immediate families: *"And when I told her that I'd put her mother into case management, I felt that that was really ... very reassuring for her. – That, uh, happens to me pretty often. If the caregivers feel reassured ... whatever the name you give it, what reassures them is that there's going to be someone to coach me or who's ... in coordinating the services my mother needs or who's going to play watchdog for the required services. ... because I just can't see it and you people know about that. ... yes, that happens to me often ...."*

Among all the resources that should support CMs in their roles, once again, the lack of time clearly stands out as a negative factor that generates many consequences. These include not enrolling as many people as hoped for in case management, difficulty in performing professional responsibilities at the same time as administrative tasks: *"I don't have enough time, with all the committee meetings I have to attend and all the others ... I don't have ... that's where I save time, by not putting them into case management ...."* Having to put time and effort into related tasks, in addition to regular interventions, increases the burden, which is already perceived as heavy in the territory. Accumulating mixed-model clients in a caseload that isn't held in check by a waiting list contributes to the perceived overload. On top of that, there is the problem of an inadequate range of services available in the territory to respond to the general public's needs and the limited availability of existing services. Respondents expressed their feelings of powerlessness; the frustration is palpable in the following quote: *"Our problem is much larger than our range of services being in adequate to respond to needs. – You know, what am I managing? What am I managing in the ISP (Individualized Service Plan)? Sometimes, I really don't have much to manage there. – I manage family mobilization. As for family exhaustion, well, that's the way it goes."* Moreover, CMs indicate that professional guidance is inadequate with a rating of 2.75 points out of 5. We do not have any interview extracts in support of that figure. Lastly, the overall result of 3.5 out of 5 on the item 5 about the CM's feeling of offering good service could be linked to the fact that concrete means or resources for providing the right service at the right time are just not there, which diminishes CM feelings of efficacy. In this regard, case managers in Sherbrooke and Coaticook expressed similar points of view.

Exploring Determinants Yielded by the Estrie Experience

Various measurements and observations were carried out when the six integrated-network components—including case management—were implemented. We linked certain data from the CMs in the three territories to determine if we could draw a relationship between the overall questionnaire scores for efficacy and certain practice conditions, namely, the organizational-integration model used to implement case management in their territories, working on a team or alone, and the proportion of cases that receive intensive interventions with respect to those who receive low intensity.

Caseloads and Organizational-Integration Models

Granit and Coaticook evident similarity in terms of the proportion of CMs hired and the percentage of clients reached compared to expectations. In Coaticook, 48 % of full-time equivalents (FTEs) required for case management at work and 48 % of clients had been reached. In Granit, with 80 % of the resources required, they reached 74.3 % of the targeted clients. Sherbrooke shows the broadest discrepancy since, with 79 % of their resources, they had reached 36.4 % of the targeted clients when the questionnaire was administered. A waiting list was set up once the client flow made it impossible to maintain the smaller caseloads.

The other point that merits notice is that the average caseload in Coaticook is very high compared to the other two territories. Moreover, Coaticook's caseload is directly related to the mixed model and the lack of a waiting list, as per territory policy.

Caseloads and Perception of the Mode of Operation

Case management centers primarily on interdisciplinary collaboration, regardless of the department to which the professionals with whom the CM interacts on a daily basis belong. The prime "zone" for interdisciplinary work is the broadened home-care team in the CLSC. When we asked CMs what operating method was used and if it suited them or if they preferred another way of working, we observed that nearly half of Sherbrooke CMs worked on a team and/or in tandem and that they were satisfied with this approach (Table 6.6). Three individuals who worked alone were satisfied with the status quo, while a fourth would have preferred another arrangement. Granit was similar, with nearly half of CMs working on a team and/or in tandem and satisfied with the situation, whereas one person was working alone and would have preferred another arrangement. Lastly, in Coaticook, 75 % of the CMs were working on team and in tandem; all were satisfied with this approach. One person, however, usually worked alone and hoped that this approach would not continue.

Out of the 22 individuals responding to this item, 14 people (64 %) stated that they worked on a team and/or according to a mixed model, including teamwork. Nine CMs (41 %), however, indicated that they were not involved in teamwork and one third of them stated they would prefer another approach.

Given the specificity of the CM role and case complexity, the interdisciplinary approach appears to have advantages and should be used in case-management models with a clinical perspective. Case discussions clarify the direction of difficult and complex cases, while enabling the case-management team to share information about the state of the network and to standardize their professional practices. Certain number of hypotheses can be made about the fact that more than 40 % of case managers made no mention of teamwork. 1) Working in tandem provides for mutual help on a daily basis, since there is no need to coordinate schedules for formal meetings. It can be used instead of or as an adjunct to teamwork. 2) Working individually could indicate that the CM is part of an "initial case-management team" that interacts primarily by telephone and maintains a very high caseload. For the three case managers in the three territories who would like another approach to work, it could also indicate a need to make recourse to teamwork systematic (under what circumstances it is indicated, what can and cannot be expected of a team discussion about clients, work objectives, the different procedures that a team meeting can adopt, etc.) in order to make all team resources available to the team and, when necessary, have recourse to outside resources.

There does not appear to be any direct link between operating mode and caseload. On the other hand, the workload (number of cases plus related organizational responsibilities), which has been subjectively described by the CMs as heavy in the three territories irrespective of the caseload, could account for the scarcity of formal and informal case discussions and could result in an individual operating mode. Similarly, the organization of clinical supervision—which appears necessary but seems inadequate, especially in the two rural territories—could doubtless improve operating as a team.

Table 6.6
Case Manager Perceptions about Operating Mode

CM (n = 22) Operating Mode (functioning = fc)	Sherbrooke (n = 14)	Granit (n = 4)	Coaticook (n = 4)
Fc perceived team (n)	Team OK* (4)	Team OK (1)	Team OK (1)
Fc perceived team and tandem (n)	Team + tandem, OK (3)	Team + tandem, OK (1)	Team + tandem, OK (2)
Fc perceived by team+ tandem+ alone (n)	Team + tandem + **alone** OK (1)		
Fc perceived tandem (n)	Tandem OK (2)	Tandem OK (1)	
Fc perceived alone (n)	**Alone-OK (3) Alone-NO** (1)**	**Alone-NO (1)**	**Alone-NO (1)**

OK*:   The CM is happy with the operating mode and does not want another approach.
NO**: The CM finds the operating mode unsatisfactory and wants another approach.

Caseloads and Perceived Intensity of Interventions

After the group interviews with the CMs, we asked them in writing if they could estimate the percentage of cases they were managing based on the intensity of the monthly interventions carried out. Major variations were observed between the CMs in the three territories. This phenomenon may reflect the actual situation. On the other hand, it may be due to their recall of the proportions. Once their responses were compiled, the medians provided a clearer idea. Table 6.7 shows that 10 % to 50 % of cases require more than 12 monthly interventions, which we consider high intensity. There is a similar proportion of 15 % to 17 % of interventions of low intensity, which means about 1 intervention per month. The large majority of cases are of moderate intensity, which translates into 2 to 12 interventions per month.

We have associated the high intensity of case-management interventions to cases in the initial assessment phase and to those involving a request for placement. The latter often requires a number of steps taken with the family as well as with various administrative authorities. Low intensity would pertain more to the culmination of putting services into place. The situation is stable and only requires regular monitoring.

Table 6.7
CM Perceived Intensity of Interventions

Intervention Intensity	Sherbrooke (median)	Granit (median)	Coaticook (median)
High intensity (> 12 interv./month)	15 %	10 %	10 %
Moderate intensity (2 to 12 interv./month)	50 %	55 %	37 %
Low intensity (about 1 interv./month)	15 %	17 %	17 %

The Coaticook results that show a smaller proportion of cases of high or moderate intensity can be explained by heavy caseloads compounded by administrative responsibilities. Statements made during the group interview appear to bear this out. The practitioner therefore would tend to reduce the proportion of cases receiving a high or moderate intensity of interventions, while ensuring a response to all clients but without needing to implement a waiting list.

Discussion

Caseload is one of many elements potentially concurrent in a given context generating a positive or negative synergy, in particular, its impact on the case manager's perceived self-efficacy. One of these contextual elements undoubtedly lies with the research project because of the high expectations formulated for the role and intervention efficacy of new case managers. The more general context of limited availability of services (both basic and specialized) increased the difficulty of task performance.

Avenues Opened by Triangulation

With our attention focused on the linkages between certain of these results and caseloads, triangulation enabled us to see a direct relationship between the overload expressed in Coaticook and the lack of time. Granit CMs cited travel distance to account for the lack of time, even with a smaller caseload. It should be emphasized that the CMs in this territory had to take extended leave and that, upon return, had to be accompanied while making the rounds of the partners in order to reestablish contact, clarify roles and expectations on both sides, and encourage collaboration centered on the needs of the elderly. The Granit territory operates with five general and/or specialized hospitals, one of which is located in the territory. Their primary-care and placement services are located at different service points. Service structure complexity is often cited in urban settings, but this territory deals with many partners, all of which are located at some distance from Granit's central institution. This particular structure, compounded by distance, introduces an additional level of difficulty. As a result, time cannot be set aside in planning logistics and coordinating services provided by case managers.

Sherbrooke's average load of 36 cases might lead to the expectation that CMs can comfortably carry out their role. This seems all the more likely because they benefit from overall needs assessment provided by the single entry point, nearby specialized services, and larger case-manager teams. Yet that is not the case. The outline below attempts to account for this, based on our overall understanding of the practice conditions in urban settings as described during the group interviews.

1. The single entry point's needs assessment team travels to the client's home to assess the precise nature of the function decline. This is an undeniable gain, since the individual can be directed towards the appropriate service. On the other hand, the fact that Sherbrooke had not yet hired the required number of CMs resulted in so much pressure that a waiting list had to be created. Its management fell to the "initial case-management team" those comprised of two professionals working basically over the telephone to ensure that certain more urgent services were actually put into place. This way of doing things could result in some people being assigned to case management several months after the request for services was made. In such cases, the CM must redo the overall assessment. As can be seen, an initial gain is not always a net gain.

2. Urban settings have more community and specialized services. CMs try to get these services for their clients but are not necessarily successful on the first attempt because there is often a wait for a particular service. For each client awaiting a certain number of services, the CM has to perform follow-up or subsequently argue the case in order to obtain a priority, when required. In cases in which there is no response to the elderly person's needs and home support is compromised, additional efforts— with family members if they are able to do so—are made to find alternatives. If this doesn't work out, a request for placement may be necessary. The lack of resources can therefore generate more demanding interventions than if there had been a response when the request was made. That has the potential for increasing the perceived burden of the caseload. This aspect concerns the handicap, that is, the discrepancy between what is required and what can be provided, both by the formal network and informal caregivers.

3. Urban settings with significant traffic through its services also have larger teams of professionals and technicians, which generates their own particular dynamics because of the large numbers of clients and practitioners. Consequently, the relations between CMs and visiting homemakers are defined in the same way from one territory to the next, regardless of the volume of clients and team size. In other words, all of the problems encountered by visiting homemakers and social-services assistants when visiting the elderly are addressed to case managers. In Sherbrooke, it appears, however, that a non-negligible number of problems to be solved (e.g. mending a pair of pants, buying shampoo) are ordinary requests that do not jeopar-

dize home support. In Sherbrooke, these problems get dumped on the desk of one case manager who, according to the work organization now in effect, is the only person who can solve them. It might be appropriate to look further into this issue to see if case-manager time (which is rare and therefore valuable) couldn't be put to better use on clinical situations requiring their competencies and to turn over daily problems to home-maker team leaders for solution. Freeing up time in this manner might enable case managers to take on a few more clients.

Conclusion

Triangulating questionnaire results with the contents of interviews with case managers enable us to see that perceived efficacy often appears tied to difficulties in obtaining services from a complex network comprised of actors who do not all have the same authority and practitioners who do not all have the same level of information about the role that case managers are attempting to fill. Moreover, disparities between the territories make it impossible to attribute the same cause to a given effect. To illustrate, the lack of time can be attributed to three very different reasons in the three territories.

The main idea that should be drawn from this matching of results relates to the strength of the environmental determinants with respect to the determinants intrinsic to efficacy. The environmental determinants in this instance represent the practice contexts (reactivity of the continuum services, the degree of information that practitioners have about the case-manager role, service availability and accessibility, etc.). They can either initiate or hinder the application of the individualized service plan. Intrinsic determinants pertain to self-perceived ability to successfully carry out a specific activity or intervention. These two categories of determinants introduce a new element into the equation. In fact, the efficacy scale for case managers should take into account the very essence of case management, which means the interactions with service providers and with the elderly and their caregivers. The success of this is not unilateral but bilateral in nature. To illustrate, a partner cannot be forced to collaborate, change his practices, communicate effectively, and so on. We even noted that, when interaction with the different departments and services ends in repeated failures, CMs feel less efficacious, even if their perception was that the interventions were carried out properly. The interaction between CMs and clients (and caregivers) did not surface as a factor of influence during triangulation. The literature, however, brings out that the difficulty connected to the characteristics of certain clients and caregivers (or the lack of a caregiver) can impede putting services into place. Consequently, Diem[1] raised the idea that the caseload comprised of the elderly must be put in relationship with the caseload's composition, that is, the characteristics of the clients comprising the load, since certain clients or caregivers are more difficult to serve than others. Diwan,[2] on the other hand, studies the time spent of CM core functions and brings out the time-consuming determinants that go beyond the physical needs of the elderly. These determinants are 1) client problem behaviors; 2) problems in the informal support network; and 3) new clients. The case managers expressed all three of these determinants.

Lastly, in looking at the results obtained in the three territories, our understanding is that the case-manager role (its basis, objectives, intervention specificity, and ties to other professions) has matured but only to part of its potential three years after implementation. The mixed model does not appear to foster intervention specificity, with the result that partners as well as case managers themselves and their colleagues still have questions about the role. In the other two territories, which use the hybrid case-management model, CMs often have a clear idea of their role. On the other hand, they find that professionals and sometimes even their home-care coworkers do not have an accurate idea of what is expected of case managers and their contribution to the integrated network. Vagueness also surrounds justification of the smaller caseload for case managers compared to their home-care colleagues.

Conclusively, the perceived self-efficacy of case managers appears markedly influenced by the network's overall state either in terms of availability of a range of continuum services or access to the required intensity of services. It is further influenced by the support or priority that case management receives within the network, which, in turn, impacts on the quality of collaboration obtained from the different providers. This variable, which could be considered context-linked, opens up a whole other status in exercising the case-management role, since the system's overall performance (continuum of services to the elderly) directly conditions the case manager's capacity to act. These findings should provide incentives to performance and service-quality evaluators to go beyond the normal indicators (e.g. number of clients served, number of interventions, waiting time, and others) and include indicators of effective collaboration between case managers and service providers as a whole, including within their own team under CLSC home-care structures. This quality of collaboration appears crucial to us.

References

1. Diem, E., Alcock, D., Gallagher, E., Angus, D., and Medves, J. Looking beyond caseload numbers for long-term home-care case managers. *Care Management Journals*. 2001; 3 (1): 2-7.

2. Diwan, S. Allocation of case management resources in long-term care: predicting high use of case management time. *The Gerontologist*, 1999; 39 (5): 580-590

3. Hébert, R., Tourigny, A., and Gagnon, M. Intégrer les services pour le maintien de l'autonomie des personnes. PRISMA – programme de recherche sur l'intégration des services pour le maintien de l'autonomie, dans

Chapitre 5: Résultats intérimaires de l'implantation de mécanismes et outils d'intégration des services aux personnes âgées en perte d'autonomie dans trois territoires de l'Estrie (Québec), EDISEM, 2004; 79-124.

4. Kanter, J. Clinical case management: definition, principles, components. *Hospital and Community Psychiatry*, 1989; 40: 361-368.

5. King, R., Le Bas, J., and Spooner, D. The impact of caseload on the personal efficacy of mental health case managers. *Psychiatric Services*. 2000; 51 (3): 364-368.

6. King, R., Meadows, G., Le Bas, J. Compiling a caseload index for mental health case management. *Australian & New-Zealand Journal of Psychiatry, 2004*; 38 (6): 455-462.

Chapter 7
Perceptions of Service Continuity among Case Managed Recipients of Services for Frail Elders during Implementation of the Integrated Services Network[*]

Anne Veil, Lynne Michaud, and Réjean Hébert

Findings of a study on the role of case managers and service continuity for dependent elders

Introduction

This component on continuity is part of a broader study called PRISMA–Estrie,[1] whose purpose is to assess the implementation and impact of three instruments/tools and three mechanisms, including case management, put in place to enhance continuity of care and services to elders who are moderately to seriously frail (Hébert, Durand, Dubuc, Tourigny, and Groupe PRISMA, 2003). Three Estrie territories that differ sociodemographically and in their health and social services networks took part in the project. In Quebec, case management constitutes a new professional role in service delivery to the elderly. The case manager's responsibilities consist of conducting comprehensive assessments of client needs, organizing and coordinating required services, advocating for clients, verifying whether services have been duly received as intended, and doing systematic follow-up. As regards continuity, case managers answer to a coordinating committee on services to elders. They must report to this committee on what has been done to solve problems and prevent situations detrimental to continuity.

Our main objective was to explore perceptions of continuity by the caregiver-receiver dyad[2] and identify the role played by case management in dyad members' service experience. Under the concept of the caregiver-receiver

[*]   This chapter is reprinted with the kind permission of *Intervention*, the journal of the *Ordre professionnel des travailleurs sociaux du Québec* (the Quebec College of Social Workers), where it appeared as: Les perceptions de continuité des services de clientèles âgées en perte d'autonomie suivies en gestion de cas dans le cadre de l'implantation du réseau de services intégrés. Anne Veil, Lynne Michaud, Réjean Hébert. Intervention, December 2006; 125: 97-108.

dyad, the client and the family caregiver are viewed as forming a dyad because their relationship and their needs are closely intertwined (Noelker, L., 2002):

1. The needs of one are closely linked to the needs of the other, especially in the case of couples. With couples, care providers sometimes wonder which member is the caregiver, since both are frail.
2. Family caregivers contact service providers to obtain or adjust assistance, often sharing this task with the case manager.
3. Some of the services delivered to clients, for example respite care, are actually intended to benefit the family caregiver.

Since then, the needs of one are framed according to the needs of the other, the family caregiver and the client must be viewed together as a dyad so that a realistic and feasible individualized service plan (ISP) can be drawn up as part of long-term service delivery.

Literature Review

Continuity is a concept invoked in several management and professional practice contexts in the field of health and social services. The way it is defined tends to reflect the perspective authors derive from their area of practice. Two fields in which literature on continuity has been widely disseminated are physical health (Shortell, 1976; Institute of Medicine, 1996; Starfield, 1998; Reid, Haggerty, and McKendry, 2002; Biem J., Hadjistavropoulos, Morgan, Biem H.B., and Pong, 2003) and mental health (Bachrach, 1981; Sparbel and Anderson, 2000; Clément, Aubé, Bolduc, Damasse, Beaucage, and Tremblay, 2003). In a recent Canadian study (Woodward, Abelson, Tedford, and Hutchison, 2004), the concept was examined in the context of home care with case management. The features of care delivery that emerge from this research as facilitating continuity can be grouped along two dimensions:

1. Management of care: planning, monitoring, and coordination.
2. Direct services to clients: unbroken, consistent, professional, competent, and timely, with ongoing monitoring and promoting a relationship of trust between clients and care providers.

The various parties do not all prioritize the different aspects of continuity the same way. For example, clients are little inclined to take service-management aspects into consideration, while they value receiving services at the right time, care-provider competency, a relationship of trust, and client involvement in decision-making.

One recent study (Reid et al., 2002) on how the concept of continuity is measured reflects current interest in Quebec and Canada in the measurement of continuity. Three types of continuity are singled out in this study: 1) informational continuity, which makes it possible to adjust care to the individual's disease; 2) relational continuity, which links past, current, and future care and gives the client a sense of coherence and predictability; and 3) management continuity, which ensures that service plans provide for complementary and appropriate services and service consistency. Another Canadian study, by Biem et al. (2003), focuses on new dimensions of continuity, including empowerment, the comfort of the clients and the clients' family caregivers, and unforeseen factors associated with changes in the individual's setting.

In line with work in the US by Shortell (1976), the Institute of Medicine (1996), and Starfield (1998), the physical health sector has been determining priorities on the basis of the need to coordinate the sequencing of medical care and focusing on communication in relation to the time factor. Later in this book, the computerized clinical chart is proposed as a means of attaining these goals. In the field of mental health in the US, Bachrach (1981), and Sparbel and Anderson (2000) have introduced dimensions related to interdisciplinary care and individualization. The work of Clément et al. (2003) in Quebec differentiates between vertical continuity (for a given service over time) and horizontal continuity, which is the product of links among several organizations and service providers. Under their seven dimensions of continuity, inspired by Bachrach (1981 and 1993) and Penchansky and Thomas (1981), access is heavily emphasized and concepts associated with best practices and clients' changing needs are linked to it. For example, goodness of fit and acceptability of service, flexibility, and the individualization of service planning and delivery in order to promote client involvement in decision-making are all identified as continuity factors in delivering services to the vulnerable target groups that concern Clément et al. Many researchers are now invoking the concept of continuity; it would appear to be taking on ever broader meaning as it is tailored to various service sectors and different target groups' specific features. We do not yet have a theoretical construct capable of incorporating all these attributes into a coherent whole.

The case manager's role is generally described as consisting of planning, research, and service monitoring to meet a client's needs in an appropriate and continuous manner. Recognized case-manager activities consist of performing assessments, coordinating services, and providing education and support (Wodarski and Williams-Hayes, 2002). A degree of consensus exists in the literature in identifying case managers as belonging mainly to two professions: social work and nursing. Nevertheless, there is much variation in the ways the role is put into effect and in case-manager practices, reflecting the diverse target groups served and the different case-management models endorsed by the employers of case managers.

From the literature, it is possible to identify several case-management models, which can be grouped under two major headings:
1. Control-type models, which subsume the brokerage model, are task focused and can thus target short-term intervention objectives in a linear perspective. These models are geared to clients able to deal directly with service providers.
2. Preventive-type models cover the patient-centered—or in our terms client-centered—model, which is associated with long-term services and

intended for moderately to seriously frail individuals. The patient-centered model is defined as a more fully developed case-management model focused on change in the relations among the various systems in order to serve the client's interests. It consists of a clinical process that includes direct intervention with clients and their families, in which the client perspective is acknowledged as the basis for arguments with a legitimate place in the decision-making process (Long, 2002).

When case managers have a geriatric caseload comprised of the moderately to seriously frail, they are required to navigate through hospital departments and medical services, rehabilitation departments, and in-home services. These may be public, private, community based, collective, or cooperative. The multiplicity of services and their fragmented nature are conducive to breaks in continuity. Case managers constantly work at the interfaces between the three spheres of health services, psychosocial services (including in-home services), and management (Couturier and Carrier, 2006).

The case-management model that has been implemented in Estrie is comparable to the patient-centered one. In the territories covered by this study, nine case managers were social workers or other psychosocial professionals. Two others were psychologists and one a nurse. Because they are trained in numerous approaches, social workers are familiar with the systemic perspective, which facilitates their psychosocial and administrative work. On the other hand, some feel less at ease with the medical matters specific to elder care (e.g., diagnoses, medications, and physical care).

Our primary concern in this article is how members of caregiver-receiver dyads perceive continuity along the whole service continuum, regardless of the sector the services used belong to or the role played by case management in the dyad members' experience. Our intent is to make a contribution to health-care, rehabilitation, and long-term in-home services delivered in a service-integration framework.

Methodology

Our study design is qualitative, and more specifically exploratory and descriptive. The multiple-case study method (Yin's typology) underpinned our approach procedure. We preferred a qualitative strategy because it allows for in-depth understanding of actor experiences. By using the marker-case intentional sampling method, we were able to choose case-managed individuals with defined problems. We established two predictable care trajectories. One was focused on psychosocial services (cognitive disorders; depression; change of life setting). The other was focused on medical services (stroke; hip fracture); that is, it included the occurrence of a critical event involving hospitalization and a rehabilitation period. Semi-directed face-to-face interviews were conducted; they were 40 to 60 minutes long. The material analyzed consisted of the verbatim interview transcripts, ISPs, and flowcharts of the services received during the year preceding the interview. Once the selection was complete, we had four cases of stroke, two cases of cognitive disorders, and four cases of changes in life settings, for a total of twelve cases studied. Interviews might be conducted with the client, the family caregiver, or both together.

To explore dyad members' perceptions of continuity and identify the role played by case management in their experience of services, we used the full slate of services the client received, dropped, refused, or was wait-listed for over the previous year, as presented in the ISP. We ensured the list so obtained was a faithful portrait of reality by validating it first through systematic phone consultation with case managers and then by asking users themselves during the interview. Analysis of the interview transcripts was paired with analysis of the service flowcharts to obtain an understanding of the caregiver-receiver dyad's situation and identify the case manager's contribution to continuity in a complex care and service situation. To be included in our sample, participants had to be aged 65 or over (whether with or without a family caregiver), live in one of the territories taking part in the PRISMA–Estrie project, speak French, present with one of the marker problems, and have been under case management for over two months. When the elderly client was not in a position to take part in the interview, we conducted it with the family caregiver who dealt with service providers.

Findings

DESCRIPTION OF PARTICIPANTS. We did not recruit any participants with fractured hips or depression. In recruiting study participants who were changing their life setting, we had no control over reasons for the change, and all of them proved to have cognitive disorders, which resulted in a high representation of such cases in the study. The case-managed target group included a significant proportion (30% or more) of individuals with varying degrees of cognitive impairment; our recruitment process was influenced by this factor.

All the elders we met with during the study were recipients of long-term services. For those with cognitive disorders, the development of frailty had been gradual, while, for those with stroke, it was sudden and entailed major adjustments in all areas of their lives. Participant prior experiences with the health and social services system were not of equal duration. In the eight cases of cognitive disorders, the caregiver-receiver dyad had long experience with home-support services, with a CLSC worker actively involved in the case as key contact. At the time of interviewing, seven of the twelve elders lived at home: one lived alone, three with family members (children/siblings), and three with their spouses. In four cases, the elders had just moved to either a private residence for the elderly or a residential and extended care centre ("centre d'hébergement et de soins de longue durée," known as CHSLD). Last, one individual was in a geriatric acute-care facility for assessment.

Table 7.1 presents participants' characteristics.

Table 7.1
Distribution of Marker Cases

Territory	Client's Age	Sex	Marker Cases	Case-Management Duration	Interview Conducted with	Number of Participants
Urban	91 yrs	F	Cognitive disorders	10 months	Family caregiver alone (daughter, aged 53)	1
Urban	69 yrs	F	Cognitive disorders	7 months	Family caregiver alone (husband, aged 74)	1
Rural, with hospital center*	94 yrs	F	Cognitive disorders	2 months	Family caregiver alone (son, aged 56)	1
Rural, with no hospital center**	70 yrs	M	Cognitive disorders	18 months	Family caregiver alone (wife, aged 68)	1
Urban	66 yrs	F	Change in life setting	21 months	Family caregiver alone (husband, aged 70)	1
Rural, with hospital center	65 yrs	M	Change in life setting	12 months	Family caregiver alone (sister-in-law, aged 54)	1
Urban	74 yrs	M	Change in life setting	8 months	Family caregiver alone (wife, aged 70)	1
Rural, with no hospital center	83 yrs	F	Change in life setting	5 months	Family caregiver alone (son, aged 44)	1
Urban	84 yrs	M	Stroke	11 months	Client with family caregiver (wife, aged 64)	2
Urban	66 yrs	M	Stroke	15 months	Client with both family caregivers (sisters, aged 70 and 68)	3
Rural, with no hospital center	78 yrs	F	Stroke	7 months	Client with family caregiver (brother, aged 83)	2
Rural with hospital center	66 yrs	F	Stroke	11 months	Cliente	1
Total Number of Participants						16

* A territory remote from major urban centers but with its own hospital.
** A rural territory located comparatively close to a major centre, with emergency facilities and no local hospitalization.

Service Flowchart: Stroke Marker Cases

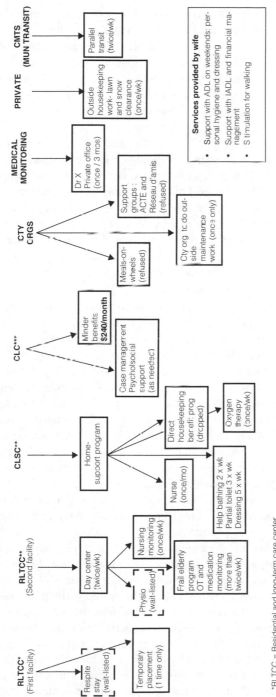

RLTCC* (First facility)

Respite stay (wait-listed) → Temporary placement (1 time only)

RLTCC** (Second facility)

Day center (twice/wk) → Nursing monitoring (once/wk)

Physio (wait-listed) → Frail elderly program OT and medication monitoring (more than twice/wk)

CLSC** → Home-support program → Direct housekeeping benefit prog (dropped) → Oxygen therapy (once/wk)

Nurse (once/mo)

Help bathing 2 x wk / Partial toilet 3 x wk / Dressing 5 x wk

CLC***

Minder benefits **$240/month**

Case management Psychosocial support (as needed)

CTY CRGS

Support groups: ACTE and Réseau d'amis (refused)

Cty org tc do outside maintenance work (once only)

Meals-on-wheels (refused)

MEDICAL MONITORING

Dr X Private office (once / 3 mos)

PRIVATE

Outside housekeeping work - lawn and snow clearance (once/wk)

CMTS (MUN TRANSIT)

Parallel transit (twice/wk)

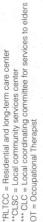

Services provided by wife
- Support with ADL on weekends: personal hygiene and dressing
- Support with IADL and financial management
- Stimulation for walking

*RLTCC = Residential and long-term care center
**CLSC = Local community services center
*** CLC = Local coordinating committee for services to elders
OT = Occupational Therapist

CASE MANAGEMENT AND SERVICE COMPLEXITY. The service flowcharts for our case-management sample show not only that a significant variety of service providers are called on to help maintain clients in the community, but also that these providers include a variety of different organizations, each with its own method of operation and specific constraints. We present one of these flowcharts here to illustrate this diversity, and indeed the heterogeneous nature of the universe case managers are called upon to navigate in ensuring clients' needs are met.

The development of frailty gives rise to the need for services that cannot subsequently be withdrawn or altered without producing significant consequences for the elderly and their family caregivers. Our interview with those whose cases required the highest level of care revealed dependency in relation to services, especially when few alternatives are within family caregivers' reach. The importance of individualizing services is especially salient, in particular in the eyes of family caregivers, who watch over their relatives' immediate quality of life and ensure that decisions are made in harmony with their relatives' known values, especially when cognitive impairment prevents clients themselves from affirming those values.

CASE MANAGEMENT AND THE PERCEPTION OF CONTINUITY. Interview analysis brought out three distinct groups based on the role played by the case manager. In the first group, the case manager had assumed full responsibility for negotiating with service providers and thereby freed up the family caregiver to a significant degree. In the second group, the family caregiver had retained an important role in negotiating with service providers and case management had come on the scene at a late stage. Last, in a single case, the dyad and the formal service providers were acting in parallel. In this single instance of parallel action, case management was not highly visible. Although management of this case had been initiated by a case manager, that person was subsequently replaced by a professional who had not been trained in case management. Our analysis did not turn up a significant health and social-services care provider, whether a case manager or other. Management of care occurred in constant reaction to the needs voiced by the caregiver-recipient dyad rather than unfolding proactively and preventing problems.

In the first group, case managers coordinate actively; they take ownership of most aspects of the dyad's problem. Most of our marker cases (seven out of twelve) fall into this group. In general, clients and family caregivers described a series of active interventions and a positive relationship with their case managers. The dyad members' main concern was to maintain the services they were receiving. Family caregivers also stressed the importance of adjusting services as soon as the client's frailty or the family caregiver's circumstances require it; they also spoke of the need to make service-delivery formulas (e.g., assistance with getting up and personal hygiene given at fixed times; bureaucratic obstacles) more flexible. Above all, they decried the difficulties presented by ongoing

Table 7.2

Client-Caregiver Dyad Members' Perceptions of Continuity in Relation to Case-Manager Interventions

GROUP 1: Case management characterized by active coordination for client-caregiver dyads

Interviewee	Marker Case Type	What Perceptions of Continuity Relate to	Stage Client is at*	CM's Profession	Focus of Intervention
Husband-caregiver aged 70 yrs	Cognitive disorders 69 yrs	Planning and adapting services as disease progresses Organizing CLSC services according to client needs and availability Caregiver agrees to delegate to case manager (trust)	Facing and of life	Pychologist	Protecting caregiver's health by contributing to coordinating and organizing
Husband-caregiver aged 74 yrs	Change in life setting 69 yrs	Intensity required in in-home services Relationship of trust and support with case manager; delegates some responsibilities	Facing end of life	Psycho-social professional	Protecting caregiver's health by contributing to procedural measures and coordination Moral support
Wife-caregiver aged 68 yrs	Cognitive disorders 70 yrs	Reassuring presence of case manager supports anxious caregiver Consistency and receptiveness of case manager: need for support in context of family tension	Facing end of life	Psycho-social professional	Advice and assistance to caregiver in regard to decision making Moral support and monitoring of caregiver's needs
Client and two sister-caregivers aged 68, 70 yrs	Stroke 66 yrs	Improvement in quality of life (especially social) makes it possible to continue living normally Better access to customized equipment	Coming to terms with the disease	Nurse	Protecting the client's health and safety Intense coordination of hospital, nursing, and medical services
Client and brother caregiver aged 83 yrs	Stroke 78 yrs	Receiving needed in-home services seven days a week in order to live at home Availability and reliability of public and private services essential Delegates certain coordination tasks – supported by case manager	Coming to terms with the disease	Psycho-social professional	Protecting brother's and sister's health and safety Coordinating all services

* Health-related stages experienced by the elderly: 1. Health maintenance 2. Recovery. 3. Coming to terms with disease. 4. Facing end of life (Tourigny, A. – PRISMA-Estrie).

Interviewee	Marker Case Type	What Perceptions of Continuity Relate to	Stage Client Is at*	CM's Profession	Focus of Intervention
Son-caregiver aged 44 yrs	Change in life setting 83 yrs	Major significance of quality of case manager's communications and follow-up (information on progression of the disease and its consequences) Emergency interventions giving rise to risk of break in continuity (e.g., family tensions, trust relationship, shared decision making)	Facing end of life	Psycho-social professional	Protecting client's safety Coordination related to change in life setting
Client and wife-caregiver aged 64 yrs	Stroke 84 yrs	Reliability of assistance personnel's assignment and skills Trust in case manager, turns to case manager willingly if problems arise If waiting time for services to be set up is excessive, caregiver exceeds her strength (injury) Need for case manager to ensure good logistics because of invasion of home by numerous care providers	Coming to terms with the disease	Psycho-social professional	Active coordination and numerous steps taken on behalf of the client and in order to protect the caregiver's health

GROUP 2: Case Management Characterized by Support to Client-Caregiver Dyads

Interviewee	Marker Case Type	What Perceptions of Continuity Relate to	Stage Client Is at*	CM's Profession	Focus of Intervention
Daughter-caregiver aged 53 yrs	Cognitive disorders 91 yrs	Knowing that trusted care providers will be there in case of need (responsiveness) Family caregiver's openness makes service continuity possible: individualized service supply, flexibility in timelines and timetables, etc.	Facing end of life	Psychosocial professional	Protecting the family caregiver, especially by being vigilant Respecting the family caregiver's wish to manage services herself
Son-caregiver aged 56 yrs	Cognitive disorders 94 yrs	Lack of access to assistance services on weekends, making respite care impossible Increase in assistance services according to circumstances (availability, flexibility) Family caregiver sees himself as a link in continuity: without his interventions, his mother would have been placed in a RLTCC years ago	Facing end of life	Psychologist	Client's safety Coordinating in-home assistance services Monitoring

Wife-caregiver aged 70 yrs	Change in life setting 74 yrs	Even though burned out, continues to coordinate everything on her own. Need for access to relevant information regarding programs and services, lack of which results in uncertainty and anxiety. Staffing stability and reliability of timetable for assistance services. Personnel's skill appreciated. Difficulty living with invasion of home by numerous care providers	Facing end of life	Nurse	Coordinating ISP services. Monitoring during placement waiting time
Sister-in-law aged 54 yrs	Cognitive disorders 65 yrs	Family caregiver takes responsibility for continuity but with difficulty. Family caregiver carries out all coordination tasks and asks little for herself. Requests by family caregiver on behalf of client (flexibility of timetabling and frequency of delivery of assistance services) not fulfilled – family caregiver falls ill. Case manager was replaced and trust has not developed with new one. Teaching needed on progression of the disease to support the family caregiver in her role	Facing end of life	Psychosocial professional	First case manager: Supporting family caregiver by listening and offering advice about strategies to use with client. Adjusting services when possible

* Health-related stages experienced by the elderly: 1. Health maintenance 2. Recovery 3. Coming to terms with disease. 4. Facing end of life

changes in assistance personnel. When conditions become more demanding or family caregivers feel overwhelmed by the scope of their responsibilities, case-management services must include support to the family caregiver. Where family caregivers are themselves frail, there is greater receptivity to the assistance that case managers suggest.

The second group of case-management interventions related to support for the family caregivers. These were observed in situations where home-support services had reached their limit, whether because the elderly individual needed an institutional setting or because death was near. In these instances, case management focused on monitoring pending institutional placement. All four clients in this group evidenced serious cognitive disorders and three family caregivers manifested pronounced burnout, even though they continued to meet their relatives' needs. Since they were accustomed to dealing directly with service providers—which they were familiar with from long experience—they sometimes preferred to use their own contacts rather than call on their case managers. It should be noted that the case managers had come on the scene late in these dyads' care trajectories. In such situations, it would appear that no alternatives can be found in the repertory of home-support services. The family caregiver is thus highly active, while the case manager's role is mainly to accompany. In some of the cases studied, the family caregiver displayed a clear ability to negotiate with the health and social services system. Yet however self-reliant caregivers may appear, case managers should still increase their vigilance, especially when the family caregiver is burned out, or trust between the dyad and the case manager is fragile or has not yet been developed.

Consideration of these two groups of clients yielded certain observations. First, the case-manager role is linked to the extent of client needs. At the threshold of the final stage of life, we observed less coordination, more actions taken to change life settings, and heightened vigilance so that the moment when it would be necessary to establish priority of access to a given service was not overlooked. In all these cases, cognitive disorders constituted the problem. In contrast, in the four cases of stroke, even though the development of frailty and environmental conditions mandated placement, if the person's need was to adjust and come to terms with her or his diseases or handicaps, the case manager maintained a coordinating role. As for continuity, this sample of individuals emphasized the importance of access, flexibility, service availability, and care personnel's reliability in terms of skills and timetable, so that clients could continue to live at home.

Another observation relates to the second group's perception of continuity as influenced in a fundamental way by disruptions of different kinds, for example in relationships, information flow, service intensity, and access to assistance programs. In these cases, the family caregivers shared the trait of not having delegated certain portions of their responsibility to the case manager and viewing themselves as an important link in the chain of service continuity for their relatives. They tended to take full responsibility on themselves.

Last, it was observed that case managers' professions did not play a systematic role in case assignment. Thus, a client with stroke might be followed by a psychosocial professional, while a client with cognitive disorders might have a nurse as case manager. In our sample, all three of the professions that case managers are drawn from were represented.

Discussion

In all cases, continuity was associated with the long-term or permanent nature of services that interviewees considered essential to the maintenance of a familiar and normal life situation. Given this, the services in question must be predictable. In dyad members' perceptions, continuity relates above all to the routine recurrence of daily assistance and the adjustment of services over time as the frailty progresses.

CASE-MANAGER ROLES AND CONTINUITY OF SERVICE. In some of our marker cases, case managers were replaced by care providers who had not received in-depth training for the role. The relative scarcity of trained case managers creates a problem in passing on the baton and entails the risk of breaks in continuity. Because of unforeseen developments and leaves, which inevitably necessitate replacements, it is hard to ensure the same care provider always deals with a given individual. In the long-term in-home services sector, the difficulties caused to the dyad by staff changes are especially significant and should be taken seriously in organizing services, since relational continuity contributes to the consistency and coherence of services (Reid et al., 2002). The specific features of the case manager's role that are associated with a proactive geriatric approach are not taken into account when replacements are made, and this in itself constitutes a break in continuity.

Our marker cases do not all display the same needs for service coordination or support to the client's close circle; and needs can change suddenly and oblige the case manager to find speedy, effective solutions. Factors that affect the scope of a case manager's interventions are: 1) the dyad's openness towards services; 2) the services' acceptability to the dyad (for example, as regards flexibility in methods of functioning and the stability and reliability of staff and timing); 3) insufficient service accessibility; 4) the ability of members of the close circle to take on the role of family caregiver and these individuals' limitations. The more limiting factors in a given case, the more demanding the case, because alternatives grow fewer. While the psychosocial interventions a case manager can offer are entirely necessary, they are subject to certain constraining factors, in particular the development of the relationship between the case manager and the caregiver-receiver dyad, which requires receptivity and a shared willingness to discuss matters related to the disease, placement, and end of life. In ISPs, attention to psychosocial needs is less in evidence than provision for concrete measures to find, negotiate, and access resources for keeping the client at home. We observed indications that psychosocial work is done but that clients do not recognize it as such because it is intertwined with the relationship itself. These interventions often affect the private areas of family life: the feelings, relationships, and events that family members experience, as well as unresolved or latent conflicts that tend to surface when important decisions have to be made.

DISTINCTIVE ASPECTS OF COGNITIVE DISORDER MARKER CASES. The cognitively impair require especially attentive monitoring, in particular those living alone or with a family caregiver who is burned out, because they tend to refuse services even though they face risks such as fire or hygiene-related and nutritional problems. Their resistance heightens the risk of disrupting their service plans. Moreover, the very symptoms of their disease prevent them from judging their circumstances appropriately, while those close to them tend to interpret their difficulties with memory and judgment as the normal accompaniment of aging. Not noticing the problem, they do not seek assistance. At the same time, the later in their decline these individuals are referred, the fewer the choices of resources available to implement, and this too is attended by the risk of a break in continuity. We observed that, besides needing to have their tangible needs for services and reassurance met, family caregivers must pass through certain stages as the client's disease and frailty progress. When these stages are not fully completed, difficulties arise, for instance, resistance to suggested solutions. Families need to adopt a position on possible approaches to take as chronic or degenerative diseases progress. Case managers must restore adequate information flow in order to help individuals progress through their present circumstances and prepare them for upcoming stages. This role should define case managers' interventions, given how closely situated they are to caregiver-receivers dyads' life settings. This form of continuity in intervention is compatible with management continuity as identified by Reid et al. (2002), who maintain that a coherent ISP contributes to all parties working towards the same goal.

In the cases studied, the case manager already had a limited range of services to offer because of Quebec's inadequate funding for home-support services. This range is even more limited for clients with moderate to serious cognitive impairment, because of such factors as the disease's lack of social acceptability, problems associated with the client's behavior, and the client's difficulty in adjusting to a setting other than home. Few programs exist that are adapted to the needs of such individuals, fewer still for those with serious impairment; yet these are the circumstances when family caregivers need such services the most. For caregiver-receiver dyads who are thus situated, the need is not just for someone to negotiate with service providers on their behalf. It is also necessary to negotiate with the clients and win their acceptance of services, staff, bathing, transfers, and so on. The experiences of our marker cases show that in cases of cognitive disorders, services to support clients in the community decrease just when needs intensify, because the system does not have sufficient resources of the kind demanding cases require. Several family caregivers expressed the fervent wish that services be adjusted at the point when frailty increases. But case managers do not have more services to offer and the status quo does not meet family needs. This dimension of the issue of continuity is not addressed in this form in the literature. It is exceptional, in that it concerns the goodness of fit between the level of need on one hand and the nature and intensity of services on the other, while also relating to the sensitivity of the system's timing, i.e., its ability to react at the right moment.

DISTINCTIVE ASPECTS OF STROKE MARKER CASES. In cases of stroke, once the more intense period of hospitalization and rehabilitation is over, the family caregiver is often observed to become the case manager's client on account of age, disease, or injury. Since stroke is sudden, in these cases caregiver-receiver dyads tend not to have much prior experience with home-support services. They thus display openness towards such services, knowing they will have a direct impact on quality of life and the ability to remain at home. In contrast to cases of cognitive disorder, these caregiver-receiver dyads themselves contribute to continuity of care. Their decision-making ability is fully present, and they express their wishes directly to their case manager and not via an intermediary. None of the stroke marker cases in our study considered transfer to an institution or a supervised setting desirable, even when their physical handicaps were pronounced. They wanted to preserve their independence and assume a share of the responsibility associated with obtaining services. They insisted on remaining informed and taking part in decisions relating to the services they received.

Through our research with caregiver-receiver dyads, we learned that their conception of continuity is strongly associated with their will and ability to remain at home rather than the service trajectory. We also discovered a previously unnoticed aspect of continuity that is more complex than others. This can be described as maintaining the fit between level of need and level of services over time. Until now, attention has largely and justifiably been focused on the risk of a break in continuity presented by the elderly person's passage from one service setting to another. Our marker cases told us that for them, an important aspect of continuity is their perception of the balance or correspondence between the caregiver-receiver dyad's needs and services. It would be useful for future research to explore this aspect as well as elders' lack of familiarity with psychosocial intervention.

Conclusion

The present role of the case manager is the forerunner of a new kind of intervention. It is one that psychosocial professionals are already attuned to, not just because their own professional role is defined to include following clients regardless of setting, but also because, in their fields, the responsibility for support tends to be shared by several service providers, which creates the need for consistency in responding to the caregiver-receiver dyad and for arbitration among all the service providers involved with a given individual. Ethically speaking, this arbitration process should reflect the needs and wishes of individuals and their families.

Notes

1. PRISMA–Estrie: A research program on integrating services for maintaining independence, which was implemented specifically in three Estrie territories that constituted an experimental zone.
2. In this article, we have made use of the concept of the caregiver-receiver dyad. It is defined as the frail elderly person under case management and that person's family caregiver, both of whom interact with service providers.

References

Bachrach, L.L. (1981). Continuity of care for chronic mental patients: A conceptual analysis. *American Journal of Psychiatry*, 138 (11), 1449-1456.

Bachrach, L.L. (1993). Continuity of care and approches to case management for long-term mentally ill patients. *Hospital and Community Psychiatry*, 44 (5), 465-468.

Biem J., Hadjistavropoulos H., Morgan D., Biem H.B., and Pong R.W. (2003). Breaks in continuity of care and the rural senior transferred for medical care under regionalisation. *International Journal of Integrated Care*, 3, 1-11, http://www.ijic.org.

Couturier, Y., and Carrier, S. (2006). L'appropriation par les acteurs professionnels de la gestion de cas. Fourth PRISMA Colloquium, Sherbrooke, Quebec, 24 May.

Clément, M., Aubé, D., Bolduc, N., Damasse, J., Beaucage, C., and Tremblay, M. (2003*). La continuité des soins auprès des personnes présentant un trouble concomitant de maladie mentale et de toxicomanie: responsabilité des usagers et perspective organisationnelle*. Report of a study funded by the Canadian Health Services Research Foundation and other partners.

Hébert R., Durand, P.J., Dubuc N., Tourigny A., and Groupe PRISMA. (2003). PRISMA: A new model of integrated service delivery for the frail older people in Canada. *International Journal of Integrated Care*, 3, 1-10, http://www.ijic.org.

Institute of Medicine. (1996). *Improving the Medicare Market—Adding Choice and Protections*. National Academy Press, Washington, 195-235.

Long, M.J. (2002). Case-management model or case manger type? That is the question. *Health Care Manager*, 20 (4), 53-65.

Noelker, L.S. (2002). Case management for caregivers. *Care Management Journal*, 3 (4), 199-204.

Penchansky, R., and Thomas, J.W. (1981). The concept of access: Definition and relationship to consumer satisfaction. *Medical Care*, 19 (2), 127-140.

Reid, R., Haggerty, J., and McKendry, R. (2002). *Dissiper la confusion: concepts et mesures de la continuité des soins*. Final report to the Canadian Health Services Research Foundation, Ottawa.

Sparbel, K., and Anderson, M.A. (2000). Integrated literature review of continuity of care: Part 1 - Conceptual issues. *Journal of Nursing Scholarship*, 32 (1), 17-24.

Shortell, S.M. (1976). Continuity of medical care: Conceptualization and measurement. *Medical Care*, 14, 377-391.

Shortell, S.M., Gillies, R.R., Anderson, D.A., Morgan Erickson, K., and Mitchell, J.B. (2000). *Remaking health care in America: The evolution of organized delivery systems*. Josscy-Bass, 2nd ed, San Francisco.

Starfield, B. (1998). *Primary care: Balancing health needs service and technology*. Oxford University Press, New York.

Wodarski, J.S., and Williams-Hayes, M.M. (2002). Utilizing case management to maintain the elderly in the community. *Journal of Gerontological Social Work*, 39 (4), 19-38.

Woodward, C. A., Abelson, J., Tedford, S., and Hutchison, B. (2004). What is important to continuity in home care? Perspectives of key stakeholders. *Social Science and Medicine* (58), 177-192.

Chapter 8
Family Physicians' Perceptions of the Integrated Services Network and Case Managers

Louis Voyer and Réjean Hébert

The problem

Over the past few years, an integrated network model called RISPA (Réseau intégré de services pour personnes âgées) has been implemented for delivering services to the elderly in Estrie. This model relies heavily on the role played by a new kind of health professional—the case manager—who is responsible for assessing the individual's needs, organizing services, and doing follow-up, among other things. The family physician is among the case manager's primary collaborators, because, besides being the patient's main medical caregiver, the family physician also provides access to specialized medical services. For an integrated services network to be efficient, therefore, family physicians must take an active part and collaborate closely with case managers. Above all, integrating the case manager role into medical practice requires that physicians subscribe to the integrated services model in general and case management in particular.

Objectives

A mail survey was conducted whose main objectives were to document the expectations of case management held by family physicians with elders among their patients at the start of RISPA's implementation (T1) and the physicians' experience of case management six months (T2) and three years (T3) later, at different stages of implementation. At T1, T2, and T3, implementation was at 22 %, 37 %, and 73 % respectively. Case managers came on the scene between T1 and T2.

Methodology

Study Population

The study population consisted of all the family physicians of the regional municipal counties (MRCs, "Municipalités régionales de comté") of Sherbrooke,

Granit, and Coaticook (n = 267). They were identified using the registry maintained by the Quebec health insurance plan (Régie de l'assurance maladie du Québec). Eligible physicians were in active practice and had elders among their patients.

The Instrument

Questionnaires on family physicians' perceptions of RISPA and case management were mailed out at each of the three study times. The first questionnaire, sent out at T1: 1) evaluated how physicians felt they would be affected by RISPA implementation; 2) assessed physician attitudes to the case-manager role and the physician's own potential role, given the new context; 3) included questions of a sociodemographic and socioprofessional nature; and 4) enabled physicians to freely express their opinions and concerns.

The second questionnaire, sent out at T2, targeted only physicians who had responded to the first and was designed to track the progress of their opinions. This questionnaire's first part was addressed to physicians who were aware that case management was already in place; its purpose was to document the frequency of physician—case manager contacts and physicians' opinions about case-manager work. The second section was addressed to all the respondents; its purpose was to identify the main obstacles to case management use and gather physicians' comments. The third questionnaire, sent out at T3, contained the same items as the T2 questionnaire.

Each questionnaire and mailed reminder was accompanied by a one-page explanatory letter. The three questionnaires were laid out following Dillman's "Tailored Design Method",[1] i.e., with a simple format, in this instance, a booklet and short questions grouped by response type. The majority of questions were closed-ended and dichotomous or Likert-scale. In all three questionnaires, statements in favor of case management alternated with unfavorable ones and respondents indicated their degree of agreement or disagreement with each statement (degrees of agreement consisted of "Strongly agree," "Agree," "Disagree," and "Strongly disagree"). The mailing of the questionnaire also followed Dillman's rules. Each mailing was individualized and contained a stamped, addressed reply envelope. A week after the questionnaire mailing, a reminder was sent to those who had not yet responded. Three weeks after the initial questionnaire mailing, a new personalized mailing, accompanied by another copy of the questionnaire, was sent to those who had still not responded.

We scored responses to our postal questionnaire for "positiveness of opinions about case management." The questionnaire contained 10 favorable and 6 unfavorable statements about case management. The respondent had 4 response choices, scored from 0 for "Strongly disagree" to 3 for "Strongly agree" for favorable statements and scored in the inverse direction for unfavorable ones. Total scores could range from 0 to 48. A high score represented a favorable view of case management. Using stepwise linear regression analysis, we identified the characteristics of physicians who were favorable to case management at the outset (T1) and three years into implementation (T3). For the regression analysis, we used the positiveness score as a dependent variable. The independent variables were sex, training type (multidisciplinary internship or family-medicine residency), number of years in practice, type of practice (solo or with no patient sharing as opposed to practice with patient sharing), number of hours worked per week, the MRC of practice, the percentage of the physician's patients consisting of elders, and the percentage of weekly hours spent in different practice settings (in private practice, in CLSCs, in residential facilities, with hospitalized patients, on house calls, in the emergency room, and so on). For T3 analysis, these four questions were added: "Have you discussed the possibility of recourse to case management with any of your patients?", "Have you heard about case managers through your patients?", "Have you referred at least one patient to a case manager?", "Has a case manager notified you that she or he was following one of your patients?" For the univariate tests, we set 0.15 as the maximum p-value for initial variables included in the stepwise regression analysis. For our final models, only variables with a beta coefficient significantly different from 0 were retained (p < 0.05). The threshold for statistical significance was 0.05.

Findings

Response Rate

At T1, the first questionnaire was sent out to 267 family physicians in 3 Estrie MRCs (237 in Sherbrooke, 10 in Coaticook, and 20 in Granit). Sixty-one physicians had no elders among their patients and were therefore excluded from follow-up. Of the 206 eligible family physicians, 124 responded, for a response rate of 60.2 %. When the second questionnaire was sent out at T2, three of the 124 physicians were no longer eligible and 17 did not respond, bringing the number of respondents down to 104. The response rate for the T2 questionnaire was 86 %. Detailed findings for T1 and T2 responses have been previously published.[2, 3] Finally, the 104 respondents were contacted again at T3, three years after [T1]. Three were no longer eligible and 14 did not respond, yielding a total of 87 respondents and a response rate of 86.1 % (see Figure 8.1).

Description of Respondents to T3 Questionnaire

Nearly 83 % of the respondents were from Sherbrooke. The majority were men (60.9 %) with over 21 years of practice (41.8 %) and who shared patient information (74.7 %). The majority of respondents (72.4 %) worked between 35 and 54 hours a week. Most of their consulting time was spent in private practice (50.1 %). Table 8.1 summarizes the characteristics of respondent physicians.

Figure 8.1
Response Rate for Three Study Times

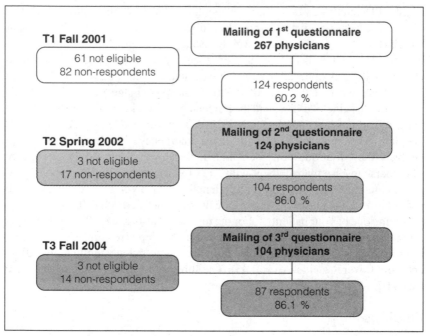

Elders account for 45.7 % of physician patients. Seventy-nine percent (79 %) of respondents had at least one patient under case management.

Responses to Mail Questionnaires

The family physicians targeted by this study were contacted before case managers came on the scene (T1) and statements on the T1 questionnaire were framed to assess physician <u>expectations</u> regarding case management (e.g., "In my opinion, case managers <u>will</u> play a role complementary to mine."). Six months (T2) and three years (T3) later, physicians were asked to present their <u>experience</u> with case managers (e.g., "Case-manager work <u>has complemented</u> mine."). Note however that the number of physicians who had had contact with case managers at T2 was limited.

Our findings from responses to the questionnaires are presented under five headings: 1) statements favorable to case management; 2) statements unfavorable to case management; 3) statements regarding the progress of case management in physician's practice; 4) characteristics of physicians who were favorable to case management; and 5) the main obstacles to case management use and suggestions for promoting it. Our findings are presented on a dichotomous response scale: we have grouped the "Agree" with the "Strongly agree" level and the "Disagree" with the "Strongly disagree" levels.

Table 8.1
Respondents' Sociodemographic Characteristics at T3 (n = 87).

Characteristics	Frequency (Percentage)
Sex	
Male	53 (60.9 %)
MRC	
Sherbrooke	72 (82.8 %)
Coaticook	6 (6.9 %)
Granit	9 (10.3 %)
Number of years in practice	
Less than 5	7 (8.1 %)
Between 5 and 10	11 (12.8 %)
Between 11 and 20	32 (37.2 %)
Between 21 and 30	34 (39.5 %)
More than 30	2 (2.3 %)
Type of practice	
Solo	17 (19.5 %)
No patient sharing	5 (5.7 %)
Patient sharing	65 (74.7 %)
Number of hours worked per week	
<25 heures	
25-34	2 (2.3 %)
35-44 h	6 (6.9 %)
45-54	38 (43.7 %)
55-64	25 (28.7 %)
>65	11 (12.6 %)
	5 (5.7 %)
Percentage of spent in different settings weekly	
Private practice consulting	50.06 %
CLSC consulting	9.97 %
Emergency room	6.50 %
Hospitalized patients	8.63 %
Residential facilities	8.82 %
House calls	6.77 %
Geriatrics	3.10 %
Research	1.61 %
Administration	1.66 %
Obstetrics	0.40 %
Public health	0.23 %
Other	2.25 %

Statements favorable to case management

Before implementation, physician expectations of case management were very high. At T1, physicians were hoping that case-manager work would complement their own (95.5 %), facilitate elder access to services (95.2 %), and facilitate their own work (95.1 %) and information gathering (94.7 %). The experience of case management after three years of implementation appears positive. Agreement levels for statements favorable to case management range from 47 % to 95.5 %. Thus, 47 % of physicians found that case-manager work had prevented needless hospitalizations and 95.5 % considered case-manager work to be complementary to their own. Nevertheless, although physicians' experience with case management was positive overall, it did not match the very high expectations observed at T1. Table 8.2 presents rates of agreement with the 10 statements favorable to case management.

Table 8.2

Comparison of Agreement with Favorable Statements before and after Case-Management Implementation

The work of case managers...	Strongly agree or agree		
	T1*	T3*	p-value**
...has complemented mine. (n = 67)	64 (95.5 %)	64 (95.5 %)	1
...has enabled the frail elderly to remain at home longer. (n = 61)	55 (90.2 %)	49 (80.3 %)	0.146
...has made it easier to access services for the elderly. (n = 63)	60 (95.2 %)	49 (80.3 %)	0.039
...has made my job easier. (n = 61)	58 (95.1 %)	45 (73.8 %)	0.001
...has helped with decision making when hospitalized patients returned home. (n = 59)	52 (88.1 %)	42 (71.2 %)	0.013
...has made it easier to collect information on new patients. (n = 57)	54 (94.7 %)	36 (63.2 %)	<0.001
...has helped reduce duplication of services. (n = 62)	54 (87.1 %)	43 (69.4 %)	0.027
...has reduced my administrative tasks. (n = 63)	42 (66.7 %)	34 (54.0 %)	0.134
...has avoided unnecessary hospitalizations. (n = 55)	44 (80.0 %)	26 (47.0 %)	<0.001
...has given me a better understanding of the living situations of my patients. (n = 66)	58 (87.9 %)	35 (53.0 %)	<0.001

* Frequency (percentage)
** McNemar test p-value.

4.3.2 Statements unfavorable to case management

A total of six statements discredited case management. Physician responses to these statements remained the same from study time to study time. Generally speaking, whether at the pre-implementation stage or three years into case management, few physicians agreed with the unfavorable statements. For example, at T3, only 10.6 % of family physicians agreed with statements that case managers made the physician's task more complicated or interfered in the patient-physician relationship. On the other hand, 54.1 % agreed with the statement that case-manager work should be done by nurse practitioners (Table 8.3). These rates of agreement are substantially the same as those observed at T2.

Table 8.3
**Comparison of Responses to Unfavorable Statements
before and after Case-Management Implementation**

Case-manager work...	Strongly agree or agree		
	T1*	T3*	p-value**
...has been and additional expense on the health care system. (n = 64)	27 (42.2 %)	22 (34.4 %)	0.405
...should have been done by nurse clinicians who deliver care directly to patients in addition to coordinating their services (n = 61)	34 (55.7 %)	33 (54.1 %)	1
...has not been very effective because resources are very limited in my area. (n = 62)	11 (17.7 %)	12 (19.4 %)	1
...has made the existing health care system more cumbersome. (n = 65)	14 (21.5 %)	9 (13.8 %)	0.227
...has interfered in my patient-physician relationships. (n = 66)	12 (18.2 %)	7 (10.6 %)	0.227
...has made my job more complicated. (n = 66)	15 (22.7 %)	7 (10.6 %)	0.057

* Rate (Percentage)
** McNemar test p-value.

The progress of case management in physician practice

Table 8.4 gives a good picture of the progress of case management 6 months and 3 years into implementation. At T3, 64.6 % of physicians stated they had discussed the possibility of recourse to case management with some of their patients. This contrasted with 39.7 % at T2. The average number of patients referred to a case manager rose, going from 3.1 to 5.2. The percentage of physicians who stated that had heard of case management from their own patients rose from 24.7 % at T2 to 61 % at T3. Moreover, at T3, nearly 80 % of physicians had been told a case manager was following at least one of their patients, whereas at T2 the percentage had been 60.3 %. The average number of such patients rose from 2.81 at T2 to 4.27 at T3.

Table 8.4
Progress of Case Management between Six Months and Three Years Following Implementation

Statement	T2	T3
Have you discussed the possibility of recourse to case management with any of your patients?	Yes: 29/73 (39.7 %)	Yes: 53/82 (64.6 %)
Have you heard about case management through your patients?	Yes: 18/73 (24,.7 %)	Yes: 50/82 (61.0 %)
Have you referred at least one of your patients to a case manager? If so, how many?	Yes: 26/70 (35.6 %) 3,1 patients (3.9)*	Yes: 43/82 (52.4 %) 5,2 patients (5.0)*
Has a case manager notified you she or he was following one of your patients? If yes, for how many patients is this so?	Yes: 44/73 (60.3 %) 2,81patients (2.49)	Yes: 65/83 (78.3 %) 4,27 patients (3.21)

* Mean (standard deviation)

Characteristics of physicians favorable to case management

We compared scores for the physicians' positiveness towards case management before implementation (T1) and 3 years into implementation (T3). Table 8.5 shows that physicians had a higher positiveness score before implementation than after 3 years.

Table 8.5
Comparison of Scores for T1 and T3 (n = 67)

	T1	T3	
	Mean (standard deviation)	Mean (standard deviation)	p-value*
Positiveness score	32.11 (7.25)	30.11 (7.88)	p = 0.038

* Paired t-test p-value

Using the positiveness score, we performed two stepwise linear regression analyses to identify the characteristics of physicians favorable to case management at the outset (T1) and three years into implementation (T3). The variables were those specified above in the "Methodology" section. The first analysis identified the characteristics of the physicians who were the most favorable to case management before RISPA implementation (T1). Univariate tests were performed for each independent variable; the p-value for a variable's inclusion in the initial regression model was 0.15. The variables selected are presented in Table 8.6. The wording in parentheses indicates what feature of a variable is associated with a high positiveness score.

Tableau 8.6
Variables Selected for Stepwise Regression Analysis for T1

Variable	p-value
Training (Family-practice residency)	p=0.060 *
Type of practice (Patient sharing)	p=0.009 *
Percentage of time spent in private practice (High)	p=0.139 **
Percentage of time spent in CLSC (High)	p=0.009 **
Percentage of time with hospitalized patients (High)	p=0.094 **
MRC of practice (Sherbrooke and Coaticook)	p=0.006 ***

* t-test p-value
** correlation test p-value
*** ANOVA p-value

The practice-type and MRC variables were closely linked; physicians in Granit do not share patients, they work solo. We therefore withdrew the MRC variable. Of the five that remained, two were retained by means of the automated stepwise procedure. Table 8.7 presents the final model for this analysis.

Table 8.7
Final Model of Stepwise Regression Procedure for T1

Variable	Beta coefficient	p-value
Percentage of time spent in CLSC (High)	0.189	p=0.039
Type of practice (Patient sharing)	0.186	p=0.042

Physicians who <u>were most favorable to case management before RISPA implementation</u> were more likely to practice in a CLSC (p = 0.039) and have a practice with patient sharing (p = 0.042). These two variables account for 8.9 % of variance.

The variables initially selected for the linear regression analysis of factors associated with positiveness towards the integrated network and case management at three years, i.e., at T3, are presented in Table 8.8.

Table 8.8
Variables Selected for Stepwise Regression Analysis for T3

Variable	p-value
Number of years in practice (High)	p=0.067 *
Percentage of time spent in CLSC (High)	p=0.001*
Percentage of time spent in emergency room (High)	p=0.094*
Question: Have you discussed the possibility of recourse to case management with any of your patients? (Yes)	p=0.014**
Question: Have you heard about case management through your patients? (Yes)	p=0.041**
Question: Have you referred at least one of your patients to a case manager? (Yes)	p=0.017**

* t-test p-value
** correlation test p-value

Three of these variables were retained by the automated stepwise procedure. Table 8.9 presents the final model.

Table 8.9
Final Model of Stepwise Regression Procedure for T3.

Variable	Beta coefficient	p-value
Percentage of time spent in CLSC (High)	0.138	p<0.001
Question: Have you discussed the possibility of recourse to case management with any of your patients? (Yes)	6.452	p=0.004
Number of years in practice (High)	1.883	p=0.04

Regression analysis indicated that three years into implementation, the family physicians who were most favorable to case management: 1) tended to practice in CLSCs (p < 0.001); 2) had discussed the possibility of recourse to case management with some of their patients (p = 0.004); and 3) had been practicing medicine for many years (p = 0.040). The first variable accounts for 15.5 % of variance; adding the second variable raises the figure to 27.1 %; and last, the three variables together account for 32.1 % of variance.

Main obstacles to recourse to case management and suggestions for promoting it

All the physicians who responded to the study, whether or not they had patients under case management, were able to state what might influence their recourse to it. At both T2 and T3, the main obstacles to recourse were forgetting to make use of case management (71.6 % at T2 and 69.1 % at T3), followed by the reflex of turning to CLSC or hospital social workers (63.3 % at T2 and 60.8 % at T3). It is worth noting, however, that some obstacles became less prominent between T2 and T3, indicating greater familiarity with case management. As may be seen in Table 8.10, there is a significant difference between T2 and T3 for the statements "I do not know how to contact case managers," "I do not yet clearly understand how case managers can help my patients," and "I was not aware this service was available to me."

Table 8.10
**Main Obstacles to Recourse to Case Management:
Comparison of T2 with T3 (n = 81)**

Obstacles to recourse to case management are that...	Strongly agree or agree		
	T2	T3	p-value*
...I forget to use them. (n = 81)	58 (71.6 %)	56 (69.1 %)	0.832
...I use social workers from a local community service centre (CLSC) or hospital rather than calling a case manager. (n = 83)	50 (63.3 %)	48 (60.8 %)	0.860
...I don't know how to contact them. (n = 84).	47 (58.0 %)	29 (35.8 %)	0.001
...I look after coordinating and nego- tiating my patients' services myself. (n = 82)	45 (57.7 %)	39 (50.0 %)	0.263
...I still don't really understand how case managers can help my patients. (n – 84)	43 (52.4 %)	30 (36.6 %)	0.015
...I don't know which of my clients could benefit from case management. (n = 85)	32 (38.1 %)	32 (38.1 %)	1.000
...I need nurse clinicians, not case managers. (n = 77)	27 (37.0 %)	27 (37.0 %)	1.000
...I didn't know this service was availa- ble. (n = 83)	25 (30.9 %)	8 (9.9 %)	0.001

* McNemar test p-value.

Family physicians suggested solutions for promoting recourse to case management. They appear to want: 1) to know more about case management and how to make it operational (they want to get to know case managers, their availability, the instruments they use, their services, and criteria for patient eligibility for case management); 2) better transmission of clinical information (the computerized clinical chart for the elderly known as SIGG [Système d'information géronto-gériatrique]); 3) for the relevant authorities to see that services to the elderly are increased and new case managers are hired; 4) standardized training for case managers. On this last point, the gerontology training centre (Centre universitaire de formation en gerontology) at Université de Sherbrooke has set up a microprogram in case management for health professionals.

Discussion

Although physicians' expectations of RISPA and case management started out very high, their experience on the ground was very positive on the whole. Physicians are growing more familiar with case managers' services and turning to them. They speak about case managers to their patients and make referrals; they hear about case managers from their patients; and they are notified by case managers about patients of theirs under case management.

Regression analysis identified the characteristics of physicians that best account for the variability in our questionnaire. At the start of implementation (T1), physicians who were the most favorable to case management tended to practice in CLSCs and to have practices with patient sharing. Three years into implementation (T3), the physicians most favorable to case management tended to practice in CLSCs, had discussed the possibility of recourse to case management with some of their patients, and had been practicing medicine for seven years. As well, we found that exposure to case management was a factor in favor of greater recourse to it. The obstacles to familiarity with case management and case managers' roles decreased over time and with recourse. Suggestions for practical solutions to enhance recourse to case managers' services testify to physicians' interest in cooperating with this new kind of professional.

References

1. Dillman, D.A. (2000). Mail and Internet Surveys: The Tailored Design Method.

2. Millette, L., Hébert, R., and Veil, A. (2004). Perceptions des omnipraticiens en regard de l'implantation des réseaux intégrés de soins et services pour personnes âgées (pp. 135-151). In R. Hébert, A. Tourigny, and M. Gagnon (Eds.), *Intégrer les services pour le maintien de l'autonomie des personnes*, Edisem.

3. Millette, L., Hébert, R., and Veil, A. (2005). Integrated service delivery networks for seniors – early perceptions of family physicians. *Canadian Family Physician* journal, 51(8), 1104-1105.

Chapter 9
The Individualized Service Plan as a Clinical Integration Tool: Qualitative Analysis in the Quebec PRISMA Experiment

Dominique Somme, Réjean Hébert, Gina Bravo, François Blanchard, and Olivier Saint-Jean

Introduction

A number of recent literature reviews emphasize the pivotal role played by case management in the efficacy of integration experiences for the elderly around the world[1-3]. The case-management process can be defined as comprising the following key steps[4-14]: case identification according to predefined criteria, standardized multidimensional assessment, individualized service plan, resource identification, implementation, monitoring, and plan reassessment. Some include the concept of advocacy, which combines advice and representation[10, 13, 15]. While case management was being developed, it became apparent that tools were needed to support the tasks of identification, assessment, and planning. To a great extent, case identification depends on the eligibility criteria for case management. As a result, the tools used in the various experience have been quite variable in nature. The assessment task led to the development of many different tools, such as the *Outil d'évaluation multiclientèles* (OEMC or multiclientele assessment tool), including the *Système de mesure de l'autonomie fonctionnelle* (SMAF or functional autonomy measurement system) in Quebec and the Resident Assessment Instrument (RAI) in the United States and then Europe. A scientific validation process applies to all of them[16, 17]. On the contrary, the planning task, which appears to be essential since it governs implementation, monitoring, and reassessment, hasn't received the same kind of attention. Yet many authors view the formulation of an individualized service plan (ISP) as an essential component in integrating services to the elderly with a loss of independence[1, 4]. For some, it represents a case-management quality criteria[12, 18]. As with assessment, the plan is both a set of processes and a product in the form of a written document placed in the person's file. To our knowledge, no planning document has ever been validated scientifically. Consequently, the tools used for planning usually derive from that used for assessment. In Quebec, the definition of ISP used by the *Ministère de la Santé et des Services Sociaux* (MSSS) refers to the process designed to achieve social integration and to provide an individualized response to the person's needs. It requires that the person or the person's representative attend a meeting targeting cooperation and collaboration[9]. This definition, like others around the world[1, 12, 14, 18] based on major consensual principles, does not, however, explicitly state how the ISP leads to clinical integration and how important developing the ISP document is to integration. This is also observed in the literature: while the ISP is often cited as an important feature of integration, its design, expected content, size, usefulness, and use are not defined[9]. The PRISMA integration experiment, in which case managers were asked to develop ISPs, enabled us to clarify these ISP aspects using qualitative methods.

Methodology

The PRISMA Program

PRISMA (Program of Research on the Integration of Services for the Maintenance of Autonomy)[4] is an integration model implemented in three experimental territories. The research program comprised, on the one hand, a study of the impact integration has on independence, satisfaction, and use of services for the elderly in experimental areas compared to the control areas and, on the other, ongoing monitoring of the model's effective implementation[19]. This program proposes a coordination-type approach to the integration model as defined by Leutz[20]. In this kind of model, all health and social-services organizations are involved, whether public, private, volunteer, or community. Each organization maintains its structure but takes part in integration by adapting its operations and resources. The outcome is that the individual no longer has to search for the proper resource for his or her needs. Rather, it is up to the integrated system to provide a continuum of services that respond to the needs of people. The PRISMA model, designed after reviewing the literature, comprises six components: 1) coordination at all levels of decision-making, 2) a single entry point, 3) case management, 4) individualized service plans, 5) a unique standardized assessment tool, and 6) a computerized clinical chart. Each of these points have been described in detail elsewhere[4, 19]. There are different case-management models[9]. In the PRISMA model, case managers (CMs) were under the responsibility of and remunerated by Quebec's public health care and services system. Each CM had to manage about 45 people. Individual eligibility corresponded to a high need for coordination given the number of caregivers and providers (greater than two, in addition to the attending physician and meal provision) or the degree of loss of independence measured with a standardized assessment instrument referred to as the SMAF (need for assistance exceeding that provided for domestic needs). CMs had to have or perform a comprehensive assessment of the individuals' needs. They had to be in close contact with patients and especially be familiar with their home settings. In interacting with patients, their circles, and attending physicians, CMs had to develop an ISP resulting from a cooperative interdisciplinary process with the various caregivers and providers. Afterwards, they were responsible for the follow-up and reassessment of the plan over time, thereby guaranteeing the diachronic continuity of management. In the PRISMA model, therefore, the ISP represented one of the key elements in effectively implementing integration on the clinical level. Since electronic medical records were gradually introduced[19], CMs soon had an electronic version of the same form. No databases (needs or services) were associated with the ISPs. No tasks were automated and the text was written in free text on paper or electronically.

Analysis Methods

Our analysis of the individualized service plan fits into the framework of cognitive ergonomics[21] in which the research objective lies in the discrepancies between what is prescribed, said, and done. The prescribed task (CMs have to develop ISPs in order to achieve clinical integration) was assessed with respect to the task actually performed (ISP production and use) and what the CMs had to say about it (which refers both to knowledge about the task prescribed and performed, and their expectations). The discrepancies between the task prescribed and performed, and what the CMs had to say are not treated here as deficiencies. Indeed, as was just said, knowledge about the necessity of ISPs for integration was vague. Accordingly, we will discuss these discrepancies as a source of information about the work carried out by the CMs related to ISPs and as a source of potential information about the very usefulness of the ISP with respect to integration.

For this study, we used a sequential schema with multiple investigative methods in order to achieve a certain level of triangulation. The research team that examines methods and interview grids was comprised of researchers in the area of health services and the social sciences. A number of professions were represented, including physicians, social workers, and psychologists.

Our analysis of the implementation context focused on the documentation used for CM training, to which we had complete access. This material was analyzed for information that would yield the most precise description of the "prescribed" task of developing the ISP, its expected contents, and its practical use. As a result, we attempted to identify the rules contained in these documents that CMs were supposed to follow to develop an ISP.

Interviews

The criteria for including CMs in the qualitative interview study about what the CMs "said" about the ISP are provided below.

• Participation in the PRISMA program
• Having a minimum caseload of five
• Having been a CM for at least 6 months
• Having signed an informed consent form for taking part in the study

All the CMs meeting these criteria were invited to take part. No CMs refused to participate.

The interview plan was developed through multidisciplinary cooperation. It was based on the theoretical framework of cognitive ergonomics and a literature survey[9]. The following issues were dealt with:

• In order to deal with CM knowledge about ISPs (that is, CM representation of the "prescribed task":
  • ISP usefulness and function(s) relative to CM work
• In order to deal with the ISP "activity" in the work of CMs from the perspective of "what is said":
  • Time-related aspects of the ISP in CM work
  • Factors fostering or hindering ISP formulation development
  • Distribution of the instrument to other system professionals

The interview plan enabled interviewers to systematically deal with the various issues and to bring out further information, if necessary. CMs could also bring up points of interest outside of the plan as long as the interview remained focused on the ISP as a CM tool. All the interviews were carried out face-to-face at the CMs' workplaces by the same person and recorded without intermediate analysis or modification of the interview plan prior to being transcribed verbatim.

Each interview was coded from a double point of view: descending, that is, starting with the interview plan described above, for the most unequivocal coding possible; and ascending, that is, starting with analysis of interview content outside of the plan in order to add value to the analysis plan while maintaining an ergonomic approach. The interviews were all coded by the same individual without cross coding. A preliminary grouping of the codes emerging from the ascending approach was made. The grouping was discussed by the multidisciplinary team and modified so as to have an adequately stable theoretical framework for analyzing the interviews. This made it possible to code the entire corpus of interviews a second time. The second encoding revealed that the first-round codes were quite stable. The codes that came up during the process served mainly to encode passages that hadn't been during the first round. Data organization and encoding was facilitated by using NVivo® software (QSR International), which can be used to encode, assign multiple codes, and reorganize the corpus according to code or category.

Record Analysis

We analyzed the contents of the 50 records managed by the 13 CMs in order to come up with a description of the task carried out. Records were selected randomly except for ensuring that there were at least two records from each CM interviewed. The drafting date had to be as close as possible without exceeding the start date of our study of ISPs, which the CMs were aware of. The elements that we looked for in the CM records were defined by the multidisciplinary team, after the "prescribed" was analyzed at a time close to when the interviews were conducted in order to grasp the significance of the ISP as a tool. As for the ISP itself, we used the date the ISP was written compared to the case-management starting date (date on which the CM signed the consent to exchange information). We attempted to determine the ISP's readability in terms of the number of lines and the various kinds of information it contained. The ISP form is structured as a series of columns (Appendix 1); the lines (rows) depend on how the CMs fill it out. As a result, a single line may contain a number of problems, objectives, and interventions and, therefore, involve a number of caregivers and frequencies. The analysis took into account the fact that the rows on the electronic ISP form are predetermined. In the case of paper forms, the numbering along the left-hand side used by certain CMs or a skipped line was considered as separators for the purpose of analysis. With the electronic ISPs, we were able to determine the number of consultations and the professional categories of the individuals with access to ISPs. We also attempted to determine to what degree the CMs followed the development rules that we identified based on our analysis of the training documentation. We also carried out a qualitative study of the vocabulary used in the ISPs by certain key caregivers, such as general practitioners and case managers. Lastly, we examined the records for indications of individualized planning (progress notes, conclusion of the standardized CM assessment).

ISP–Assessment Comparison

The assessment instrument used in Quebec is the Multiclientele Assessment Tool (MCAT), which includes 25 dimensions assessed as to whether or not the patient was experiencing a problem (or if means were used to compensate for the difficulty) (Appendix 2). functional autonomy was assessed with the SMAF[22], which examines 29 dimensions of independence based on whether the does or does not have a disability and, if so, whether it appears as a handicap (Appendix 3). Both types of items therefore make it possible to identify difficulties and often many of the resources that respond to these difficulties at the time of assessment. We therefore compared the contents of each ISP with that of the most recent standardized assessment in order to determine how well the ISP corresponded to the summary of all the problems arising in the assessment (with or without solution), and if the ISP contained all the resources cited in the assessment as compensating for the person's handicap or difficulty. If so, the ISP could be viewed as a portrait of the person's services, even if they didn't respond to all of the needs.

Results

Contextual Analysis (the "prescribed")

No ISP documents were created when the integrated networks were implemented. Indeed, the forms serving for planning home support services, called the "individual service allocation plan" (Appendix 1), were used. This document was designed at the same time as the Multiclientele Assessment Tool to provide for planning professional services. Evolving out of similar documents in nursing, it had already been used as a guide in multidisciplinary team work well before the creation of integrated networks. On the other hand, it was not designed for higher-level coordination (that is, of more than one group of professionals).

The training documents whose contents are analyzed here were prepared for regional use (regional board). Document 1 had a regional scope (November 2001). Documents 2 (2001) and 3 (2003) were developed specifically to train CMs at a single site. Document 4 (1999) is not training material, but rather a collection of general objectives providing a framework for training delivered to CMs in 2001. All of these documents have an indirect or direct connection to the book by D. Boisvert on the individualized service plan[23]. Two of the four documents cite Boisvert's work as their prime reference (documents 2 and 3). The reference cited by the other two was a 1992 document from the department that was also based on Boisvert's book (documents 1 and 4)[23]. Moreover, document 1 used the same order of steps in ISP development as Boisvert's book. The ISP definitions given in all four documents refer to a "process." None of the documents dealt with the opportunities and means that a CM can or must use in his or her work. These documents give prominence to major consensual values (such as fairness, justice, equality, solidarity, social integration, and primacy of the individual), whose definitions constituted part of the training (documents 1 and 2). Two documents stressed the importance of organizing the multidisciplinary meeting (as in Boisvert's book[23]). Two documents gave specific rules for drafting the *Problem* section (documents 1 and 3). The form proposed in document 4 gives the impression that each ISP focused on treating a single problem per client. As for the *Objective* section, the rule was to record observable or measurable behaviors with a threshold and an observation delay (documents 1 and 3); action verbs had to be used (documents 2 and 3). Document 3 included a four-page list of verbs to use as help in drafting the objective. Moreover, it was indicated that instructional verbs (maintain, reduce, promote, improve, etc.) should be avoided (document 3). No specific training was provided about the other sections on the form. The changing nature of needs and services was not dealt with. ISP use by network members was not explained. The written comments of the people who received training in Sherbrooke—which were kept—revealed dissatisfaction related to the ISP, although the overall training was deemed very satisfactory. They felt that the ISP training was too theoretical: "How do you adapt a tool made for planning services over the medium and long term to a clientele whose health and needs change rapidly?" or "Why does someone in the network still not use an ISP after several years of training and awareness?"

Interviews: What Was Said

When it comes to using the ISP, CMs indicated that it usually comes after planning, since the ISP is described as the last step in a record that has achieved a certain level of stability (*"The ISP is the final act.... That's how I see it, once I have all the information I require...." CM 5*). (*"I don't put anything into the ISP until the client's situation has stabilized. Once the client is set up, I use the ISP." CM 3*). We should point out that 12 out of the 13 CMs made the same kind of comments. The remaining one said that he didn't use the ISP at all (*"It's a step that I often skip...because it just doesn't seem useful to me...it's just one more step if you have to write up the intervention plan or ISP." CM 12*).

Moreover, the CMs cited motives for producing the ISP that reinforced the impression of it being an administrative task. Indeed, CMs stated that: *"It's one of our tasks. We knew when we were hired...that it had to be done" (CM 5)* or *"One goes into every file." (CM 3)* or *"Well, there is an ISP, but it hasn't been finished.... I'm going to update it because I have to submit it to the allocation committee next week."(CM 6)*. Nine CMs mentioned the nature prescribed by case management as motivation for developing the ISP. Some people perceived that the research program itself had an influence: *"If I hadn't read the research now, I'm not sure that there would be ISPs in the records" (CM 1)*. Five CMs mentioned the research protocol either directly or indirectly by referring to the PRISMA model as a motivation for developing the ISP.

The CMs were not in agreement among themselves about the expected contents of an ISP (*"I put down all services." CM 10*); (*"No, I didn't put down everything, and I won't in the future." CM 8*); (*"Every handicap and disability must be included in the ISP." CM 5*). It is interesting to point out that the highly elaborate ISPs did not always conform to the expressed intentions. Consequently, CM 5 only managed to follow his rule of mentioning all needs in 2 out of the 12 ISPs analyzed, while CM 8 complied with the same rule in 3 cases out of 4.

The CMs were concerned by the fact that few people in the network appear to want to read ISPs. CM 8, whose ISPs have the highest average access rate (average of 3 in addition to the CM), stated: *"I've already looked at the history. Not too many people are going to do that."* The CMs also took different positions about the usefulness of the ISP for the CM (*"The first thing I do...is to see what's in the plan." CM 12*); (*"Sometimes, I'll look at the file, but rarely the ISP." CM 1*). Plan access could serve CMs as reminders of the services in place, the steps already taken, or as help in managing schedules. Given that the ISP aims at determining an individual's needs and planning the services to respond to them, it's paradoxical that the only clinical motivation cited by two CMs were related to limiting services for people who are deemed overly demanding (*"The ISPs for manipulative people...contain tons of details...because they tend to always ask for more." CM 7*).

The ISP has been described as an element fostering multidisciplinary-team joint action. With the exception of the latter function, the others could be replaced by reviewing some progress notes or concluding the assessment without an ISP. Consequently, no functions related to CM clinical work appeared to specifically devolve to the ISP.

All the CMs presented the ISP as being very strongly related to their work: (*"It's THE case manager's tool." CM 11*). No CMs raised the idea of case management without an ISP. On the contrary, the difficulties encountered were explained by the innovativeness of integration (*"An integrated network...and case management are new." CM 7*); lack of partner computer access (*"The system...must be accessible elsewhere." CM 7*); lack of definition of confidentiality rules (*"I tell myself to be careful not to put too much into the ISP, because the information can be shared." CM 13*). They also emphasized a lack of clarity about the concept (*"No one has a clear idea of what the ISP is all about." CM 7*). Four CMs had highly similar perceptions: *"Everything goes into our ISPs today, like disciplinary intervention plans and service plans. Everything is thrown together." (CM 10)*. CMs also pointed out the lack of training or, more exactly, the inappropriateness of training: (*"I don't think they were clear enough about ISP contents." CM 13*).

CMs felt that the form used for ISPs had problems, specifically its lack of clarity (*"It's clear to me, but I don't think it is for the others." CM 5*); its static appearance (*"You know that you can't exchange with an ISP. An ISP doesn't budge." CM 9*); and the burden of writing (*"I often wrack my head trying to write the objective." CM 9*). The clash of these expectations with reality resulted in uneasiness among CMs: *"My own plans bother me sometimes...but I don't know what else to do." (GC 10)*. There were, in fact, many expectations and they concerned, in particular, the concept itself (*"What use is it? Why are we doing this? What should it contain?" CM 10*); training (*"I think that training on this is needed." CM 10*); and form simplification (*"I think that ISPs should be easy to develop." CM 1*).

File Analysis

Our analysis involved all of the ISPs (n=101) in the 50 files. The average time between the start of management and the first ISP varied greatly: 0 to 598 days for the 50 ISPs. The average lapse was relatively high (117 d). There was also variability in CM attitude regarding ISPs because the averages varied from 11 to 308 d, depending on the CM. Yet the CMs themselves were not consistent with ISP production, except for two who appeared to try to do the ISP within the first 30 days. These two CMs, who worked at the same location, had been instructed by their superior that the files had to conform to the integration model (therefore, containing an ISP). Another CM at the same site, however, turned in an average production time for the first ISP of 71 d from the start of case management (ranging from 0 to 267 d). The time lapse between assessment and ISP production was similarly variable: 0 to 524 d, for an average of 68 d, with 2 averages falling between 5 and 250 d, depending on the CM. Lastly, the lapse between assessment and ISP production shortened: 138 d in 2001–2002 and 39 d in 2003.

The average number of lines in the ISP averaged 5.5, although the variability was high (1 to 19). In addition, several issues were often put on the same line, since the average number of issues was 7.1, varying from 1 to 20. The complexity of reading the ISP increased in the Objective column, which contained an average of 6.9 objectives per ISP. It was even more so with the number of interventions (average of 10.6, ranging from 2 to 33) not directly related to the number of caregivers, since many interventions were performed by the same caregiver. To illustrate, in ISP 2, File 47, the visiting homemaker carried out the following: *Help with hygiene, help with clipping nails, meal preparation, support with home maintenance, and grocery shopping.* In contrast, several caregivers had to provide the same intervention (e.g., ISP 2, File 38: 7 caregivers provided spouse respite: the day care center, the temporary placement center, two social workers from these organizations, the case manager, a community organization, and a private resource).

The access count for the 77 electronic ISPs ranged from 0 to 30 (an average of 11 times in the 6 months following ISP drafting). CMs accounted for the large majority (91 %) of ISP accesses, specifically the writer in 70 % of cases. For the remaining 9 %, administrative purposes were the reason for at least 5 instances of access: program managers (n=2) and archivists (n=3). Access by other caregivers within the assistance system was rare. ISPs were mailed to the concerned family physicians in 27 cases out of 101. No other recipients were mentioned in the file.

No specific guideline was followed in writing up problems or needs; the recommended structure was never used. None of the 699 objectives appearing in the ISPs could be considered as observable or measurable behaviors with a threshold and observation delay, as presented during training. In contrast, 80.7 % of the objectives corresponded to directions for actions continuing over time expressed with verbs that were supposed to be avoided (compensate, improve, maintain, monitor, learn, etc.). The family physician (FP) was mentioned in 73 of the 101 ISPs. Since the document is structured so that the caregiver is mentioned depending on the problems identified, the FP sometimes repeatedly appeared in the same ISP. It is also possible that he was not the only caregiver cited on a single line for problem. As a result, we analyzed such ISPs on a per-line basis. When mentioned on an ISP line, the problems that the FP should be able to resolve were health issues in 58 cases out of 80, loss of independence in 17 cases, and psychosocial disorders in 5 cases. The objectives were often quite vague, related to the medical profession in a general way (*"Provide medical management," "Maintain state of health"* and *"The patient will have the required medication and care"*). More specific objectives were used much more rarely (*"Reduce the micturitional frequency and redness associated with incontinence"*).

We also studied the ISP lines in which the CM was mentioned as caregiver. There were often multiple problems, possibly of different types, but mainly psychosocial and related to the loss of independence, such as *"Precarious recovery of fractures"* or *"Needs help in managing appointments and contacts with the system."* Moreover, we also noted that the objective was very often a fairly general description of the CM's function: *"Enable service use and reduce management burden," "The patient will have advice enabling him to live in his home as long as possible," "Maintain a presence and be supportive, while providing support to the natural caregiver."* A more individualized description of the task was rarely encountered. It is interesting to note, however, that, when it occurred, the objective was always health related and did not always correspond to the CM's previous profession: *"Avoid increasing pain, avoid falls or increased pain during bathing"* (CM was initially a nurse); *"Investigate incontinence and identify adequate compensation"* (CM was initially a psychologist); *"Ensure that the patient has adequate dietary intake (no weight loss), monitor problem with constipation"* (CM was initially a social worker). Frequency was stated in the form of *"as needed,"* without describing the process for detecting the need recurrence in 37.5 % of cases. As a result, this didn't make it possible to have an accurate schedule for delivery or the actual frequency of service.

The qualitative analysis of the files highlighted the fact that individualized planning indeed existed but was not supported by the ISP, which means that it provided only partial representation. Indications that individualized planning actually occurred appear in the progress notes (*"Contact with family physician reveals that pain-clinic physicians did not recommend infiltration and suggested morphine...He is in agreement with swimming and the day care center..."*). Assessment conclusions also appeared (*"As for housekeeping, Mr. X refused system help; he will ask his family to play a greater role.... He accepts help with grooming and some financial aid to purchase these services."*).

ISP-Assessment Comparison

Three ISPs were written with no trace of a previous or current assessment; 7 were written after a limited assessment to determine loss of autonomy. It was therefore possible to compare ISP and assessment data in nearly all of the cases. The comparison of ISP and multiclientele assessment data highlighted that the ISPs as a whole did not inventory people's problems (Table 9.1) or the services they used (Table 9.2). The problems most often missing from the ISPs related to health; the services most often omitted were nonprofessional in nature. We attempted to find out if CMs adhered to the same writing logic from one ISP to the next. Based on our analysis of the ISPs (Tables 9.1 and 9.2), two types of logic might have been used: the CM either closely followed a comprehensive list of needs or of all needs except those directly related to professional health services or the CM closely followed a list of all services or all professional services. We therefore classified ISPs based on whether they surveyed problems or services (Table 9.3). This led to the observation that 46 out of 101 ISPs appeared to follow no rule for concerning services or problems. In addition, in 25 cases, the writer inventoried all professional services around the person. Afterwards, we attempted to determine if the same individual drafted all the ISPs that seemed to correspond to a standard. None of the 13 CMs consistently followed the same rule in drafting all his or her ISPs. Nevertheless, while 7 followed no rule in more than 50 % of their ISPs, 2 CMs inventoried needs in more than 50 % of their ISPs and 4 the list of professional services.

Discussion

We are reporting here on a qualitatively problematic implementation of ISPs in an experiment in which quantitative assessment alone indicated successful implementation of the tool. Indeed, despite the fact that the files contained ISPs for the most part, our analysis brought to light that it was barely put to practical use and that its usefulness remained rather theoretical. Specifically, the motivations underlying its development and use were vague when written. The clinical file as a whole attested to real individualized planning carried out by CMs, but the ISP appeared to play an accessory role in the process at best. The conceptual framework guiding the trainers[23] was based on another clientele (specifically, individuals with intellectual impairments) with needs and disabilities that remained stable over long periods of time. Moreover, the dynamic nature of the ISP was not essential for this target group. The form itself was developed for planning a fairly limited number of interventions over a relatively short period of time (intervention plan derived from nursing and adapted to the care team's work). It appears limited in use for a longer term with a significant number of problems and caregivers. Consequently, the ISPs were primarily produced to document the file or for administrative purposes, although they can occasionally serve a clinical purpose in summarizing the file. Nevertheless, CMs expressed a need for a planning tool, which they thought that the ISP should have been.

It should be noted that any tool or instrument used in an integrated system often has both clinical as well as management and guidance functions. This is the case with assessment tools (SMAF) that are tied to classification systems (case mix) (Iso-SMAF profiles[24]) and therefore served in managing resources (personnel, budget, etc.) as well as in planning services and developing integrated networks. From this viewpoint, the fact that ISP information was not used for management and guidance is symptomatic of its inappropriateness for integration in its current form. When integration was being developed in Quebec, the choice of assessment tools gave rise to very serious rethinking that, in particular, led to the CTMSP being dropped for failing to take into consideration certain environmental factors deemed essential for integrated networks[25].

Our results put into question the ISP's adequacy as a clinical integration tool. If CM feedback is taken into consideration, then there appears to be a need to support and facilitate this complex task of individualized planning within an integrated service network. The functions most highlighted in training and the literature as well as CM expectations of the ISP center on coordination (not only in terms of time but also in consistency between interventions) and continuity of information (conciseness and accuracy). There was also an expectation that the writing task would be simplified and that the dynamic aspect of the tool would present as a CM "instrument panel," rapidly indicating the needs, the services in place, and those either pending or unavailable (and the solution arrived at). With such a tool, the objectives do not need to be observable behaviors with a threshold and a waiting time, but rather overall directions. That is premised on the directions being taken into account by each caregiver or team of caregivers when drafting its intervention plan. Modifying the drafting guideline in this way would respond to certain CM concerns about making the ISP much more user friendly. Moreover, it is based on an intuitive adaptation of CMs who were already using such verbs in more than 80 % of cases when drafting their objectives. It could be noted in passing that a instrument panel documenting the discrepancies between the needs of people and the services actually offered by the integrated network would be useful for management and guidance purposes, which is what makes it a comprehensive integration tool. Of course, certain prerequisites seem necessary. The CMs insist, in particular, on adequate training for themselves and the other network caregivers in order to develop the habit of seeking out the information in ISP. In the regard, computerizing the tool also appears necessary as does improving access to the electronic tool with networks.

Based on the quality criteria for qualitative research developed by Mays et al.[26], our study presents many factors making it possible to judge its validity. The qualitative methods we have deployed (contextual analysis, documentary analysis, and discussions) enabled us to triangulate our research methods on our objective and, through congruence analysis, increase our degree of confidence in our results. This triangulation also enables the reader to judge our level of interpretation of the corpus. The principal investigator's field lies far outside that of this study. A hospital geriatrician from France, he joined the research group when the impact and implementation study was in its third year. He brought an unbiased perspective of the ISP since he had no prior knowledge of Quebec's health and social-services fabric. Indeed, while French legislation refers to the planning task in developing an assistance plan, responsibility for it never falls on a hospital physician. Such plans in France are purely social in nature and do not involve physicians. Lastly, unlike Quebec health-care providers, their French counterparts have no tradition of viewing the plan and techniques for developing it as being important. The researcher's distance from the study topic and from the people who provided opinions reduces the personal and intellectual bias inherent in this type of research.

We approached the study from the standpoint developed in the literature that CMs needed ISPs to do their jobs. By paying particular attention to the opposite of this presumption, we came to the conclusion that the instrument currently used in the networks examined was not directly useful to CMs in their planning tasks. We also tried to get respondent validation by presenting our research results initially to small groups of professionals (CMs) and then larger groups (conference open to the public, with invitations to CMs, and managers of the health and services network), and finally conferences on the provincial and international levels. During these encounters, our results appear to have revealed the working reality of CM in the three target territories of our study and well beyond.

Our study's main limitation is that it involves a single planning tool. Nevertheless, this is the only tool recognized under the regulations governing Quebec's health and social services system. Moreover, it is structurally quite similar to tools presented in the various case-management manuals from around world (in particular, France[27] and the United States[14]). We are not aware of other tools that have been developed and scientifically validated to help CMs with individualized planning. Our work provided for reflection in Quebec about the individualized planning practices and producing recommendations about the tool's evolution[28]. We think that the PRISMA experiment offers many strengths that make these results significant for other integration contexts. All of the study zones attempted to implement integration according to the PRISMA model defined a priori, with one of the constituent criteria being the use of the ISP. Consequently, it could be considered that there was initially a certain degree of homogeneity in the implementation of each aspect of the model, including the ISP. This homogeneity of intent is nevertheless carried out in the contrasting study sites (rural, rural centered on a town, and urban). In our study, we do not highlight the influence that location at one site or another can have on ISP effectiveness. Conversely, practices can differ slightly anecdotally depending on instructions regarding the drafting date or systematically entering the FP as caregiver. Moreover, while the CMs came from different professional backgrounds (social workers, nurses, psychologists), the influence of background on ISPs was not brought out. Lastly, the fact that the CMs came from different organizations in the Quebec health and social-services system (hospitals, local community service centers, and community organizations, in particular) had no impact on these parameters. Consequently, our conclusions should be applicable to a very broad range of integration contexts.

Conclusion

ISPs appear to constitute a significant instrument for CMs, which should help in performing individualized planning, being dynamic, and providing for information exchange. The forms with five major columns (other than the date), as used in the PRISMA experiment and in other care contexts, do not appear to be satisfactory. As the result of strong push towards implementation, there has been an increase in the number of files containing ISPs. That, however, does not reflect an individual's needs or his or her services in general. CM motivation in filling out such instruments is mainly administrative in nature; the level of use by the individual or the system in low. Because of the discrepancy between the potential usefulness expected by CMs and actual use, a working committee met under the mandate of the *Ministère de la Santé et des Services sociaux* with a view to developing concrete proposals for modifying the instrument. Were a new tool implemented, our results emphasize the importance of providing adequate training in its use. Moreover, we consider that our qualitative methodology based on the conceptual framework of cognitive ergonomics would be appropriate for assessing its usefulness in implementing genuine and effective clinical integration.

Table 9.1
Comparison of the Number and Type of Problems and Handicaps in the ISP and Multidimensional Assessment

Problems or Handicaps	Indicated in the ISP	Not in the ISP but in the Assessment	Total
Health Problems	141	225	366
Prevention Problems (diet, tobacco, alcohol, safety)	2	29	31
Problems with Loss of Independence (handicap or instability of the resource offsetting the handicap)	424	271	695
Psychosocial Problems	132	132	264
Financial Problems	11	15	26
Other Problems	6	23	29
Total	**716**	**695**	**1411**

Table 9.2
Comparison of the Number and Types of Caregivers in the ISPs and Multidimensional Assessment
(The family physician is a given in both cases, which is analyzed in the text.)

Service Providers other than Family Physician	Indicated in the ISP	Not in the ISP but in the Assessment	Total
Patient	17	67	84
Family and Significant Others	159	513	672
Private Resources	109	176	285
Community Organizations	67	14	81
Public Services (medical and social)	461	81	542
Public Institutional Resources (day care center, temporary placement)	116	5	121
Others and Poorly Defined	29	14	43
Total	**958**	**870**	**1828**

Table 9.3
**Breakdown of the 101 ISPs as Responding to Drafting Guidelines
related to Services (columns) or Needs (rows)**

	All Services	All services except the Patient and Casual Assistance	No Rules/ Services	Missing information or Service	Total
All Needs	1	1	8	0	10
All Needs except Health	0	2	8	1	11
No Rules/Needs	4	22	46	5	77
Missing Assessment	1	0	0	2	3
TOTAL	**6**	**25**	**62**	**8**	**101**

References

1. Kodner DL. The quest for integrated systems of care for frail older persons. *Aging Clin Exp Res*. 2002; 14: 307-13.

2. Kodner DL and Kyriacou CK. Fully integrated care for frail elderly: two American models. *Int J Integr Care*. 2000; 1: e08.

3. Johri M, Beland F, and Bergman H. International experiments in integrated care for the elderly: a synthesis of the evidence. *Int J Geriatr Psychiatry*. 2003; 18: 222-35.

4. Hebert R, Durand PJ, Dubuc N, and Tourigny A. PRISMA: a new model of integrated service delivery for the frail older people in Canada. *Int J Integr Care*. 2003; 3: e08.

5. Applebaum RA and Wilson NL. Training needs for providing case management for the long-term care client: lessons from the National Channeling Demonstration. *Gerontologist*. 1988; 28: 172-6.

6. Bernabei R, Landi F, Gambassi G, Sgadari A, Zuccala G, Mor V, *et al.* Randomised trial of impact of model of integrated care and case management for older people living in the community. *Bmj*. 1998; 316: 1348-51.

7. Newcomer R, Harrington C, and Kane R. Challenges and accomplishments of the second-generation social health maintenance organization. *Gerontologist*. 2002; 42: 843-52.

8. Tourigny A, Durand PJ, Bonin L, Hébert R, and Rochette L. Evaluation de l'efficacité d'un réseau de services intégrés pour les personnes âgées vulnérables, in Intégrer les services pour le maintien de l'autonomie des personnes, Réjean Hébert, Tourigny André, and Gagnon Maxime, Editors. Québec (QC): EDISEM, 2004: 57-78.

9. Somme D, Hébert R, Bravo G, and Blanchard F. Le plan de services individualisé (PSI). Concept et utilisation à travers les expériences québecoises et internationales d'intégration des services aux personnnes âgées, in Intégrer les services pour le maintien de l'autonomie des personnes, Réjean Hébert, Tourigny André, and Gagnon Maxime, Editors. Québec (QC): EDISEM, 2004: 281-299.

10. Challis D, Darton R, Johnson L, Stone M, and Traske K. An evaluation of an alternative to long-stay hospital care for frail elderly patients: I. The model of care. *Age Ageing*. 1991; 20: 236-44.

11. Pacala JT, Boult C, Hepburn KW, Kane RA, Kane RL, Malone JK, *et al.* Case management of older adults in health maintenance organizations. *J Am Geriatr Soc*. 1995; 43: 538-42.

12. Riley PA, Fortinsky RH, and Coburn AF. Developing consumer-centered quality assurance strategies for home care. A case management model. *J Case Manag*. 1992; 1: 39-48.

13. Capitman J and Sciegaj M. A contextual approach for understanding individual autonomy in managed community long-term care. *Gerontologist*. 1995; 35: 533-40.

14. Moxley DP. The practice of case-management. *Sage Human Services Guide*. Newbury Park (CA): Sage Publications Inc, 1989.

15. Genrich SJ and Neatherlin JS. Case manager role. A content analysis of published literature. *Care Manag J*. 2001; 3: 14-9.

16. Landi F, Tua E, Onder G, Carrara B, Sgadari A, Rinaldi C, *et al.* Minimum data set for home care: a valid instrument to assess frail older people living in the community. *Med Care. 2000*; 38: 1184-90.

17. Hébert R, Guilbeault J, Desrosiers J, and Dubuc N. The Functional Autonomy Measurement System (SMAF): A clinical-based instrument for measuring disabilities and handicaps in older people. Geriatrics Today: *J Can Geriatr Soc*. 2001; 4: 141-7.

18. Geron SM and Chassler D. Advancing the state of the art: establishing guidelines for long-term care case management. *J Case Manag*. 1995; 4: 9-14.

19. Hebert R and Veil A. Monitoring the degree of implementation of an integrated delivery system. *Int J Integr Care*. 2004; 4: e05.

20. Leutz WN. Five laws for integrating medical and social services: lessons from the United States and the United Kingdom. *Milbank Q*. 1999; 77: 77-110, iv-v.

21. de Montmollin M. L'ergonomie. 3e ed. Reperes 43. Paris: *La Decouverte*, 1996.

22. Hebert R, Carrier R, and Bilodeau A. The Functional Autonomy Measurement System (SMAF): description and validation of an instrument for the measurement of handicaps. *Age Ageing*. 1988; 17: 293-302.

23. Boisvert D. Le plan de services individualisé: participation et animation. Éd. rev. et corr. ed. Cap-Rouge, QC: *Presses inter Universitaires*, 1995.

24. Dubuc N, Hebert R, Desrosiers J, Buteau M, and Trottier L. Disability-based classification system for older people in integrated long-term care services: the Iso-SMAF profiles. *Arch Gerontol Geriatr*. 2006; 42: 191-206.

25. Collectif. Comité aviseur sur l'adoption d'un outil d'évaluation intégré des besoins des personnes en perte d'autonomie et de détermination des services requis notamment en institution ou à domicile. Québec, (QC): Ministère de la santé et des services sociaux, 2000.

26. Mays N and Pope C. Qualitative research in health care. Assessing quality in qualitative research. *Bmj*. 2000; 320: 50-2.

27. Collectif. Notice d'information sur l'allocation personnalisée d'autonomie. Paris, (France): Ministère des affaires sociales, du travail et des solidarités, Ministère de la santé de la famille et des personnes handicapées, 2001.

28. Collectif. Groupe de travail sur la planification des services. Cadre de référence sur la planification des services. Québec, (QC): Ministère de la santé et des services sociaux, 2006.

Acknowledgements

This project was made possible through the financial support of PRISMA, the Canadian Health Services Research Foundation, the *Ministère des Affaires Étrangères français* as part of the *Bourse Lavoisier* program and *Assistance-Publique Hôpitaux de Paris*.

Appendix

Appendix 1
Titles of Document Columns Used at the Outset of Implementation to Produce Individualized Service Plans

DATE	N°	PROBLEMS	OBJECTIVES	MEANS	WORKERS	SERVICES
		How are the problems manifested and what is the source of the difficulty?	What are the expected results of the intervention?	What intervention is needed to correct the problems or difficulties and attain the set objectives?	Who will provide the services?	Number of times or frequency of intervention

Appendix 2
Sample Item from the Multiclientele Assessment Tool

3. PSYCHOLOGICAL HEALTH (depressed, suicidal, paranoid, delirious, violent, manic, etc.)

Difficulties experienced or specific observations: ☐ No _____

☐ If so, specify: _____

Comments: _____

Problem identified   No — N   Yes — Y

Appendix 3
Sample Item from the Functional Independence Measurement System

1. EATING

0   Feeds self independently _____
    -0.5 With difficulty

-1 Feeds self but needs stimulation or supervision OR food must be prepared or cut or pureed first

-2 Needs some assistance to eat OR dishes must be presented one after another

-3 Must be fed totally by another person OR has a naso-gastric tube or a gastrostomy

☐ naso-gastric tube   ☐ gastrostomy

Does the user presently have the human resources (help or supervision) necessary to overcome this disability?   0 | –   +

☐ Yes _____
☐ No _____   -1
Resources*: ☐ ☐ ☐   -2
-3

Comments (e.g., technical aids used): _____

Chapter 10
Implementation and Operation Costs for an Integrated Service Delivery Network for the Frail Elderly in Estrie

Suzanne Durand, Danièle Blanchette and Réjean Hébert

Highlights

With a degree of implementation of the Integrated Service Delivery Network for the Frail Elderly (ISDN) of 85 %, the implementation cost in an urban area is $27 per person age 65 or older (in 2002 dollars). In rural areas with degrees of implementation of 69 % and 78 %, the cost varies between $37 and $47.

When the same degrees of implementation are considered, the annual differential costs incurred through the operation of ISDN components amount to $52 per person age 65 or older in urban areas (in 2002 dollars). The costs range from $41 to $49 in rural areas.

Examining the implementation and operation costs of an integrated services delivery network for the elderly (hereafter, ISDN) is an integral part of economic impact study of ISDN in Estrie, which is presented in Chapter 13 herein. Economic impact is evaluated using differential analysis based on comparing the costs of all the health and social services delivered in the three experimental regional county municipalities (hereafter, MRC) involved in the study (Sherbrooke, Granit, and Coaticook; this order will be followed consistently throughout when citing figures and numbers herein) and the three control MRCs (Lévis, Montmagny, and L'Islet). One essential component of this differential analysis is the identification of the costs related to the new ISDN program[1]. Most of the studies on integrating services that we consulted[2, 3, 4, 5, 6] pay little attention to implementation costs. The costs for organizing and setting up a program must be evaluated[1, 7]. Doing so provides better information to executives and managers about the activities deemed essential to instituting an ISDN and the related costs.

We begin by briefly presenting several methodological aspects described in detail in a previous text[8]. Then, we analyze the results for the three experimental MRCs, their accumulated implementation costs as of March 31, 2005, and their annual operation costs for the fiscal years (hereafter, FY) ended on March 31,

2003, 2004, and 2005 (hereafter, designated as 2003, 2004, and 2005). The results are then discussed.

Methodological Aspects

The economic impact study (Chapter 13) gave precedence to the societal perspective, as recommended in the literature on health economy[1]. This perspective entails taking into consideration all the costs borne by all public, private, and volunteer sources. With respect to implementation and operation, however, only the costs exclusively defrayed by public sources are reported herein because the costs underwritten by private and volunteer sources were not deemed large enough to be taken into account.

Many of the features of the context under which ISDN in Estrie was implemented underscore the difficulties encountered during the study and justify opting for microanalysis to evaluate costs attributable to ISDN:

- ISDN implementation began in 2000 and had not been entirely completed by March 31, 2005[9].
- The health and social services system was concurrently undergoing reorganization.
- The six ISDN components were deployed at different paces.
- The budgets granted for ISDN implementation and operation also indistinctly covered improvement to the range of services, which was not an ISDN component.
- Since supplemental budget were limited, the MRCs reallocated part of their operation budgets to ISDN.

For the purposes of the microanalysis, we asked the program heads and financial officers in the three experimental MRC, many regional institutions, and the Agence de la santé et des services sociaux de l'Estrie (hereafter, the Agency). Both the additional resources and reallocations were identified based on questionnaires, interviews, and analysis of financial statements. The value of these resources, used to translate them into costs, was carried out according to their opportunity cost[1, 10] which generally corresponds to market value[1, 10, 11]. A major part of the resources devoted to ISDN are human resources. In this case, the market value corresponds to the overall remuneration, which includes both salary and benefits. FY 2002 constant costs are used for comparison unaffected by inflation[1].

Compiling per-person costs varies according to ISDN component. Table 10.1 presents the breakdown methods of the six components: interinstitutional coordination (hereafter, coordination), single entry point, case management (CM), computerized clinical chart (CCC) supported by the Système d'information géronto-gériatrique (gerontogeriatric computer system or SIGG), the individualized service plan (ISP) and common instruments. Since ISDN is not for the institutionalized (admitted to a CHSLD), coordination and single entry point costs are divided between people age 65 or older living at home (individual or collective residences). CM and CCC target people in this group who are at risk of losing autonomy. In the case of these two components, the *effective* per-person costs were therefore established using an average number of people receiving case management during the target period. We also compiled *theoretical* per-person costs using a standard load of 45 cases[12]. These *theoretical* costs give an idea of the outcome if the MRC reached the targeted caseload of an average of 45 cases per case manager. The ISP cost was integrated into that of CM. As a result, ISDN generated no specific costs related to common instruments.

Table 10.1
Cost Breakdown Method for Each ISDN Component

Component	Breakdown Method — Denominator
Coordination	Number of elderly persons age 65 years or over living at home in an individual or collective residence
Single entry	
CM	*Effective*: Average number of people receiving case management during the target period
CCC	*Theoretical*: 45 cases (multiplied) by the number of case managers on duty during the target period (FTE)
ISP	Cost integrated into CM costs
Common instruments	No costs attributable specifically to ISDN

Since MRC characteristics influence implementation and operation costs, we present and analyze them before describing these costs.

MRC Descriptive Results

Table 10.2 summarizes several characteristics of the three MRCs under study as well as the data used as denominators in calculating the various per-person costs.

Sherbrooke is a central city in which the following are located: a) Many university and regional institutions, a local community service center (French acronym: CLSC), and a residential and long-term care center (French acronym: CHSLD), which were merged in 2005, and a general and specialized hospital (French acronym: CHSGS); b) regional institutions, rehabilitation center (RC), an intensive functional rehabilitation unit (IFRU), and a short-term geriatric unit (STGU); and c) a local day center and a day hospital. Granit, a rural MRC, has a health complex [carrefour de la santé, which became a Centre de santé et de services sociaux (health and social services center) or CSSS in 2005] that carries out the functions of a CHSG, CLSC, and CHSLD. If needed, the residents of this territory seek services and care at regional institutions in Estrie or a neighboring administrative region. Coaticook, the second rural MRC, also has

Table 10.2
MRC Description

Feature	Sherbrooke	Granit	Coaticook
MRC Type	Urban	Rural	Rural
Institutions in the territory	University CHSGS, CLSC, and CHSLD; RC, IFRU, STGU, day center, and day hospital	Carrefour santé: CHSG, CLSC, and CHSLD	Carrefour santé: CLSC, CHSLD, and 6-bed ER
Degree of implementation in 2004	85.2 %	77.6 %	69.3 %
Number of elderly living at home	17 941	3 197	2 210
CM model	hybrid	hybrid	mixed
FTE in CM (hybrid model) 2003* 2004* 2005*	6.00 8.17 14.00	1.93 2.42 2.80	0.75 0.76 1.14
Average number of people receiving CM (average caseload) 2003* 2004* 2005*	179 (30) 199 (24) 485 (35)	55 (29) 75 (31) 100 (36)	15 (20) 25 (33) 40 (35)

* Year represents the fiscal year ended on March 31 of the designated year

a health complex (which became a CSSS in 2005) that carries out the function of a CLSC and CHSLD in addition to its six emergency beds. If needed, MRC residents seek services and care at regional institutions in Estrie.

In the case of all three MRCs, the coordination, single entry, and CM components became operational in the second half of 2002, which is considered the starting year of ISDN and the initial year of the impact study. The impact study ended in the fourth year, that is, 2005, which is why we compiled implementation costs up to March 31, 2005. While a component may be considered operational, it is not necessarily at 100 %. The implementation study conducted by Veil and Hébert[9] yielded biannual measurements of the degree of implementation from July 2001 until July and November 2004 (taking into account the six components). We consider the last measurements available (see Table 2) as a measurement of the degrees of implementation as at March 31, 2005. These figures indicate degrees of ISDN implementation of 85 %, 78 %, and 69 % in Sherbrooke, Granit, and Coaticook.

The number of elderly people living at home (individual or collective residences) in each MRC totaled 17,941, 3,197, and 2,210, respectively. These figures were arrived at using 2002 demographic projections from the Ministère de la Santé et des Services sociaux and the Agency's "image" bank.

The Sherbrooke and Granit MRCs decided on the hybrid CM model, under which the case manager practices case management with eligible individuals, while carrying out interventions related to his or her initial profession (mainly social work or nursing) with this clientele. Coaticook, on the other hand, opted for the mixed model, in which the case manager intervenes in both his or her roles (CM and his or her profession) with clients eligible for CM and in his or her original profession with clients who are ineligible for CM. For the sake of consistency in determining full-time equivalent (FTE) figures for CM, we converted the mixed model to the hybrid model by only considering the time case managers devoted to clients eligible for CM in Coaticook. In the case of Sherbrooke and Granit, the FTE was established according to the length of time the individual held a case-management position.

We began studying operation costs in FY 2003, which was the first year during which the major components (coordination, single entry, and CM) were operational throughout the entire year. Consequently, the study of operation costs reflect FY 2003 to 2005, which is why Table 2 provides FTE data for CM and the average number of people receiving CM for these FYs.

The average number of people receiving CM during the target period is the arithmetic mean of the number of active files at the end of each of the 13 periods of the given year. Changes in the average caseload bring out an interesting break-in curve. From the first to the third year, the caseloads in Sherbrooke and Granit rose from about 30 to about 35. The trend in Coaticook was somewhat slower during the first year with a load of 20 cases, but it caught up to the other two MRCs in the last year with 35 cases.

A standard caseload had been estimated to be 45 cases per manager[12]. The discrepancy between the standard and the average load of 35 cases during third year gives rise to two questions. Is it plausible to assume that the standard caseload of 45 could be achieved if ISDN were fully implemented? Is the standard caseload actually representative of the hybrid case-management model? In responding to the first question, the differences between the degrees of implementation given in Table 2 tend to indicate that the caseload is affected more by the break-in period than the degree of implementation. Indeed, the three MRCs achieved an average caseload of 35 during the third year, despite their different degrees of implementation. As for the second question, it is already fueling discussions between experts and practitioners. Moreover, it is dealt with in several other chapters in this book.

Implementation Costs

Implementation costs are non-recurrent and associated primarily with activities to put into place ISDN components. The resources involved are grouped into several categories, including per-person costs, and presented in Table 10.3. Costs related to committees, supervision, and coordination include the remuneration of participants at roundtable and follow-up committees dedicated to ISDN and the remuneration of program heads for ISDN-specific activities. The consultation expenses are professional fees related to service organization. Recruitment and training expenses include remuneration and other associated expenses. Installation, furniture, and equipment expenses consist of amounts spent on providing office space, basic furniture, and computer equipment for people holding positions created for or reassigned to ISDN. Lastly, computer-system costs consist of the MRC's share for developing and deploying SIGG.

Table 10.3
**Detailed Implementation Costs Cumulated as of March 31, 2005
(per person in 2002 dollars)**

Component / Type of Expenditure	Sherbrooke	Granit	Coaticook
Total coordination cost*	**$6.18**	**$7.09**	**$4.98**
Committees, supervision, and coordination	3.55	1.91	4.98
Consultation	0.98	5.18	---
Installation, furniture, and equipment	1.65	---	---
Total single entry cost*	---	**7.47**	**4.93**
Committees, supervision, and coordination	---	---	2.47
Consultation	---	5.97	1.11
Recruitment and training	---	1.47	1.17
Installation, furniture, and equipment	---	0.03	0.18
Total CM *effective* cost**	**340.11**	**368.11**	**318.55**
Committees, supervision, and coordination	7.20	14.00	56.00
Consultation	8.44	100.00	---
Recruitment and training	114.72	81.69	67.67
Installation, furniture, and equipment	209.75	172.42	194.88
Total CCC *effective* cost**	**483.02**	**709.95**	**1 232.23**
Committees, supervision, and coordination	5.93	45.50	113.75
Recruitment and training	37.78	249.14	341.95
Installation, furniture, and equipment	45.36	154.08	275.00
Information system	393.95	261.23	501.53

* The denominators are 17,941, 3,197 and 2,210 elderly at home, respectively (see Table 2).
** The denominators are 485, 100, and 40 CM files, respectively (see Table 2).

For both of the components for which the costs are distributed among all elderly people living at home (coordination and single entry) the cost per person is relatively low. Implementing the single entry was both the most and least costly. It cost $7.47 in Granit but entailed no additional costs in Sherbrooke.

We noted that the *effective* per-person costs for CM varied little among the MRCs, ranging from $318 to $368. On the other hand, comparison of these costs for the CCC reveals clear differences, which, without doubt, largely depend on the population differences between the three MRCs. Sherbrooke, the

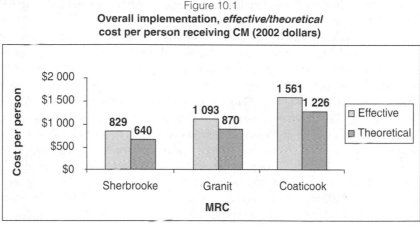

Figure 10.1
**Overall implementation, *effective/theoretical*
cost per person receiving CM (2002 dollars)**

MRC with the highest number of the elderly living at home, has an effective cost per person of $483, followed by Granit at $710 and Coaticook, the least populated, at $1,232.

Based on these detailed costs, we calculated on overall cost, including coordination and single entry, for each elderly person living at home. Consequently, implementation of these two components cost the equivalent of $6.18 per person in Sherbrooke, $14.56 in Granit, and $9.91 in Coaticook. We attributed the cost of the four components to people who had received CM. We compiled an *effective* cost per person by adding the four per-person costs (as mentioned in Table 10.3) and, for the purposes of comparison, we compiled a *theoretical* cost per person. The latter is based on breaking down CM and CCC costs using a theoretical number, namely 45 cases per FTE in CM (according to Table 10.1, respectively, 14, 2.80 and 1.14 FTEs). The *theoretical* numbers of people (cases) are therefore 630 for Sherbrooke, 126 for Granit, and 51 for Coaticook. Figure 10.1 compares *effective* costs per person with the *theoretical* costs per person.

Consequently, ISDN implementation costs the equivalent of $829 to $1,561 per person receiving CM, according to an average caseload of 35 (*effective* cost). If the theoretical load of 45 cases were reached, the cost would rise from about $640 $ to $1,226 (*theoretical* cost). All these data appear to confirm the significant influence of the number of people to receive CM, because, as Table 10.3 illustrates, CCC implementation costs are the most important.

Other than the cost per person for CM implementation costs, we compiled an average CM cost per FTE, which can provide an order of magnitude for budget purposes. The cost for each MRC per FTE is $11,782, $13,147, and $11,177.

Operation Costs

Operation costs refer to recurrent expenses for new activities introduced as a result of ISDN implementation. They are mainly for human resources and related costs. In this section, we look at the annual costs per person during FY 2003, 2004, and 2005.

The coordination and single entry, distributed across all the elderly living at home, generated no significant costs. The annual per-person costs for coordination varied from $0.84 to $2.06. In the third year (2005), they were $1.79, $0.98, and $1.65. Variations in the *single entry* component were slightly higher, with annual costs ranging from $0.70 to $3.40, with those in the last year at $3.40, $0.71, and $0.74. Altogether during fourth year of ISDN implementation (2005), coordination and single entry operation costs amounted to $5.19 in Sherbrooke, $1.69 in Granit, and $2.39 in Coaticook per elderly person living at home.

As for CM, Figure 10.2 depicts the trend of annual *effective* costs per person. The break-in curve is interesting: costs that drop consistently in Granit ($1,954, $1,728, and $1,436) and in Coaticook ($3,349, $2,207, and $1,954). In Sherbrooke, the increased costs in 2004 ($2,587) compared to 2003 ($2,356) can be accounted for by the hiring of seven new case managers in February 2004. According to a program head, they need at least six months to achieve a normal level of productivity. The situation recovered in 2005 when costs dropped to $1,774.

Figure 10.2
CM operation, annual *effective* cost per person receiving CM (2002 dollars)

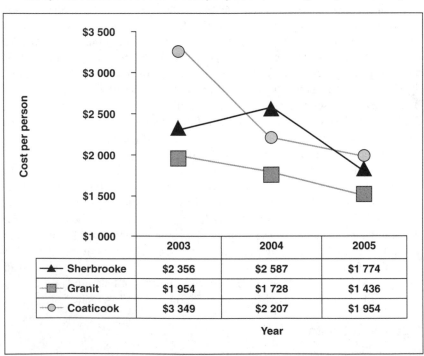

	2003	2004	2005
▲ Sherbrooke	$2 356	$2 587	$1 774
■ Granit	$1 954	$1 728	$1 436
◯ Coaticook	$3 349	$2 207	$1 954

Year

Discrepancies between MRCs can be partially accounted for by case-manager level of experience, since this directly influences case managers remuneration, which represents 92 % of CM operation costs in Sherbrooke, 89 % in Granit and 95 % in Coaticook. This rationale is supported by comparing CM operation costs broken down according to CM FTEs. The 2005 costs per FTE were $61,472, $51,298, and $68,574, respectively.

SIGG, which supports the CCC, was deployed during FY 2003. The costs incurred during this year were for implementation, which is why operation costs began in FY 2004. The annual *effective* costs per person receiving CM in 2004 and 2005 are presented in Figure 10.3. The break-in impact (increased average caseload) accounts for the reduction in costs between 2004 and 2005. FY 2005 costs, which are, respectively, $32, $132, and $289, highlight the advantage of deploying a computer system such as SIGG for a larger population, as discussed in the section on implementation costs.

Figure 10.3
CCC operation, annual *effective* costs per person receiving CM (2002 dollars)

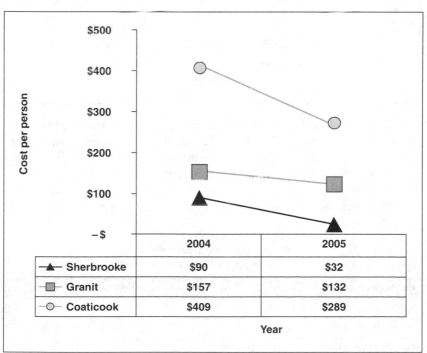

	2004	2005
—▲— Sherbrooke	$90	$32
—■— Granit	$157	$132
—O— Coaticook	$409	$289

Year

For FY 2005, we compiled overall operation costs (for components) per person receiving CM. As with implementation, we compiled an *effective* cost based on an average caseload of 35 and a *theoretical* cost based on a standard caseload of 45. Figure 10.4 provides a comparison of these annual *effective* and *theoretical* costs. The figure shows that the annual *effective* costs per person receiving CM ranges from $1,570 and $2,246, whereas the annual *theoretical* costs per person fall between $1,247 and $1,762. These figures illustrate the results that could be achieved if the MRC were able to handle an average of 45 cases per case manager FTE.

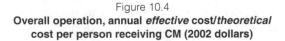

Figure 10.4
Overall operation, annual *effective* cost/*theoretical* cost per person receiving CM (2002 dollars)

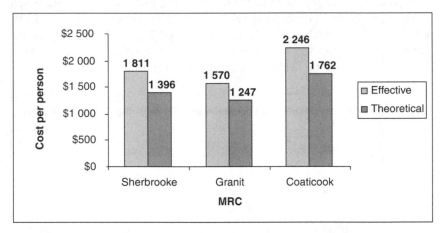

The different breakdown methods described in Table 10.1 adhere to rationale of the economic impact study (Chapter 13) and support the breakdown of implementation and operation costs presented up to this point. Nevertheless, we propose a rule of thumb for financial planning comprising a uniform breakdown based on the number of people aged 65 or older, which is readily available. Table 10.4 presents implementation costs and operation costs per person separately.

Table 10.4
Implementation and Operation Costs, Broken Down across the Entire Elderly Population (2002 dollars)

Description	Sherbrooke	Granit	Coaticook
Number of people age 65 or older	18 715	3 299	2 297
Overall implementation costs	$510 108	$154 355	$83 928
Implementation costs per elderly person	**$27**	**$47**	**$37**
Overall operation costs in 2005	$969 276	$162 274	$95 018
Annual operation costs per elderly person	**$52**	**$49**	**$41**

According to this table, implementation ranging in completeness from 69 % to 85 % cost from $27 to $47 per person age 65 or older. We should point out that implementation is a non-recurring cost related to implementing a new program. Annual operation costs vary from $41 to $52.

Discussion

The data about implementation and operation costs presented herein are specific to the contexts in each of the MRCs under study. The implementation costs cover the period from the start of implementation to March 31, 2005, when ISDN was partially implemented in the three MRCs (69 % to 85 %). The costs for full implementation, however, are not available and there are no extrapolation methods that would be relevant under these circumstances, since the costs are not predictable or incurred progressively. The same holds true for operation costs, which deal with the second, third, and fourth years of ISDN implementation.

A variety of factors influence implementation and operation costs. It was not possible to measure these factors or their impacts on costs:

- MRC nature (urban or rural)
- Population size for each MRC
- Types of health and social services establishments in the MRC's territory and the distance to regional institutions
- Service organization prior to ISDN implementation
- Range of services offered and resources available in the MRC prior to ISDN implementation
- Choices made about certain ISDN components, specifically the structure of inter-institutional coordination and the CM model
- Profiles of individuals managed by case managers

The implementation and operation costs described herein are all provided in constant 2002 dollars. They were compiled within the framework of the economic impact study for the Estrie ISDN (Chapter 13). The specific context for implementing such ISDNs accounts for the decision to use microanalysis to assess costs. This context and the significant number of unmeasurable factors that influence costs represent barriers in using the results to define standards.

To our knowledge, no other experiment in integrating services has been subject to such an in-depth economic evaluation. As a result, we have nothing that our data can be compared to. Both the implementation and operation costs identified appear reasonable. Table 10.5 provides information to compare the unit cost of certain services with ISDN costs.

In producing this table, we compiled an overall cost, including an annual implementation cost, which corresponds to the breakdown of overall implementation costs over a period of 7 years (according to experts in health and social services, programs are revised every 5 to 10 years), plus operation costs

Table 10.5
**ISDN Implementation and Operation Costs Compared
to the Cost of Services (2002 dollars)**

ISDN costs	
Implementation (amortized over 7 years) and operation costs per person age 65 or older	$47 to $56 per year $0.13 to $0.15 per day
Services	
Family physician	$37 per visit
Medical specialist	$65 per visit
Emergency department	$261 per visit
Day hospital	$261 per day
Short-term geriatric unit	$546 per day

for FY 2005. We obtained an annual overall cost ranging from $47 to $56 per person aged 65 or older, which yields a daily cost of $0.13 to $0.15. The costs for the different services were taken from the chapter about average costs (Chapter 21). It can be seen that only the cost for consulting a family physician ($37) is less expensive than the annual overall ISDN cost. The remaining services measured either in visits (medical specialist and emergency department) or in days (day hospital and days hospitalized in a short-term geriatric unit) cost considerably more ($64 to $546).

These figures provide information needed to determine the relative size of ISDN costs. The savings that ISDN could generate have been determined by comparison with the costs of services delivered in the experimental and control MRCs. These comparisons are part of the economic impact study (Chapter 13).

References

1. Drummond, M.F., O'Brien, B.J., Stoddart, G.L. and Torrance, G. W. (1998). *Méthodes d'évaluation économique des programmes de santé.* Paris: Économica.

2. Béland, F., Bergman, H., Dallaire, L., Fletcher, J., Lebel, P., Monette, J., Denis, J.-L., Contandriopoulos, A.-P., Cimon, A., Bureau, C., Bouvier, L., and Dubois, D. (2004). *Évaluation du Système intégré pour personnes âgées fragiles (SIPA): Utilisation et coûts des services sociaux et de santé.* Ottawa, Canada: Fondation canadienne de la recherche sur les services de santé.

3. Bernabei, R., Landi, F., Gambassi, G., Sgadari, A., Zuccala, G., Mor, V., Rubenstein, L. Z., and Carbonin, P. (1998). Randomised trial of impact of model of integrated care and case management for older people living in the community. *British Medical Journal, 316* (7141), 1348-1351.

4. Challis, D., Darton, R., Johnson, L., Stone, M., and Traske, K. (1991). An evaluation of an alternative to long-stay hospital care for frail elderly patients: 2. Costs and effectiveness. *Age and Ageing, 20*, 245-254.

5. Eng, C., Pedulla, J., Eleazer, G. P., McCann, R., and Fox, N. (1997). Program of all-inclusive care for the elderly (PACE): an innovative model of integrated geriatric care and financing. *Journal of American Geriatrics Society, 45*(2), 223-232.

6. Pinnel Beaulne Associates Ltd. (1998). *CHOICE Evaluation project, Evaluation summary, Final report.* Edmonton: PBA Pinnel Beaulne Associates Ltd.

7. Bourgueil, Y., Brémond, M., Develay, A., Grignon, M., Midy, F., Naiditch, M., and Polton, D. (2001). *L'évaluation des réseaux de soins, enjeux et recommandations.* Centre de recherche d'étude et de documentation en économie de la santé (CREDES), Groupe Image-Ensp.

8. Durand, S., Blanchette, D., and Hébert, R. (2004). Aspects financiers liés a l'intégration des services de maintien de l'autonomie - Volet «Implantation et fonctionnement». *In* Hébert, R., Tourigny, A., et Gagnon, M. *Intégrer les services pour le maintien de l'autonomie des personnes,* Québec: Edisem; 251-266.

9. Veil, A. and Hébert, R. (2005). Évaluation de l'implantation des mécanismes et outils d'intégration des services aux personnes âgées en perte d'autonomie: Résultats de mise en œuvre. *In Actes du 3ᵉ Colloque PRISMA: L'intégration des services: un moyen essentiel pour améliorer la réponse aux besoins des personnes âgées.* Sainte-Foy, March 23 and 24.

10. Gold, M. R., Siegel, J. E., Russel, L. B., and Weinstein, M. C. (1996). *Cost-effectiveness in health and medicine.* Oxford, New York: Oxford University Press.

11. Robinson, R. (1993). Economic evaluation and health care: cost and cost-minimization analysis. *British Medical Journal, 307* (6906), 726-728.

12. Hébert, R. and Veil, A. (2004). Monitoring the degree of implementation of an integrated delivery system. *International Journal of Integrated Care* (www.ijic.org), 4 (September), 1-11.

Chapter 11
The Effectiveness of the PRISMA Integrated Service Delivery Network: Preliminary Report on Methods and Baseline Data[*]

Réjean Hébert, Marie-France Dubois, Michel Raîche, Nicole Dubuc, and the PRISMA-Estrie Group

Abstract

Purpose: The PRISMA study analyzes an innovative coordination-type integrated service delivery (ISD) system developed to improve continuity and increase the effectiveness and efficiency of services, especially for older and disabled populations. The objective of the PRISMA study is to evaluate the effectiveness of this system to improve health, empowerment and satisfaction of frail older people, modify their health and social services utilization, without increasing the burden of informal caregivers. The objective of this paper is to present the methodology and give baseline data on the study participants.

Methods: A quasi-experimental study with pre-test, multiple post-tests, and a comparison group was used to evaluate the impact of PRISMA ISD. Elders at risk of functional decline (501 experimental, 419 control) participated in the study.

Results: At entry, the two groups were comparable for most variables. Over the first year, when the implementation rate was low (32 %), participants from the control group used fewer services than those from the experimental group. After the first year, no significant statistical difference was observed for functional decline and changes in the other outcome variables.

Conclusion: This first year must be considered a baseline year, showing the situation without significant implementation of PRISMA ISD systems. Results for the following years will have to be examined with consideration of these baseline results.

---

[*] This chapter is reprinted with the kind permission of *International Journal of Integrated Care,* where it appeared as: Hébert R, Dubois M-F, Raîche M, Dubuc N, & the PRISMA-Estrie Group. The effectiveness of the PRISMA integrated service delivery network: preliminary report on methods and baseline data. *International Journal of Integrated Care* 2008; 8(feb): (www.ijic.org) e1-15.

Key words
health services for the aged, integrated service delivery systems, frail elderly, program evaluation

Purpose

While health services for the elderly have improved significantly over the last decades these improvements have led to fragmentation of services, particularly in specialized care. Acute geriatric evaluation units, geriatric rehabilitation services, and home services for the elderly are now usual parts of health-care systems. At the same time, other organizations such as voluntary agencies, meals on wheels and privates home services, as well as clinicians are all strongly engaged in the maintenance of elders' independence. Even if each of these partners improves their services, the spread of intervening parties exposes the older person to a lack of continuity, an important consequence of fragmentation[1-3]. Repeated evaluations with different tools, communication problems between clinicians, services and organizations, loss of efficiency of the uncoordinated interventions, and inappropriate use of costly hospital and institutional services are some of the other consequences resulting from the fragmentation of services. Lack of coordination could be considered as a new risk factor for functional decline[4].

Integrated service delivery (ISD) systems have been proposed to improve effectiveness and efficiency of health-care systems, particularly for patients with multiple needs and complex interactions with many professionals and organizations. It is hypothesized that ISD systems could improve continuity of care as well as client health and satisfaction, while reducing the use of costly resources, like hospitals and institutions. Although there are some indications of the effectiveness of ISD systems for clients such as frail older people[5], their real effectiveness at the population level remains to be demonstrated.

Theory

According to Leutz, there are three levels of integration in health care: 1) linkage; 2) coordination; and 3) full integration[6]. ISD refers to systems targeting either coordination or full integration. In fully integrated ISD systems, a central organization is responsible for all services, either under one structure or by contracting some services with other organizations.

Many variants of full integration ISD programs have been developed. In the United States, the California On Lok project[7] gave rise to the PACE (Program of All-Inclusive Care for the Elderly) projects[8]. In Canada, the CHOICE (Comprehensive Home Option of Integrated Care for the Elderly) project in Edmonton is an adaptation of the PACE projects[9]. These programs are built around Day Centres where the members of the multidisciplinary team who evaluate and treat the clients are based. The Social HMO in the United States[10] and the SIPA ("Système de services intégrés pour personnes âgées en perte d'autonomie") project in Montreal are also integrated services but do not include a day center[11]. However, home-care services are provided by personnel hired by or under contract with the organization. All these fully integrated models are nested within the usual health and social services in a particular area but run parallel to them. This could generate problems in a universal publickly funded heath care system as in Canada. They do not involve significant changes to the structure or processes of existing services, except in negotiating protocols for referring clients to ISD programs and providing some services not covered by ISD. Capitation budgeting is usually a key component of these programs. Evaluation of these fully integrated programs[5, 12] showed that they have an impact on the number and duration of short-term hospitalizations, the number of admissions to long-term care institutions, drug use, mortality, and the cost of services.

Targeting the other level of integrated care—coordination—involves the development and implementation of defined structures and mechanisms to manage the complex and evolving needs of patients in a coordinated fashion. Every organization keeps its own structure but agrees to participate in an "umbrella" system and to adapt its operations and resources to the agreed requirements and processes. At this level, the ISD system is not simply nested within the health-care and social services system but is embedded within it. It could then be more easily implemented without duplication in the Canadian universal publickly funded health care system. The PRISMA (Program of Research to Integrate the Services for the Maintenance of Autonomy) project in the Province of Quebec is an example of this type of integrated care[1]. The mechanisms and tools developed and implemented by PRISMA are: 1) coordination between decision-makers and managers at the regional and local levels, 2) use of a single entry point, 3) a case-management process, 4) individualized service plans, 5) a single assessment instrument coupled with a management system based on client disabilities, and 6) a computerized clinical chart allowing communication between institutions and clinicians for client monitoring purposes. The full description of the PRISMA ISD model can be found in a previous paper published in this Journal [1]. Since this coordinated system model was developed to fit into a publicly funded health-care system, capitation budgeting is not an essential component and system funding can be included as part of the agreement between organizations.

After a preliminary study in the Bois-Francs region in the Province of Quebec showed positive results on institutionalisation rates, desire to institutionalise and caregiver's burden[13], the group is now extending this model to three other areas in the Eastern Townships region of Quebec that present different types of environment: Sherbrooke, an urban setting with a large university regional hospital and many health and social organizations; Granit, a rural setting with a local acute-care hospital, and Coaticook: rural without an acute care hospital. The evaluation of the implementation focuses on the process of implementing the mechanisms and tools, and how they function. A measure of the degree of implementation has been designed and allows for monitoring the implementation process. This quantitative index includes a series of weighted indicators for each of the components of the PRISMA ISD model and is fully described in a previous paper published in this Journal[14].

The study's objective is to evaluate the effectiveness of the PRISMA ISD network to improve the health, empowerment, and satisfaction of frail older people, and to modify health and social-services utilization, without increasing the caregiver's burden. This paper reports the study's methodology and baseline data. Baseline data include the results of the first year (T1), when the PRISMA ISD implementation rate was only 32 %[14].

Methods

Study design

Effectiveness is being evaluated using a quasi-experimental design (pretest, 2 annual posttests with control group). In contrast to the Bois-Francs pilot project in which effectiveness was measured on subjects who were service users, this study measures effectiveness by selecting a sample of older individuals "at risk" of functional decline and of becoming clients of the services. While this approach employs a different sampling strategy and requires a larger sample size, it enables us to measure the real populational effectiveness and to estimate the system penetration rate (accessibility).

The three control areas were selected based on the similarities of their demographic variables (% of people over 65, over 75, etc.) and health services (% of elders living in institutions, hospitalization rate of elders, ratio of general practitioners to the aged population, etc.) with the experimental areas according to the Matusita technique used by Junod[15]. This technique calculates a distance between each experimental area and each candidate control by combining the differences between the two areas over different indicators. The area closest to each experimental area is then chosen. The three control areas were selected in the same region (Chaudière-Appalaches) located on the south shore of the St. Lawrence River near Quebec City.

Participants

Using a list from the Quebec Health Insurance Board covering all the population, samples were selected in each of the three experimental and control areas. Inclusion criteria were to be aged 75 and over, to live on a yearly basis in one of the six areas, to be able to speak and understand French, and to be identified as at risk of functional decline. Older adults institutionalized in long-term-care facilities were excluded because they are unexposed to PRISMA ISD in the experimental zone. Older people usually living more than 2 months outside the country (e.g. moving to southern climes for the winter) were excluded. The fourth inclusion criterion was verified using the Sherbrooke Postal Questionnaire already developed and validated by our team[16]. The responses to this questionnaire or failure to return it establishes a risk of presenting a significant functional decline over the next year. We used a cutoff score of 3 and over (out of 6) to identify subjects at risk. Since the annual incidence of functional decline in this group is estimated to be 48 %[16], it is probable that the great majority of subjects selected in this way will contact the health and social-services network during the two planned years of the study.

After being informed about the study and agreeing to participate, the subjects were evaluated at pretest (T0) and one year later (T1), and will be reassessed in another year (T2). The study has been approved by the ethics review board of the Sherbrooke University Geriatrics Institute. Every subject received information and signed a consent form.

Outcome measures

The outcome measured are disabilities, cognitive functioning, satisfaction with the services received, client empowerment, caregiver burden, utilization of health services and social services, and drug use. Economic analysis is also performed. Sociodemographic data include age, sex, years of schooling, and type of housing.

The **Functional Autonomy Measurement System (SMAF)**[17]] is a 29-item scale based on the WHO classification of disabilities[18]. It measures functional ability in five areas: activities of daily living (7 items), mobility (6 items), communication (3 items), mental functions (5 items), and instrumental activities of daily living (8 items). Each item is scored on a 5-point scale from 0 (independent) and 0.5 (with difficulties) to 3 (dependent), for a maximum score of 87, with higher scores representing decreased functional ability. The SMAF must be administered by a trained health professional who scores the individual's functional ability after questioning the subject and proxies, observing, and sometimes testing the subject. A reliability study showed that the intraclass correlation coefficients for total SMAF scores was 0.95 for test-retest and 0.96 for inter-rater reliability[19]. The responsiveness of the scale has been studied and the Guyatt index was 14.53. Using both an internal method and an external criterion, the minimal metrically detectable and clinically important change of the SMAF score has been established at 5 points[20]. A case-mix classification system based on the SMAF has also been developed using cluster analysis techniques[21]. The 14 Iso-SMAF profiles generated ranged from profiles 1, 2, and 3 (disabilities in instrumental activities of daily living mainly) to profiles 13 and 14 (totally dependant for most functions).

Functional decline was defined as the occurrence one of the following during the year: 1) an increase of 5 points or more on the SMAF; 2) admission to a nursing home or long-term care hospital; or 3) death. This definition was used in previous studies to measure the effectiveness of health programs[22].

Cognitive status was assessed with the **Mini-Mental State Examination (MMSE)**[23], widely used in clinical settings and research. The MMSE comprises 11 questions assessing orientation to time and place, attention, immediate and short-term recall, language, and the ability to follow simple verbal and written commands. It provides a total score that varies from 0 (worst) to 30 (best).

The **Health Care Satisfaction Questionnaire (HCSQ)**[24] developed by our team consists of 26 statements, each answered on two four-grade scales, one for perception and the other one for importance. Combining the two scales results in scores ranging from -8 to 16 for each statement. The total score is obtained by averaging scores over all statements. A factor analysis revealed three different factors explaining 52.8 % of the total variance: satisfaction with the relationship with professionals (12 items), satisfaction with the delivery of care and services (6 items), and satisfaction with the organization of care and services (5 items). Cronbach coefficients for internal consistency were 0.93 for the total scale and 0.93, 0.74, and 0.78 for factors 1, 2, and 3 respectively. The intraclass correlation coefficient for test-retest reliability was 0.72 (95 % CI: 0.52–0.84).

The **Health Care Empowerment Questionnaire (HCEQ),** also developed by our team, has 10 statements with response scales mirroring those of the satisfaction questionnaire[25]. The total score varies from 1 to 16 and factor analysis revealed three dimensions explaining 68 % of the total variance: patient's involvement in the decisional process (3 items), patient's involvement in interactions with professionals (4 items), and patient's degree of control in regard to care and services received (3 items). Cronbach coefficients for internal consistency were 0.83 for the total scale and 0.79, 0.79, and 0.89 for factors 1, 2, and 3, respectively. The intraclass correlation coefficient for test-retest reliability was 0.70 (95 % CI: 0.48–0.83).

The **Zarit Burden Interview**[26-27] is a 22-item scale measuring the subjective load experienced by the informal caregiver by asking him/her how frequently (from "0=never" to "4=almost always") they feel various emotions in their relationship with the care-receiver for a total score out of 88. Reference values have been generated based on a representative sample of caregivers of community-dwelling people with dementia[28]. Scores between 8 and 17 represent moderate burden; between 18 and 32, high; and over 32, severe. The **caregiver's desire to institutionalize** was measured by a four-item questionnaire adapted from Morycz[29] used and translated in the Canadian Study on Health and Aging[30].

Bimonthly phone calls allow for collection of data on the **use of health and social services**. Every subject or his/her caregiver was given a calendar with a guideline, and was trained to adequately collect the required information. We chose this method because of the variety of information needed. No single source contains hospital data, home-care data, and private and voluntary services data. This type of data collection has been successfully used in other studies led by our team[22]. A reliability study was performed and showed good to excellent stability for the different measures of use[31]. The bimonthly calls and the calendar minimize memory bias and make it possible to maintain regular contact with subjects. Public, private, and voluntary services were collected. We recorded the number of visits to the emergency room (ER), the percentage followed by a hospitalization or by return to the ER within 10 days. We recorded number of hospitalizations, length of stay, and rehospitalization within different time frames (10, 30, and 90 days). The number of day surgeries was also tracked as were visits to health professionals (general practitioners, medical specialists, nurses, social workers, physiotherapists, occupational therapists, speech therapists, etc.). Specialized geriatric care was specifically noted as well as acute-care geriatric assessment and visits to intensive functional rehabilitation units. Community services included visits to day hospitals and day centers, and the use of help for personal care and home maintenance. Finally, voluntary services included data on meals-on-wheels, respite care, community transportation, and caretaking.

The **economic evaluation** includes the costs of public and private services, with equivalent costs calculated for voluntary services. The number of use for each service is multiplied by standards costs to produce total costs and detailed costs for each service and type of provider. The objective is not to measure the efficiency of a particular organization, but to determine standard costs for each service for comparison of costs between the experimental and control zones. Implementation costs are considered and are applied in the experimental zone. Drug use and costs were obtained from the Quebec Health Insurance Board and included in economic evaluation.

Data collection

Each subject was interviewed face-to-face at the outset and yearly afterward by the same interviewer. Given the design of the study, the interviewers were not blinded to the intervention group. The interviewers were health professionals with a specific training for administering the selected instruments for this study. A primary informal caregiver was also identified and a self-administered questionnaire including the Zarit Burden Interview and the Desire to institutionalize questionnaire was either left to him/her or sent by mail with a pre-stamped return envelope. Subjects (or their primary caregiver if cognitive problems were identified) were contacted by telephone every other month to collect data on health and social services use.

Data Analysis

Descriptive statistics were computed for each group and subgroup (areas within groups). For baseline data and services use during the first year, groups were compared using Chi square tests, when variables were categorical, or Student's t test, when continuous. For highly skewed distributions, Wilcoxon's rank sum test was preferred. In order to analyze first-year changes on outcomes, an analysis of covariance comparing post-test scores was performed, adjusting for baseline scores.

Results

From the 19,981 people over 75 years old living in one of the 6 areas (3 experimental, 3 control), 4,881 were randomly selected in two waves and sent a postal questionnaire. From these, 2,308 were not at risk of functional decline and 554 were not eligible (e.g. institutionalized, dead, living 2-6 months outside the country) or had a wrong address, leaving 2,019 identified at risk and asked to participate in the study. Of these 2,019 subjects, ineligibility was discovered at personal contact in 346 cases, while 753 refused to participate, mainly for reasons of lack of interest or time, or poor health. A total of 920 subjects agreed to participate and were evaluated at baseline. Their principal informal caregiver was also invited to participate in the study.

The subjects refusing to participate were compared to study participants on the available variables. They were not different for age, sex, level of education, self-perceived health, and health-care services received during the previous year. Participants reported more hospitalizations during the previous year than those refusing and a greater number were "extremely satisfied" regarding health services received.

The mean age of the 920 participants in the longitudinal study was 83 years, two thirds were women, 44 % were married, and the average level of education was 6.5 years. Table 11.1 presents the characteristics of both groups at baseline. Although subjects from the experimental group were slightly but significantly (p=0.016) older than those from the control group, there was no significant difference in the mean SMAF scores at baseline. Significantly more subjects from the control group were homeowners or tenants (p=0.001) and had received home care during the previous year (p=0.001). They were also significantly more satisfied with services (p=0.014) and showed higher empowerment (p=0.049). There was no statistically significant difference between the two groups for all other variables. Appendix 11.1 details the baseline data for subjects in each subgroup of both the experimental and control groups. Figure 11.1 shows the distribution of the Iso-SMAF profiles for the two groups. Two thirds of the subjects were presenting disabilities mainly in the instrumental activities of daily living (Iso-SMAF profiles 1 to 3). The remaining were suffering from more severe disabilities (profiles 4 and over).

Table 11.1
Characteristics of both groups at baseline

Variable	Experimental group	Control group	p value
Baseline characteristics of the subjects	(n = 501)	(n = 419)	
Age on January 1st 2001	83.29 (4.87)*	82.50 (5.08)	0.016
Female	321 (64.1%)	252 (60.1%)	0.221
Married	216 (43.1%)	185 (44.2%)	0.752
Years of education	6.51 (3.06)	6.62 (3.23)	0.597
Excellent or good health status[§]	320 (64.4%)	258 (62.2%)	0.489
Homeowner or tenant (vs. boarder)	303 (60.5%)	299 (71.4%)	0.001
Has an informal caregiver	452 (90.2%)	369 (88.1%)	0.294
Has been hospitalized at least once in the last 6 months	148 (29.7%)	120 (28.6%)	0.735
Has received home care services in the last 6 months	104 (20.8%)	126 (30.1%)	0.001
Disability (SMAF)	18.54 (11.80)	19.93 (12.92)	0.009
Cognitive functioning (MMSE)	24.83 (4.88)	24.34 (5.86)	0.177
Satisfaction with health services	7.55 (2.38)	7.98 (2.81)	0.014
Empowerment	7.76 (2.46)	8.10 (2.75)	0.049
Baseline characteristics of the informal caregiver	(n=409)	(n=306)	
Female	296 (72.4%)	241 (78.8%)	0.051
Relationship with the Spouse Child Other	138 (33.7%) 206 (50.4%) 65 (15.9%)	113 (36.9%) 151 (49.4%) 42 (13.7%)	0.579
Living with the care-receiver	182 (44.6%)	201 (65.9%)	<0.001
Burden (Zarit Burden Interview)	17.28 (14.88)	20.11 (16.29)	0.016
Desire to institutionalize [†]	62 (16.3%)	45 (17.0%)	0.823

* Mean (sd) for continuous variables; n (%) for categorical variables
[§] Subjective health status compared to others of the same age.
[†] Has thought about it somewhat seriously, has discussed it with someone, has visited an institution, or has applied for placement.

Figure 11.1
Iso-SMAF profiles at baseline, by group and by sub area

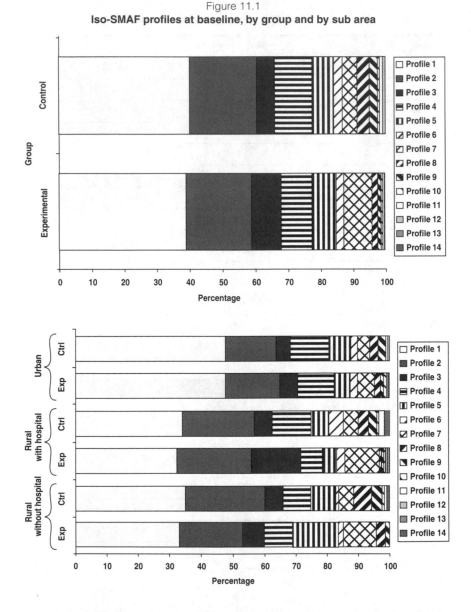

During the first year, 62 subjects died at home, 41 were institutionalized, and 32 were lost to follow-up (Figure 11.2). Overall, there was a significant increase ($p < 0.001$) on disability with mean SMAF scores of survivors going from 17.39 to 19.23. However, there was no difference between the two groups or between the subgroups. Overall, 33.1 % of subjects in both groups presented

Figure 11.2
Participant flow through the first year of the PRISMA study

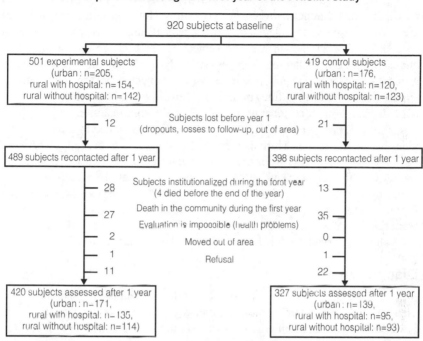

Table 11.2
First year changes on outcomes

First year changes on outcomes (a negative sign indicates decline)§	Experimental group (n = 420)	Control group (n = 327)	p value
Functional independence	-1.84 (6.08)*	-1.83 (6.26)	0.918
Cognitive functioning	-0.12 (2.75)	-0.68 (4.49)	0.020
Satisfaction with health services	0.23 (2.65)	0.15 (2.89)	0.542
Empowerment	-0.51 (2.75)	-1.14 (3.09)	0.065
Burden (any caregiver)	2.50 (12.82)	1.70 (12.83)	0.858
Burden (same caregiver)	2.29 (12.30)	1.58 (12.32)	0.883
Desire to institutionalize † (any cg)	from 16.1 % to 18.9 %	from 16.8 % to 21.1 %	0.720

* Mean (sd) for continuous variables; n (%) for categorical variables
† Has thought about it somewhat seriously, has discussed it with someone, has visited an institution, has applied for placement, or has institutionalized.
§ p-values are derived from an analysis of covariance comparing post-test scores, adjusting for baseline scores.

a functional decline over this period (7.3 % dead, 4.7 % institutionalized, and 21.1 % increased by more than 5 points on the SMAF) (Figure 11.3). There was no significant difference between the two groups. However, comparing the rural areas with hospitals revealed signicantly fewer deaths in the control subarea (p<0.05). Table 11.2 compares the subjects from both groups on one-year changes to the other outcome variables. The only significant difference between groups was on cognitive functioning on which subjects from the control group experienced a greater decline (p=0.020). This difference (less than 1 point on MMSE), however, does not appear to be clinically significant.

Table 11.3 and Appendix 11.2 show the utilization of health and social services over this first year. Thirty percent of the subjects in both groups were hospitalized. More subjects from the experimental group visited the emergency room over the year (47 % vs. 30 %), but their visits were less likely to be followed by a hospital admission (25 % vs. 67 %). There was also significant differences between the two groups on the utilization of other services. Subjects from the experimental areas displayed more frequent use of health professionals, voluntary services, home help for personal care, and day care.

Discussion

Since the PRISMA model is embedded within the health-care and social services system, its implementation requires a global system change. Doing so, however, would make it impossible to use a randomized controlled trial design to demonstrate its impact. We thus turned to a quasi-experimental design comparing three areas where a PRISMA ISD network was implemented to three comparable areas where such an implementation was not expected. To ensure comparability of the experimental and control areas on sociodemographic variables and health-services use, we opted for a standardized technique (Matusita distance[16]).

Subjects from the two groups and the six subgroups were comparable at baseline on most sociodemographic data and outcome variables. There was also no difference on functional decline during the first year. This result was expected since the implementation rate of the ISD in the experimental areas was then less than 33 %[14]. The attrition rate was around 5 % (14 in the study group and 23 in the control group) and mostly explained by the subjects' refusals to continue the study.

The utilization of health care and social services by subjects from the two groups was quite different. This was expected since it is what prompted the Estrie area to move towards new ways of delivering services. There was a greater use of the emergency room and a lower rate of hospitalisation after ER visit. This is probably an indicator of an inappropriate use of the emergency department in the experimental area for minor conditions. This area evidences a greater utilization of costly services (e.g., hospital, emergency room) and the

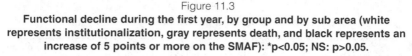

Figure 11.3
Functional decline during the first year, by group and by sub area (white represents institutionalization, gray represents death, and black represents an increase of 5 points or more on the SMAF): *p<0.05; NS: p>0.05.

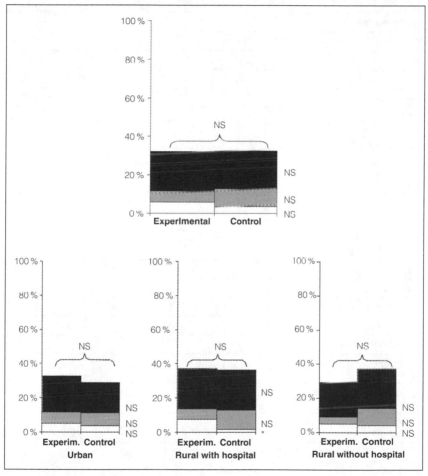

challenge of the PRISMA ISD network is to change this pattern and promote a better use of services. The objective is to ensure that the older frail subjects get the right services, at the right time, by the appropriate organization, and at the least cost.

Study participants present a moderate level of disabilities (mean SMAF score of 19/87 at entry) and one third shows significant disabilities in performing ADL (Iso-Smaf profile > 4). The functional decline rate over the first year (33 %) was less than expected from the previous studies that have used the Sherbrooke Postal Questionnaire (decline around 48 % in one year). This could

Table 11.3
Use of resources for both groups during the first year

Variable	Experimental group ($n_{pers-yrs}$ = 440,92)	Control group ($n_{pers-yrs}$ = 356,21)	p value
Emergency room (ER) visits			
At least one visit to the ER	207.5 (47.1%)[¥]	105.9 (29.7%)	<0.001
Among users:			
• Number of visits	2.15 (2.1) [1.07]	2.04 (1.9) [1.04]	0.652
• % followed by a hospitalization	41.95 (42.6) [25.0]	57.68 (45.8) [66.7]	0.003
• % return within 10 days (when there was no hospitalization)	11.26 (23.2) [0.0]	9.42 (24.5) [0.0]	0.618
Hospitalization			
At least one hospitalization	145.2 (32.9%)	98.7 (27.7%)	0.113
Among users:			
• Number of hospitalizations	1.89 (1.6) [1.1]	1.88 (1.7) [1.1]	0.937
• Length of stay (in days)	9.46 (11.1) [6.0]	9.97 (12.1) [7.0]	0.734
• % re-hospitalized within 30 days or visited the ER within 10 days	14.24 (23.3) [0.0]	8.86 (20.6) [0.0]	0.066
• % re-hospitalized within 90 days	17.41 (25.5) [0.0]	13.51 (24.2) [0.0]	0.235
Day surgery			
At least one day surgery	16.5 (3.8%)	18.2 (5.1%)	0.351
Number of days living at home	351.74 (41.34) [365]	354.53 (36.54) [365]	0.311
Services for frail older people			
At least one visit to the **day hospital** or **day center**	53.1 (12.1%)	26.4 (7.4%)	0.030
At least one use of **help for home maintenance**	261.3 (59.3%)	191.9 (53.9%)	0.127
At least one use of **home help for personal care**	178.4 (40.5%)	117.7 (33.1%)	0.031
At least one use of **services for frail older people** [†]	123.2 (28.0%)	102.6 (28.8%)	0.789
Voluntary services			
At least one **meal** delivered home or one community meal	50.1 (11.4%)	23.6 (6.6%)	0.022
At least one day of **respite care** (hospital or nursing home)	7.1 (1.6%)	13.5 (3.8%)	0.052
At least one hour of **caretaking**	11.3 (2.6%)	18.5 (5.2%)	0.051
At least one use of **voluntary services**[‡]	92.4 (21.0%)	47.6 (13.4%)	0.005

Health professionals			
At least one visit to or by a **GP**	420.1 (95.3 %)	342.2 (96.1 %)	0.589
At least one visit to an **MD specialist**	272.4 (61.8 %)	228.0 (64.0 %)	0.518
At least one visit to or by a **nurse**	320.7 (72.7 %)	203.1 (57.0 %)	<0.001
At least one visit to or by **another health professional** (OT, PT, social worker, …)	192.7 (43.7 %)	126.6 (35.5 %)	0.020

¥ Mean (sd) [median] for continuous variables; $n_{pers-yrs}$ (%) for categorical variables;
† Acute care geriatric assessment, intensive functional rehabilitation, home help for personal care or home maintenance, day hospital or day center.
‡ Meals delivered at home, community meal, accompaniment, community transportation.

be due to the improvement of health services in the area over the years or a trend of overall health improvement in new cohorts of older people. Nevertheless, the fact that 30 % of the participants were admitted to a hospital during the baseline year indicates the frailty of this sample and the probability that they will become clients of the ISD network over the study period.

The PRISMA ISD implementation rate was less than 33 % during the first year. We hypothetized that this type of intervention cannot have an impact if the implementation rate is not at least 70 %. After the first year, we faced the reality that it would be impossible to reach a degree of implementation over 70 % by the end of the second year. As a result, we decided to extend the current study and recruit additional participants to reach sufficient statistical power. With this modification in the study plan, we will now be in a position to effectively detect the impacts of a more fully implemented PRISMA ISD network in the upcoming years. The danger of not extending the study would have been to base conclusions on the impacts of a very partially implemented PRISMA ISD network.

Conclusion

PRISMA is an innovative coordination-type ISD model. Since it is embedded within the usual health-care and social services system, this model could be more appropriate for Canada's universal and publicly funded health-care system than the fully integrated models tested so far. Nevertheless, it requires a shift from the traditional institution-based approach to a client-centered approach and tremendous efforts in coordination at all levels of the organization. The ongoing study will provide data on its impact on client groups and costs.

We are also studying implementation by looking at the process and functioning of the model. The objectives are to document if the model is implemented as planned and to identify the facilitating factors and obstacles to its implementation. An economical analysis will also be performed to calculate the implementation and functioning costs and compare them with the saved costs (if any) in utilization of services. The cost-benefit ratio of such a system will then be documented.

References

1. Hébert R, Durand PJ, Dubuc N, Tourigny A, and the PRISMA Group. PRISMA: a new model of integrated service delivery for the frail older people in Canada. International Journal of Integrated Care [serial online] 2003 March 18:3. Available from: http://www.ijic.org.

2. Tinetti ME, Fried T. The end of disease era. The American Journal of Medicine 2004;116(3):179-85.

3. Bergman H, Béland F, Lebel P, Contandriopoulos AP, Tousignant P, Brunelle Y, et al. Care for Canada's frail elderly population: fragmentation or integration? Canadian Medical Association Journal 1997 Oct 15;157 (8):1116-21.

4. Raîche M, Hébert R. Coordination des services aux personnes âgées en France et au Québec: enjeux, expériences et champs de recherche traitant de leur évaluation [Coordination of services for older people in France and Quebec: concerns, experiences, and research fields for evaluation]. Santé, société et solidarité - Revue de l'Observatoire franco-québécois de la santé et de la solidarité 2003; Numéro hors série:57-66. [in French].

5. Kodner DL, Kyriacou CK. Fully integrated care for frail elderly: two American models. International Journal of Integrated Care [serial online] 2000 Nov 1;1. Available from: http://www.ijic.org.

6. Leutz WN. Five laws for integrating medical and social services: lessons from the United States and the United Kingdom. Milbank Quarterly 1999;77(1):77-110.

7. Yordi CL, Waldman J. A consolidated model of long-term care: service utilization and cost impacts. Gerontologist 1985 Aug;25(4):389-97.

8. Branch LG, Coulam RF, Zimmerman YA. The PACE evaluation: initial findings. Gerontologist 1995 Jun;35(3):349-59.

9. Pinnell Beaulne Associates Ltd. CHOICE Evaluation project. Evaluation summary. Final report, November 26. Edmonton, Alta: Pinnell Beaulne Associates Ltd; 1998.

10. Leutz W, Greenberg R, Abrahams R, Prottas J, Diamond LM, Gruenberg L. Changing health care for an aging society: planning for the Social Health Maintenance Organization. Lexington, Mass., USA: Lexington Books; 1985.

11. Béland F, Bergman H, Lebel P, Clarfield AM, Tousignant P, Contandriopoulos AP, et al. A system of integrated care for older persons with disabilities in Canada: results from a randomized controlled trial. The Journals of Gerontology. Series A, Biological Sciences and Medical Sciences 2006 Apr;61(4):367-73.

12. Johri M, Béland F, Bergman H. International experiments in integrated care for the elderly: a synthesis of the evidence. International Journal of Geriatric Psychiatry 2003 Mar;18(3):222-35.

13. Tourigny A, Durand P, Bonin L, Hébert R, Rochette L. Quasi-experimental study of the effectiveness of an integrated service delivery network for the frail elderly. Canadian Journal on Aging 2004 Fall;23(3):231-46.

14. Hébert R, Veil A. Monitoring the degree of implementation of an integrated delivery system. International Journal of Integrated Care [serial online] 2004 Sept 20; 4. Available from: http://www.ijic.org.

15. Junod B, Wietlisbach V. Méthodes et stratégies d'évaluation du programme national suisse de recherche sur la prévention des maladies cardio-vasculaires. [Methods and evaluation strategies from a Swiss national research program on cardiovascular disease prevention]. Revue Épidémiologie et Santé publique 1981;29: 15-25. [in French].

16. Hébert R, Bravo G, Korner-Bitensky N, Voyer I. Predictive validity of a postal questionnaire for screening community-dwelling elderly individuals at risk of functional decline. Age and Ageing 1996 Mar;25(2):159-67.

17. Hébert R, Guilbault J, Desrosiers J, Dubuc N. The Functional Autonomy Measurement System (SMAF): a clinical-based instrument for measuring disabilities and handicaps in older people. Geriatrics Today: Journal of the Canadian Geriatrics Society 2001 Sep;4:141-7.

18. Hébert R, Carrier R, Bilodeau A. The Functional Autonomy Measurement System (SMAF): description and validation of an instrument for the measurement of handicaps. Age and Ageing 1988 Sep;17(5):293-302.

19. Desrosiers J, Bravo G, Hébert R, Dubuc N. Reliability of the revised functional autonomy measurement system (SMAF) for epidemiological research. Age and Ageing 1995 Sep;24(5):402-6.

20. Hébert R, Spiegelhalter DJ, Brayne C. Setting the minimal metrically detectable change on disability rating scales. Archives of Physical Medicine and Rehabilitation 1997 Dec;78(12):1305-8.

21. Dubuc N, Hébert R, Desrosiers J, Buteau M, Trottier L. Disability-based classification system for older people in integrated long-term care services: the Iso-SMAF profiles. Archives of Gerontology and Geriatrics 2006 Mar-Apr;42(2):191-206.

22. Hébert R, Robichaud L, Roy PM, Bravo G, Voyer L. Efficacy of a nurse-led multidimensional preventive programme for older people at risk of functional decline. A randomized controlled trial. Age and Ageing 2001 Mar;30(2):147-53.

23. Folstein MF, Folstein SE, McHugh PR. "Mini-mental state". A practical method for grading the cognitive state of patients for the clinician. Journal of Psychiatric Research 1975 Nov;12(3):189-98.

24. Gagnon M, Hébert R, Dubé M, Dubois M-F. Development and validation of the Health Care Satisfaction Questionnaire (HCSQ) in elders. Journal of Nursing Measurement 2006 Winter;14(3):190-204.

25. Gagnon M, Hébert R, Dubé M, Dubois M-F. Development and validation of an instrument measuring individual empowerment in relation to personal health care: the Health Care Empowerment Questionnaire (HCEQ). American Journal of Health Promotion 2006 Jul-Aug;20(6):429-35.

26. Hébert R, Bravo G, Girouard D. Fidélité de la traduction française de trois instruments d'évaluation des aidants naturels de malades déments. [Reliability of French translation for three evaluation instruments related to demented natural caregivers]. Canadian Journal on Aging 1993;12(3):324-37. [in French].

27. Zarit SH, Orr NK, Zarit JM. The hidden victims of Alzheimer's disease: families under stress. New York: New York University Press; 1985.

28. Hébert R, Bravo G, Préville M. Reliability, validity and reference values of the Zarit Burden Interview for assessing informal caregivers of community-dwelling older persons with dementia. Canadian Journal on Aging 2000;19(4):494-507.

29. Morycz RK. Caregiving strain and the desire to institutionalize family members with Alzheimer's disease. Possible predictors and model development. Research on Aging 1985 Sep;7(3):329-61.

30. Canadian study on health and aging working group. CSHA Working Group. Canadian Study on Health and Aging: study methods and prevalence of dementia. Canadian Medical Association Journal 1994;150(6):899-913.

31. Dubois M-F, Raîche M, Hébert R, Gueye NR. Assisted self-report of health-services use showed excellent reliability in a longitudinal study of older adults. Journal of Clinical Epidemiology 2007 Oct;60(10):1040-5.

PRISMA (Program of Research to Integrate the Services for the Maintenance of Autonomy) is a Canadian partnership between two research teams (Research Centre on Aging in Sherbrooke and Laval University Geriatric Research Team in Quebec City) and several health organizations in the Province of Quebec: Ministry of Health and Social Services, five Regional Health and Social Services Agencies (Estrie, Mauricie–Centre-du-Québec, Laval, Montérégie, Quebec City), and the Sherbrooke Geriatric University Institute. PRISMA is funded by the Canadian Health Services Research Foundation, the Fonds de la recherche en santé du Québec (FRSQ), and the partnering organizations. The effectiveness study reported in this paper is funded by the Canadian Institutes of Health Research, the Ministry of Health and Social Services, and the Estrie Regional Health and Social Services Agency.

* **The PRISMA-Estrie Group: List of members (all are from Canada)**
From the *Research Centre on Aging, Sherbrooke Geriatric University Institute / Faculty of Medicine and Health Sciences, Université de Sherbrooke*: Gina Bravo, Chantal Caron, Johanne Desrosiers, Michel Tousignant; / *Faculty of Administration:* Danièle Blanchette; from the *Laval University Geriatric Research Team*: André Tourigny, Lucie Bonin, Pierre Durand; from the *Research Centre on Aging, Sherbrooke Geriatric University Institute*: Myriam Bergeron, Marie-Claude Boissé, Suzanne Durand, Maxime Gagnon, N'Deye Rokhaya Gueye, Valérie Guillot, Nathalie-Audrey Joly, Isabelle Labrecque, Dany Simard, Anne Veil, Karine Veilleux; from the *Health and Social Services Centre – Sherbrooke Geriatric University Institute*: Céline Bureau; respectively from the Coaticook (JB) and Granit (RB, PR, MB) *Health and Social Services Centre*: Johanne Bolduc, Robert Bellefleur, Pierre Richard, Mariette Bédard; from the *Estrie Health and Social Services regional Agency*: Linda Dieleman; from the *Québec Ministry of Health and Social Services*: Lysette Trahan and William Murray.

Appendix 11.1

Characteristics of both groups at baseline, by sub area

Variable	Urban environment		Rural environment with hospital		Rural environment without hospital	
	Experimental	Control	Experimental	Control	Experimental	Control
Baseline characteristics of the subjects	(n = 205)	(n = 176)	(n = 154)	(n = 120)	(n = 142)	(n = 123)
Age on January 1, 2001	83.16 (4.62)*	82.11 (4.84)**	82.74 (4.56)	82.93 (4.85)	84.09 (5.44)	82.63 (5.61)**
Female	151 (73.7 %)	102 (58.0 %)***	75 (48.7 %)	77 (64.2 %)**	95 (66.9 %)	73 (59.4 %)
Married	73 (35.6 %)	85 (48.3 %)**	88 (57.1 %)	45 (37.5 %)***	55 (38.7 %)	55 (44.7 %)
Years of education	7.42 (3.29)	7.87 (3.60)	5.68 (2.66)	6.01 (2.62)	6.08 (2.76)	5.48 (2.56)*
Excellent or good health status§	127 (62.3 %)	113 (65.3 %)	101 (66.0 %)	72 (60.0 %)	92 (65.7 %)	73 (59.8 %)
Homeowner or tenant	128 (62.4 %)	126 (71.6 %)*	103 (66.9 %)	82 (68.3 %)	72 (50.7 %)	91 (74.0 %)***
Has an informal caregiver	177 (86.3 %)	151 (85.8 %)	143 (92.9 %)	105 (87.5 %)	132 (93.0 %)	113 (91.9 %)
Hospitalized in the last 6 months	53 (25.9 %)	55 (31.3 %)	44 (28.6 %)	35 (29.2 %)	51 (36.4 %)	30 (24.4 %)**
Home care services in the last 6 months	32 (15.6 %)	49 (27.8 %)***	34 (22.2 %)	35 (29.2 %)	38 (27.0 %)	42 (34.2 %)
Disability (SMAF)	17.44 (11.96)	18.72 (11.58)	19.22 (11.56)	21.51 (14.53)	19.38 (11.79)	20.11 (12.98)
Cognitive functioning (MMSE)	25.31 (4.57)	24.81 (5.80)	24.15 (5.28)	24.04 (5.71)	24.87 (4.81)	23.94 (6.08)
Satisfaction with health services	7.64 (2.55)	7.91 (3.02)	7.47 (2.20)	8.39 (2.65)***	7.50 (2.32)	7.66 (2.61)
Empowerment	8.08 (2.63)	8.36 (2.92)	7.81 (2.16)	7.81 (2.30)	7.28 (2.43)	8.03 (2.91)
Baseline characteristics of the informal caregiver	(n = 161)	(n = 125)	(n = 127)	(n = 80)	(n = 121)	(n = 101)
Female	105 (65.2 %)	101 (80.8 %)***	102 (80.3 %)	61 (76.3 %)	89 (73.6 %)	79 (78.2 %)
Relationship with the care-receiver Spouse	44 (27.3 %)	49 (39.2 %)	69 (54.3 %)	29 (36.3 %)	25 (20.7 %)	35 (34.7 %)
Child	90 (55.9 %)	60 (48.0 %)*	42 (33.1 %)	40 (50.0 %)**	74 (61.2 %)	51 (50.5 %)*
Other	27 (16.8 %)	16 (12.8 %)	16 (12.6 %)	11 (13.8 %)	22 (18.2 %)	15 (14.9 %)
Living with the care-receiver	64 (39.8 %)	83 (66.4 %)***	77 (60.6 %)	52 (65.0 %)	41 (34.2 %)	66 (66.0 %)***
Burden (Zarit Burden Interview)	18.88 (16.41)	19.23 (14.49)	15.79 (13.90)	20.72 (17.71)**	16.74 (13.64)	20.73 (17.32)*
Desire to institutionalize †	29 (19.3 %)	19 (18.5 %)	15 (12.6 %)	9 (12.9 %)	18 (16.2 %)	17 (18.5 %)

First year changes on outcomes (a negative sign indicates decline)	(n = 171)	(n = 139)	(n = 135)	(n = 95)	(n = 114)	(n = 93)
Functional independence	-1.83 (6.44)	-1.33 (5.76)	-1.49 (5.89)	-1.48 (5.36)	-2.26 (5.77)	-2.92 (7.61)
Cognitive functioning	0.02 (2.46)	0.04 (4.57)	0.14 (3.01)	-1.02 (4.44)**	-0.64 (2.79)	-1.41 (4.29)
Satisfaction with health services	-0.21 (2.87)	0.39 (3.30)**	0.75 (2.37)	-0.36 (2.66)**	0.30 (2.51)	0.30 (2.35)
Empowerment	-0.76 (3.72)	-1.02 (3.86)	0.09 (2.68)	-0.65 (3.30)	-0.29 (2.57)	-0.63 (3.33)
Burden (any caregiver)	3.29 (13.62)	2.31 (12.46)	3.59 (11.11)	-0.84 (12.75)**	0.39 (13.30)	3.00 (13.21)**
Burden (same caregiver)	3.33 (13.70)	2.05 (12.55)	2.54 (10.65)	-1.16 (11.96)	0.78 (12.01)	3.15 (12.12)**
Desire to institutionalize ‡ (any cg)	18.4 % to 24.0 %	17.5 % to 25.0 %	13.1 % to 16.2 %	12.3 % to 10.5 %	16.1 % to 15.1 %	19.4 % to 25.0 %

¥ Mean (sd) for continuous variables; n(%) for categorical variables;

* p<0.10; **p<0.05; ***p<0.01

§ Subjective health status compared to others of the same age.

† Has thought about it somewhat seriously, has discussed it with someone, has visited an institution, or has applied for placement.

‡ Has thought about it somewhat seriously, has discussed it with someone, has visited an institution, has applied for placement, or has institutionalized.

⁻ p-values are derived from an analysis of covariance comparing posttest scores, adjusting for baseline scores.

Appendix 11.2
Use of services for both groups, by sub area, during the first year

Variable	Urban environment		Rural environment with hospital		Rural environment without hospital	
	Experimental (npers-yrs = 182.99)	Control (npers-yrs = 152.24)	Experimental (npers-yrs = 136.44)	Control (npers-yrs = 101.65)	Experimental (npers-yrs = 121.49)	Control (npers-yrs = 102.32)
Emergency room (ER) visits						
At least 1 visit to the ER	78.8 (43.1%)¥	46.0 (30.2%)**	68.7 (50.3%)	31.8 (31.3%)***	60.0 (49.4%)	28.2 (27.6%)***
Among users:						
- Number of visits	2.06 (2.3) [1.06]	2.20 (2.2) [1.03]	2.24 (2.1) [1.05]	1.98 (1.9) [1.03]	2.17 (1.9) [1.22]	1.84 (1.5) [1.09]
- % followed by a hospitalization	41.65 (43.3) [25.0]	53.12 (42.3) [50.0]	46.64 (42.9) [40.0]	55.80 (47.3) [50.0]	36.97 (41.4) [0.0]	67.23 (49.7) [100]***
- % return within 10 days	9.08 (20.4) [0.0]	12.38 (28.6) [0.0]	13.94 (26.1) [0.0]	5.31 (22.1) [0.0]	11.12 (23.2) [0.0]	8.91 (17.1) [0.0]
Hospitalizations						
At least 1 hospitalization	46.9 (25.6%)	43.9 (28.8%)	57.4 (42.1%)	26.2 (25.8%)***	40.8 (33.6%)	28.6 (28.0%)
Among users:						
- Number of hospitalizations	1.88 (1.6) [1.1]	2.26 (2.1) [1.2]	1.82 (1.5) [1.0]	1.65 (1.5) [1.0]	2.01 (1.6) [1.1]	1.50 (1.1) [1.0]
- Length of stay (in days)	11.21 (12.2) [7.0]	10.71 (9.9) [7.0]	8.49 (9.1) [6.0]	7.78 (6.4) [7.0]	8.80 (12.1) [5.0]	10.83 (17.7) [6.0]
- % re-hospitalized within 30 days or visited the ER within 10 days	12.70 (21.2) [0.0]	11.15 (19.6) [0.0]	11.88 (21.9) [0.0]	9.32 (24.4) [0.0]	19.29 (27.1) [0.0]	4.96 (18.5) [0.0]**
- % re-hospitalized within 90 days	17.20 (25.2) [0.0]	19.15 (27.0) [0.0]	14.56 (23.5) [0.0]	7.99 (19.5) [0.0]	21.59 (28.5) [0.0]	9.72 (22.7) [0.0]*
Day surgery						
At least 1 day surgery	4.8 (2.6%)	3.0 (2.0%)	5.9 (4.3%)	8.4 (8.3%)	5.9 (4.9%)	6.8 (6.6%)
Number of days living at home	353.3 (37.9) [365]	353.2 (35.1) [365]	351.7 (37.4) [365]	356.6 (34.5) [365]	349.4 (49.7) [365]	354.5 (40.6) [365]
Services for frail older people						
At least 1 visit to the **day hospital** or **day center**	18.3 (10.0%)	13.5 (8.9%)	18.6 (13.6%)	4.9 (4.8%)**	16.3 (13.4%)	7.9 (7.7%)
At least 1 use of **help for home maintenance**	113.8 (62.2%)	83.6 (54.9%)	73.3 (53.8%)	57.0 (56.1%)	74.2 (61.1%)	51.3 (50.1%)
At least 1 use of **home help for personal care**	65.6 (35.9%)	46.5 (30.5%)	58.2 (42.6%)	37.7 (37.1%)	54.6 (44.9%)	33.6 (32.8%)*

At least 1 use of **services for frail older people** †	37.3 (20.4 %)	43.5 (28.6 %)*	45.3 (33.2 %)	26.0 (25.6 %)	40.6 (33.5 %)	33.1 (32.4 %)
Voluntary services						
At least 1 **meal** delivered home or one community meal	23.9 (13.0 %)	15.2 (10.0 %)	13.1 9.6 %	3.9 (3.8 %)	13.1 (10.8 %)	4.6 (4.5 %)*
At least 1 day of **respite care**	1.7 (0.9 %)	4.8 (3.1 %)	0.1 0.1 %	4.0 (4.8 %)**	5.2 (4.3 %)	3.8 (3.7 %)
At least one hour of **caretaking**	3.8 (2.1 %)	1.7 (1.1 %)	4.6 4.4 %	3.3 (8.2 %)	2.8 (2.3 %)	8.5 (8.3 %)**
At least one use of **voluntary services** ‡	49.0 (26.8 %)**	25.0 (16.4 %)**	24.3 (17.3 %)	13.6 (13.4 %)	19.1 (15.7 %)	9.0 (8.8 %)
Health professionals						
At least 1 visit to or by a **GP**	175.9 (96.1 %)	143.0 (97.2 %)	128.8 (94.4 %)	94.5 (93.3 %)	115.4 (95.0 %)	99.3 (97.0 %)
At least 1 visit to a **MD specialist**	125.8 (68.8 %)	114.8 (75.4 %)	82.7 (60.6 %)	52.3 51.5 %	63.8 (52.5 %)	60.9 (59.5 %)
At least 1 visit to or by a **nurse**	117.1 (64.0 %)	83.5 (54.9 %)*	107.3 (78.6 %)	55.5 (54.6 %)***	96.3 (79.3 %)	64.1 (62.6 %)***
At least 1 visit to or by **another health professional**	84.4 (46.1 %)	59.5 (39.1 %)	55.4 (40.6 %)	36.3 (35.7 %)	52.9 (43.5 %)	30.8 (30.1 %)**

¥ Mean (sd) [median] for continuous variables; $n_{pers-yrs}$ (%) for categorical variables;   *p<0.10; **p<0.05; ***p<0.01

† Acute care geriatric assessment, intensive functional rehabilitation, home help for personal care or home maintenance, day hospital or day center.

‡ Meals delivered at home, community meal, accompaniment, community transportation.

Chapter 12
Impact of the PRISMA-Estrie Integrated Service Delivery Network on the Elderly and their Informal Caregivers

Réjean Hébert, Michel Raîche, Marie-France Dubois, Nicole Dubuc, Michel Tousignant, N'Deye Rokhaya Gueye, and the PRISMA-Estrie group

Highlights

- We present here the extension of our impact study.
- The chapter presents our findings for the four years of the study for sets of variables examined in relation to both the elderly and their caregivers: in relation to the elderly, the variables were functional decline, death, disabilities, level of handicap, institutionalization, satisfaction with services, and empowerment; in relation to caregivers, the variables were the caregiver burden and caregivers' wish to institutionalize elders.
- When differences are observed, the chapter presents concise overviews according to MRC.

Introduction

Service integration represents an intervention in service organization designed to benefit the elderly and their informal caregivers. This chapter reviews the impact of the implemented integrated service delivery (ISD) network on the elderly and their informal caregivers. In the previous chapter (11), we presented the study methodology and the baseline data from the study's first year. These data allowed for a description of the situation at the outset in the experimental and comparison zones; subsequent developments are to be viewed in their light. In the present chapter, we review the impact of the four years of the study on the elderly and those close to them.

It should be recalled that what we were measuring is impact on population. That is, it is not possible to determine whether a given component of the ISD for the elderly (hereafter, RISPA; French *réseau integré de services pour personnes âgées*) produced a given impact on a given individual in Estrie. Rather, what can be determined is RISPA's impact on the population once implemented as a whole, according to degree of implementation as measured over the course of the study (see Chapter 2.) The Estrie experimental group was exposed to integration levels of 69 % to 85 % from Year 3 of the study.

Methodology

Study Extension

Under the initial study design, it was expected RISPA would be almost fully implemented over the course of the study's first two years. However, the calculation of degrees of implementation during the implementation study made it clear after Year 1 that the target would not be reached by the end of Year 2. It thus became imperative to extend the impact study in order to be able to assess the effects of a more fully implemented integrated services network. Otherwise, we risked reaching conclusions based on less than 50 % implementation.

In light of this anticipated delay in implementation, the research team decided at the end of 2002 to ask subjects to extend their participation in the study for two years. These initial participants constituted what we called Cohort A. The high levels of mortality and institutionalization made it likely that, at the end of four years of the study, based on that cohort alone, we would not have adequate statistical power to draw conclusions about RISPA's effects. We therefore recruited a second cohort of participants, Cohort B, during 2003 and early 2004. Figure 12.1 presents our final summary diagram of the study. As seen there, 829 participants stayed in the in-home study until the end, a sufficient number to allow us to draw conclusions on the impact of RISPA once implemented.

Figure 12.1
Diagram of Extended Study

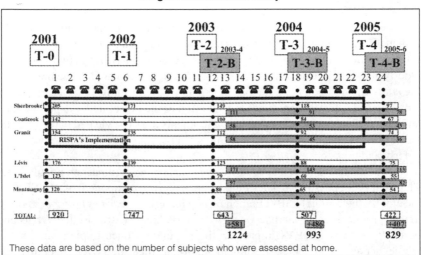

These data are based on the number of subjects who were assessed at home.

Subjects in Cohort B were recruited in exactly the same way as those in Cohort A had been (see Chapter 11), except that the age criterion for study participation was raised by two years to reflect the two years the study had already been under way. We used the same postal-questionnaire technique to identify elders at risk of functional decline.[1] Over the two waves of recruitment among the 20,000 individuals aged at least 75 who lived in the six MRCs covered by the study, 7,790 randomly chosen individuals received the questionnaire (MRC: *municipalité régionale de comté*, or regional municipal county). Of those identified as being at risk of functional decline, 1,501 (920 in 2001 and 581 in 2003) were recruited for the study (see Figure 12.2). For the Coaticook MRC we cannot refer to a sample; rather, the whole population was studied, since all the 1018 non-institutionalized individuals aged 75 and over as of 2001 (and 77 and over as of 2003) received the postal questionnaire.

Figure 12.2
Diagram of atudy-population selection – 2001 and 2003

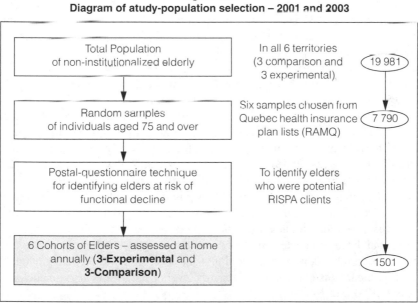

Variables Measured in Relation to Elders and Their Informal Caregivers

The variables measured, for which our findings are presented in this chapter, were:

- Death or institutionalization, institutionalization being defined as admission to a residential and long-term care centre (CHSLD; French *centre d'hébergement et de soins de longue durée*), whether public, private and under agreement, or private and not under agreement.

- Functional autonomy, measured using the Functional Autonomy Measurement System (SMAF; French name *Système de mesure de l'autonomie fonctionnelle*),[2] which measures disabilities and handicap level.
- Satisfaction with health services delivered, measured by means of Gagnon and colleagues'[3] satisfaction questionnaire.
- Empowerment of the elderly, measured by means of Gagnon and colleagues' empowerment questionnaire[4].
- The informal caregiver's burden, measured by means of the Zarit[5, 6] Caregiver's Burden Inventory.
- The informal caregiver's desire to institutionalize the elder, measured by means of the questionnaire on desire to institutionalize[7] as used and translated in the "Canadian Study on Health and Aging[8]."

Over the course of the study's four years, these variables were measured with the methodology which is presented in Chapter 11 of this book, where details are given about the measurement instruments used, their properties, and measurement scales. Here, we will provide some further details regarding SMAF and how it can be used to measure handicap level. SMAF allows for gathering information on resources (informal caregivers and public, private, or community-based service providers) that offer the user assistance, partial aid, and full aid. With this information it is possible to arrive at a handicap score, which indicates the extent to which needed services are not being provided. When subjects have all the resources they need, the handicap score is zero. A subject must be receiving assistance that fully meets quality and safety requirements to receive a handicap score of zero. If a subject only has access to a portion of the resources needed or has no resources at all with which to compensate for disabilities, the handicap score is equal to the disability score.

Using all the variables measured, it is possible to measure progress in each experimental and comparison territory, compare their progress over the study's four years, and identify any differences. Note, however, that the measurement of the handicap score was introduced into the study at T-1. We don't have that information for T-0, when the initial in-home interview was relatively lengthy. Thus comparisons of progress as regards level of handicap can be made only between T-1 and T-4.

Types of Statistical Analyses

Survival Curves

Survival probability is analyzed with Kaplan-Meier curves. Subjects with whom contact had been lost and those still alive at the most recent time of measurement were removed as of the date of the most recent information available. We used the same kind of analysis to monitor admission to CHSLDs and referred to it as the probability of maintenance in home. Thus, subjects who died at home, those with whom contact had been lost, and those who were still living at home at the study's end were removed. Then, comparisons and tests were done between findings for the experimental and the comparison zones with respect to the proportion of subjects still alive or not yet institutionalized. Cohorts A and B were evaluated separately in these analyses, since they began participating in the study two years apart and since 100 % of both cohorts consisted of subjects living at home. Each one subsequently lost subjects to death and institutionalization. The two groups were compared using a Cox regression designed to estimate a hazard ratio with a confidence interval (CI) of 95 %.

Proportion of Subjects Experiencing Functional Decline

Functional decline is a composite variable consisting of one of these three events: 1) death; 2) institutionalization; or 3) loss of five SMAF points or more over a period of a year. The threshold of SMAF points was determined during previous studies to constitute a clinically and metrically significant difference.[9] Decline is a dichotomous variable. Each year, it is possible to determine the proportion of subjects in each group that has declined or not. The difference between groups was analyzed with a chi-square test.

Continuous Variables

Under this study's initial two-year plan, comparisons between the experimental and comparison groups were to have been conducted for continuous variables (e.g., SMAF scores) by means of repeated measures analyses of variance. However, analyses of this kind require complete follow-up for all subjects. Once the study was extended by two years, this kind of analysis became inappropriate, since a large proportion of subjects died or were institutionalized over the course of the study.

Growth models, also known as multilevel models of change, were used to examine the evolution of continuous variables over the course of the five years of the PRISMA-Estrie study. These models take into account intra- and inter-individual changes; they also allow for adding subjects during different assessment waves (which makes it possible to analyze Cohorts A and B simultaneously even though they joined the study at different times). These growth models also allow for using all the information obtained from subjects who died or were institutionalized during the course of the study. When the straight line or curve of evolution is determined for a continuous variable like SMAF, subjects that were measured only once are included in the estimate of the intercept. All subjects measured more than once are taken into account in estimating the slope. To determine the shape of SMAF's evolution using the four measurement times distributed over five years, cubic, quadratic, and linear models were compared. We retained the one that fit the data best.

Recall that what interested us was the impact of implementing integrated networks on evolution trajectories. Since the implementation of the integrated network's various components took place on fixed dates, it is more appropriate to examine subject evolution in relation to those dates than in relation to artificial measurement-wave numbers (0, 1, 2, 3, 4) linked to very different dates for different subjects. Therefore, we opted to use the number of days from January 1, 2001, as the measure of time for our growth models.

Findings

We present here our findings for the study's four years. It should be recalled that differences in favor of the comparison zone were observed during the study's first year for variables measured among the elderly and their natural caregivers. Subjects in the comparison zone were more satisfied with health services delivered to them than those in the experimental zone. The result was precisely the same for the empowerment scores. Certain differences must be taken into account in interpreting the analyses. More people lived in collective housing in Estrie at the start of the study (35.1 % in Estrie versus 22.2 % in Chaudière-Appalaches, $p < 0.001$). Collective housing included family-type facilities, private lodging houses with nine residents or fewer, private residences for the elderly, and intermediate-type facilities. Of these types of collective housing, private residences for the elderly were the kind that most participants lived in. At T-0, in the comparison zone, more subjects lived with their informal caregivers (who were usually female).

To make it easier to present our findings, we have assigned the code letter X to the experimental group (in the Estrie health administration region) and the code letter C to the comparison group (in the Chaudière-Appalaches health administration region). The three p values found in the curves indicate the results of the three statistical tests for evolution over four years. The first two values relate to each group's evolution in relation to itself (e.g., "If there has been an increase, is the increase significant?"); the third relates to a comparison of each group's evolution to the others. A p value of less than 0.05 indicates a significant result. We also compared the groups for each year. Significant results are indicated above the abscissa.

General Evolution in the Experimental and Comparison Groups

Figure 12.3 presents the general evolution of the experimental and comparison groups. Subjects who were institutionalized, had died, were impossible to assess (e.g., because they were dying or hospitalized for an extended period), were in an unknown condition (e.g., had dropped out, had moved away from the study zone, were lost sight of), or who refused to participate are indicated for each measurement time and group.

Probability of Death and Living at Home

The analyses revealed no significant differences between the experimental and comparison zones for proportions of deaths. This applies to both cohorts A and

Figure 12.3
General evolution of experimental and comparison cohorts

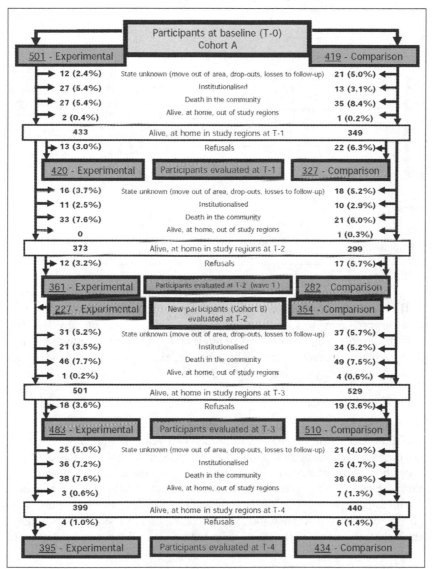

B (see Figure 12.4). In any case, it was not expected that any noticeable effect on mortality attributable to RISPA would be observed in the course of the study's four years.

Admission to CHSLDs could have been affected by RISPA's implementation. However, no significant difference was observed between the experimen-

Figure 12.4
Survival Curves

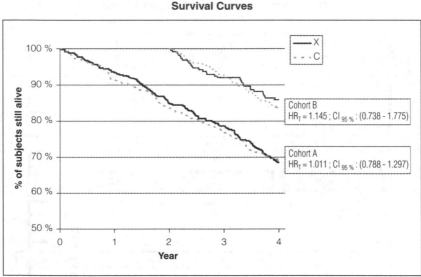

tal and the comparison zones, although small trend reversals could be observed in the A cohorts over the four years (see Figure 12.5). A trend favorable to the experimental zone was observed among individuals who initially had Iso-SMAF[10] profiles with high indices of required level of care (profiles 4 and up). Although institutionalization may have been slightly delayed at the end of Year 3, by the end of Year 4, it had not been avoided.

Functional Decline

To highlight the effects of different implementation stages on results, we compared the study's first two years to its last two years. It was thus possible to contrast the implementation period with the period when the effects of implementation could be counted on showing up. Of course, deceased and institutionalized subjects were no longer exposed to RISPA. Living and non-institutionalized subjects, whether they had lost five SMAF points or not, were still exposed to RISPA. Therefore, results for the study's last two years relate to these subjects and to the B cohorts recruited two years following the start of the study.

During the first two years, no significant difference was observable between the experimental and comparison zones. In contrast, a significant difference of 6.3 % in the experimental zone's favor could be observed during the last two years. The difference derives mainly from the five-point SMAF difference (p = 0.027; see Figure 12.6).

Figure 12.5
Probability of living at home

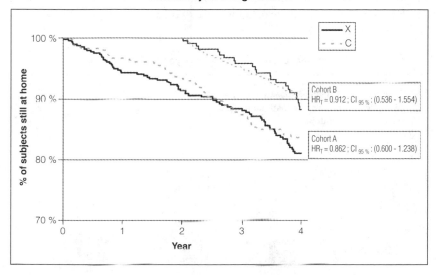

Figure 12.6
Functional decline in first two years as contrasted with last two years

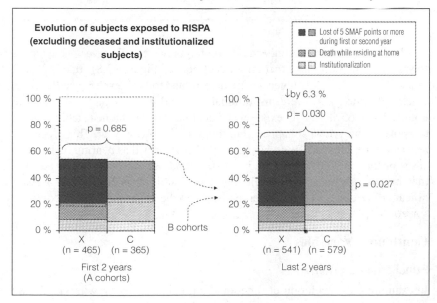

These significant differences observed during the study's first two years can also be seen in trends for years 3 and 4, when the effects of implemented RISPA are factored out of the data for those two years (see Figure 12.7).

Figure 12.7
Functional decline over the four years of follow-up

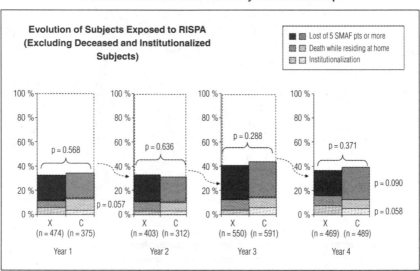

If we study the results under a different light, we can observe what happens to subjects who have not experienced decline (see Figure 12.8). Taking Year 1 as an example, 35 % of subjects were determined to have experienced decline, whether because they were institutionalized, had died, or had lost 5 SMAF points. About 65 % had not experienced decline: They remained stable and it is possible to observe what happened to them the following year. This process is repeated for each year. This analysis could be described as bearing on incident cases of functional decline. One interesting finding, even taking into account that this analysis relates to a smaller number of subjects, is that, in Year 4, a significant difference, 14 %, is observed between the experimental and comparison zones (p < 0.001).

Continuous Variables

Functional Autonomy

In examining the evolution of functional autonomy using growth models, we observe that subjects in the experimental and comparison groups experienced a significant increase in disabilities (see Figure 12.9). No significant difference is observable between the two zones.

Figure 12.8
Functional decline over the four years of follow-up

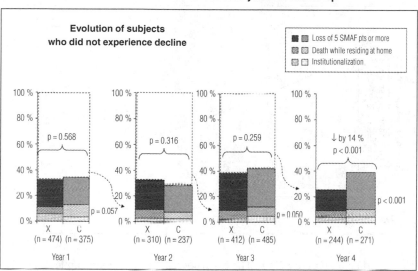

Figure 12.9
Evolution of functional autonomy (disabilities)

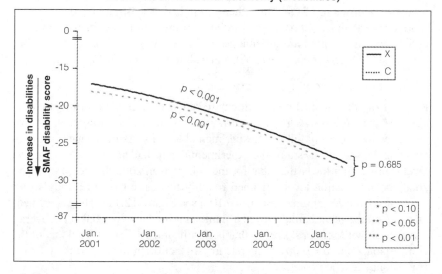

Handicap Scores

At the outset, subjects in the experimental group had handicap scores significantly greater than for the comparison group ($p < 0.001$). In comparing the evolution of the two groups, we observe significantly different trajectories

Figure 12.10
Evolution of handicap scores

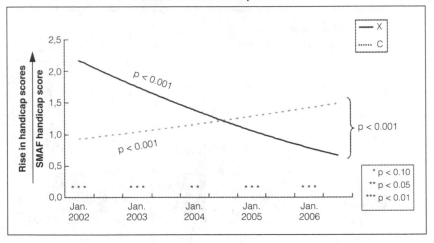

(p < 0.001) (see Figure 12.10). The experimental group's handicap levels underwent progressive reduction over the course of the study (p < 0.001), whereas that of the comparison group rose slightly (p < 0.001). Descriptive analyses carried out at the last measurement time show that 35 % of subjects in the experimental group, as opposed to 67 % in the other group, had at least one handicap, i.e., a score higher than zero. For subjects in both groups, the items for which unmet needs occur most often are grooming (25 %), washing (13 %), vision (11 %), hearing (16 %), bowel function (5 %), and walking outside (5 %).

Satisfaction with Health Services

Results from the satisfaction questionnaire can be examined according to overall score or by the *service delivery* and *service organization* subscales, the two subscales most closely linked to experimental actions. As mentioned in Chapter 11, at the start of the study, the experimental zone had an overall satisfaction level significantly lower than that for the comparison zone. In the comparison zone, the satisfaction level remained roughly the same over the study's four years (non-significant reduction, p = 0.107; see Figure 12.11). The experimental zone, on the other hand, showed a significant increase (p < 0.001) in overall satisfaction with services, a result that is significantly different from that of the comparison zone (p < 0.001). The rise in satisfaction in the experimental zone corresponds to a percentage of 5 %.

A look at the results for *service delivery* shows significantly reduced satisfaction in the comparison zone and a trajectory in the opposite direction in the experimental zone, resulting in significantly different evolution profiles for the two zones (see Figure 12.12-A).

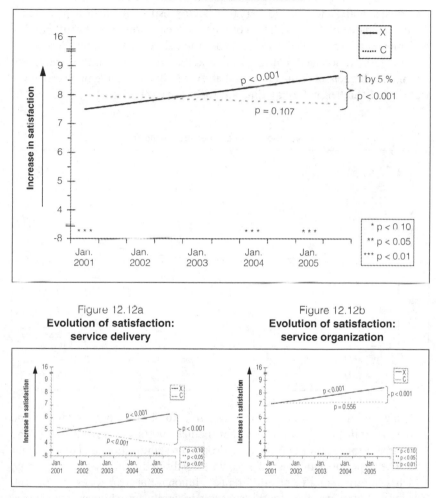

Figure 12.11
Evolution of overall satisfaction

Figure 12.12a
**Evolution of satisfaction:
service delivery**

Figure 12.12b
**Evolution of satisfaction:
service organization**

A look at the results for *service organization* shows that the departure points were identical in the two zones (see Figure 12.12-B). The satisfaction level is seen to remain constant in the comparison zone, whereas it rose significantly in the experimental zone. This yields significantly different evolution profiles when the two zones are compared.

Empowerment of the Elderly

Results from the empowerment questionnaire can be examined according to overall score or by the *level of control* and *involvement in decision making* subscales, the two subscales most closely linked to experimental actions. At the outset, a significant difference in overall empowerment is observed between the two zones (see Figure 12.13). Subsequently, reduced empowerment can be observed in both zones, but recovery then occurs, especially in the experimental zone. Comparison of the evolution of the two zones shows significantly different trajectories ($p < 0.001$): In the experimental zone, the initial downward slope is less pronounced; but the decline is then reversed, with the trajectory ending at a higher score than it started at. At the study's end, empowerment is significantly higher in the experimental zone ($p = 0.003$).

Figure 12.13
Evolution of overall empowerment

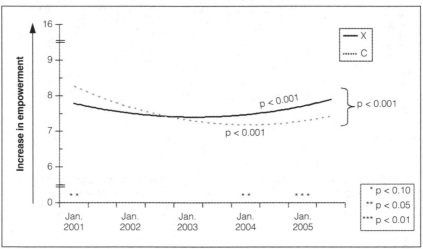

In examining results for *level of control*, we observe that the level at the start was significantly lower in the experimental zone (see Figure 12.14-A). The comparison zone shows a pronounced drop, then stabilization, and then a slight rise. The experimental zone goes down slightly and then rises significantly, which results in a significantly different evolution for the two zones ($p < 0.001$). The level of empowerment for this subscale is significantly higher in the experimental zone at the study's end ($p < 0.001$).

An examination for the results for *involvement in decision making* reveals no significant difference between the two zones at the outset (see Figure 12.14-B). We then see a decline in levels of empowerment in both zones for this subscale; but then there is recovery, especially in the experimental zone. Comparison of the evolution of the two zones shows significantly different trajectories ($p < 0.001$): In the experimental zone, the initial downward slope is less pronounced; the decline is then reversed and there is a slight climb towards the end of the study. For this subscale, the degree of empowerment is

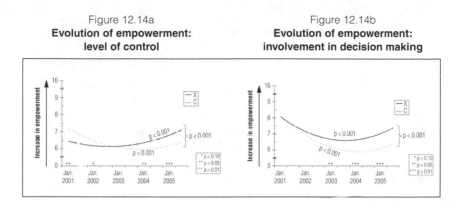

Figure 12.14a
**Evolution of empowerment:
level of control**

Figure 12.14b
**Evolution of empowerment:
involvement in decision making**

significantly higher in the experimental zone than in the comparison zone at the end of the study ($p = 0.001$).

Caregiver's Burden and Desire to Institutionalize

The number of informal caregivers who responded to the questionnaire on burden and desire to institutionalize at each measurement time is presented in Table 12.1.

Table 12.1
**Number of Informal Caregivers Who Responded to the Questionnaire
at Each Measurement Time**

	T-0	T-1	T-2	T-3	T-4
Experimental Group					
Number of subjects	501	420	588	483	395
Number of caregivers	405	351	509	415	333
%	80.8 %	83.6 %	86.6 %	85.9 %	84.3 %
Comparison Group					
Number of subjects	419	327	636	510	432
Number of caregivers	305	263	482	359	308
%	72.8 %	80.4 %	75.8 %	70.4 %	71.3 %

The caregiver's burden was significantly lower in the experimental zone at the start of this study. Close examination of this finding shows that the difference is produced by experimental subjects living in private settings (in their own house or apartment or as sole lodgers). The burden score for such subjects was 15.1, as compared with experimental subjects living in collective settings (for all intents and purposes, private residences for the elderly). These subjects had a burden score comparable to that for the comparison zone, which was 18.6. Supplementary analyses revealed no associated factors (e.g., disabilities). During the four subsequent years, the comparison zone showed a trend to a slight

Figure 12.15
Evolution of caregiver's burden

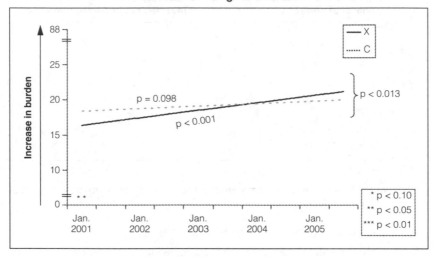

increase in burden, but it wasn't significant ($p = 0.098$). During the same period, the experimental zone showed a significant increase in burden ($p < 0.001$); its score came to equal that of the comparison zone (see Figure 12.15).

The findings for caregiver's burden must be examined jointly with those for the caregiver's desire to institutionalize the elder. (The ways this desire is known are that the caregiver has mentioned it to someone, has visited a facility, has made an application for placement, or has already institutionalized the elder.) In theory, an informal caregiver who has experienced an increased perceived burden might be expected to present with an increase in the desire to institutionalize; but this was not the case. At the start, there was no difference between the two zones in levels of desire to institutionalize. Subsequently, levels of desire to institutionalize rose in exactly the same way in the two zones (see Figure 12.16), with no significant difference being observed throughout the study.

Findings by MRC

We examined our findings by MRC (or territory), i.e., by comparing the paired MRCs of Sherbrooke and Lévis (urban settings), Coaticook and L'Islet (rural settings with no local hospital), and Granit and Montmagny (rural setting with local hospital). However, account should be taken of the fact that the comparisons relate to smaller subgroups, which reduces the statistical power for the detection of significant difference. Overall, the majority of comparisons by paired locations reflect the results obtained in comprehensive comparisons of the experimental and comparison zones. We here present only the findings for

Figure 12.16
Evolution of caregiver's desire to institutionalize elder

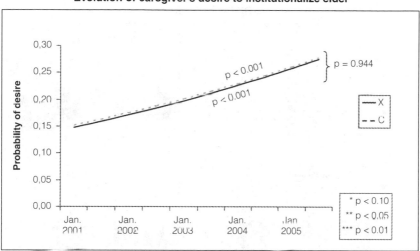

the paired cities for which noteworthy significant and distinct differences are observable.

A breakdown of the effect on functional decline shows differing results by MRC (see Figures 12.17 and 12.18). The reduction in the rate of functional decline observed overall is evident, especially in Sherbrooke – Lévis; the other MRCs did not present these differences.

The subscale for *service organization* in the satisfaction-measurement instrument shows noteworthy effects by MRC (see Figure 12.19). All the experimental MRCs saw a significant rise in satisfaction levels for service organization. However, for two pairs of territories, levels were not comparable at the outset: They were significantly higher in Lévis than Sherbrooke and lower in L'Islet than Coaticook. A significant positive effect of RISPA is observable in Sherbrooke and Granit, whereas there is no significant impact in Coaticook when it is compared with its twinned location of L'Islet.

Discussion

Discussion of Variables Measured

Two recent Quebec studies on service integration have reached completion and can therefore be compared with our study's results on elders and those close to them. According to the three-level approach to integration developed by Leutz[11] (linkage, coordination, full integration), the PRISMA-Estrie study, like the Bois-Francs study,[12, 13] related to a coordination model, while the SIPA study (SIPA stands for *services intégrés pour personnes âgées en perte d'autonomie*, or

Figure 12.17
**Evolution of functional decline in subjects exposed
to RISPA, by territory**

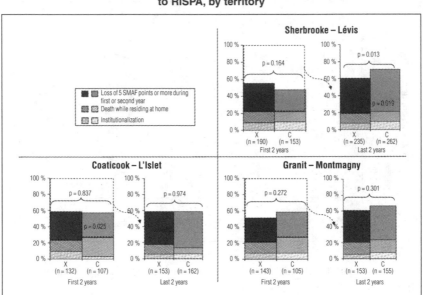

Figure 12.18
**Evolution of functional decline in subjects exposed
to RISPA, by year, by territory**

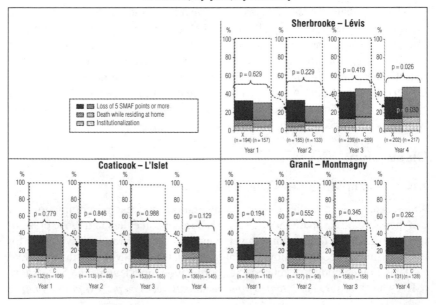

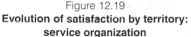

Figure 12.19
**Evolution of satisfaction by territory:
service organization**

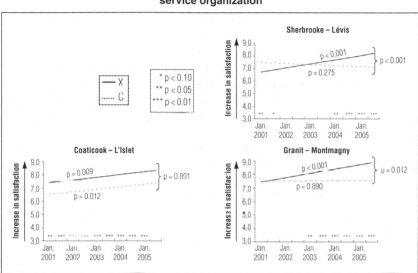

system of integrated care for older persons) related to a full-integration model[14]. To our knowledge, no study conducted elsewhere in the world with published results deals with a coordination model. Studies on the other types of integration are available, however. These have been conducted in different countries and environments that differed at the outset as to degree of integration. It should be kept in mind that Quebec already has integrated structures for several components of its system, since both health and social services are under a single government department. This is not the case elsewhere in the world.

Since care of the elderly has undergone profound transformation in the course of recent decades and new cohorts of elders have arisen, with characteristics different from those of their predecessors, we will focus our discussion on integration studies for the past 15 years. The On Lok studies in San Francisco's Chinatown (On Lok is Cantonese for happy or peaceful home),[15] American social health-maintenance organizations (known as S/HMOs),[16, 17] and the British Darlington study[18] provided the inspiration for later integration projects. In the USA, the Program of All-inclusive Care for the Elderly (PACE) has yielded a substantial literature in recent years, with often contradictory and controversial findings[19–23]. Two projects that unfolded in Italy[24, 25] have yielded interesting findings about a network that was highly fragmented at the outset.

In our own study, we observed significant differences in functional decline in the last two years for all subjects exposed to RISPA. Supplementary analyses show trends among the least independent subjects (Iso-SMAF profiles of 4 and higher) after three years; for the Year 4, however, lack of statistical power allowed for detection of no more than a trend. In the Bois-Francs study,[12, 13] a significant difference (p = 0.04) was observed in functional decline (defined as it is in the present study) in the experimental zone after one year. However, difference did not remain significant after Year 2 or Year 3. The effect was observed especially among the least independent participants (SMAF > 15.5). We observed RISPA had a positive and significant effect on incident cases of functional decline during Year 4. The most plausible explanation for this unexpected finding is the introduction during the study of the PRISMA-7 disability-case-finding procedure in the experimental zone[26]. To our knowledge, no other study exists that provides data on functional decline that could be used for comparison purposes.

We did not observe a significant difference in mortality rate between the experimental and comparison groups. The Bois-Francs[12, 13] and SIPA[14] studies did not report significant differences in mortality, either. The same is true for studies on PACE[19, 20] and the Italian study that included a comparison group[24]. Effects on mortality were not, in any case, expected in any of these studies.

We did not observe a significant impact on institutionalization. The Bois-Francs studies[12, 13] showed a downward trend in residential placement in the experimental zone (p = 0.06) after three years. The SIPA study[14] reported no significant differences in institutionalization levels after 22 months of following the experimental and comparison cohorts. The Italian study that included a comparison group[24] observed no significant differences in institutionalization levels. The PACE studies sometimes reported positive effects (reduced rate of institutionalization), but doubts have been expressed about the comparability of the comparison group[19, 20]. Delays in admission to residential facilities (CHSLDs) can be seen as desirable if home support services are significant and provide support to the close circle. But, as will be seen in the next chapter (13), in our study, we did not observe a different increase in in-home services use from that of the comparison zone. This means that, while institutional placement can be delayed, it cannot be avoided, at least for the short term. Clearly, one factor that influences the CHSLD admissions rate is bed availability. Available data on rates of placement (which come from Quebec's department of health and social services or MSSS for *Ministère de la Santé et des Services sociaux*) are from the Estrie and Chaudière-Appalaches regions as a whole and are not specific as to the MRCs studied. Following institutional mergers in 2005–2006 and municipal mergers in 2002, data by MRCs studied are either no longer available or no longer comparable for the whole period of the study. Close examination of the evolution of placement rates as compared between experimental and comparison zones did not reveal trajectories for placement rates that could have resulted in significant differential effects between the zones.

We observed no significant difference between the experimental and comparison zones in the evolution of functional autonomy. This was also the case in the Bois-Francs[12, 13] and SIPA[14] studies. The PACE study produced contradictory data,[19, 20] while the Italian study reported a significant difference that favored the experimental group with respect to six activities of daily living and seven instrumental activities of daily living, measured using a different instrument and with responses of "dependent" or "independent."[24] Findings in our own study for functional decline (death, institutionalization, or loss of five SMAF points) appear to us to indicate that there are small increments of differences that are not significant taken in isolation but are significant when grouped together. The functional decline variable had been used in previous studies[27, 12, 13] and allows for taking account of deaths and institutionalizations in examining the evolution of autonomy. Since institutionalization and death are linked to functional autonomy, we thus avoid losing sensitive information and being left with a more general view of the evolution of function. However, it remains the case that no significant effect was observed on functional autonomy examined in isolation.

To our knowledge, no other study about service integration presents findings on the evolution of handicap levels and reduction in handicap levels. The results presented in our study, showing a significant reduction in handicap levels in the experimental zone, are thus highly interesting and original.

The decision to develop a new questionnaire to measure satisfaction was made following a review of existing instruments. This review highlighted the fact that few instruments are intended for the elderly and that those that do exist are characterized by a ceiling effect (saturation of scales: the individuals surveyed are all highly satisfied). A ceiling effect makes it impossible to measure improvement in a situation. We have no comparative data emerging from other studies that used our questionnaire, which was recently developed. Using other measurement instruments, the Bois-Francs[12, 13] and SIPA[14] studies reported no significant differences in elder satisfaction that could be attributed to RISPA (on completion of the study). The Italian studies did not report findings on satisfaction. The PACE studies reported significant and positive effects on user satisfaction in the experimental group,[19, 20] though measured with a different instrument. The supply of CLSC health services was not significantly increased during our study and any increase that did occur was no different between the experimental and comparison zones. Accessibility problems were reported and persist in both zones. In light of this, the positive and significant effect on satisfaction with services in the experimental zone implies that health services are being made use of in a way that is more satisfactory for elders, despite access difficulties. One reason for this is service organization, as findings for the subscale related to that topic show.

One of RISPA's objectives has been to restore decision-making power to users to the extent possible. RISPA aims to enhance users' capacity to manage their health-services organization themselves. The questionnaire on empowerment was developed because no instrument existed with which our study's specific objectives could be achieved; and it was intended to measure the evolution of this value as translated into services integration. Since the questionnaire is of recent design, few data are available for purposes of comparing our empowerment results. The Bois-Francs study[12, 13] had measured certain perceptions about level of control over services, which is one component of empowerment. Significant gaps favoring the experimental zone were observed after one year; but no significant gap or effect was observed at the end of the study's three years. The PACE studies found that experimental subjects expressed greater confidence in their capability to control their lives and face daily problems. The results obtained in those studies argue in favor of the value of elder empowerment being given some degree of rootedness in the context of RISPA, in particular in Estrie.

The Bois-Francs study[12, 13] showed that the experiment had a positive effect on caregiver's burden (p = 0.05) after three years. At the outset, the experimental and comparison groups' scores for burdens were comparable. No significant difference was observed under the SIPA study[14] and no findings on this variable were reported in other studies. Most studies in which direct action was taken respecting the caregiver's burden did not manage to show any change owing to the intervention. It should be borne in mind that the present study did not include intervention specifically related to the caregiver's burden. Our findings, which first appear negative, would appear to contradict the findings related to desire to institutionalize, where no significant difference or trend was observed. In the Bois-Francs study,[12, 13] a trend was observed (p = 0.08) showing a positive effect over the three years on desire to institutionalize. The results were significant following both Year 1 (p = 0.02) and Year 2 (p = 0.04). These findings agree with effect on caregiver's burden for both these years (p = 0.05 and p = 0.04). The seeming inconsistency in our findings for caregiver's burden and caregiver's desire to institutionalize needs to be viewed, then, from a different perspective. There are two possible explanations for these results.

The first is that the difference observed at the outset between the experimental and comparison zones was simply followed by a regression to the mean, that is, by the tendency for results that deviate from the mean at the start to come closer to it later. Thus, the experimental subjects that started the study at a lower burden level simply saw their score approach that of the comparison group. Experimental subjects who lived in individual homes and had a low burden score at the start of the study were in fact those who experienced the highest increase in burden. By the end of the study their scores matched those of experimental subjects living in collective settings.

The second possible explanation for the increase in burden in the experimental zone emerges from an examination of other findings of our study. A significant effect was observed on reduction in handicap levels in the experimental zone. Preliminary analyses indicate that this reduction in handicap levels goes along with an increase in number of hours of assistance provided by members of the close circle to compensate for disabilities. Thus members of the close circle are more involved in compensating for the subject's disabilities; this greater involvement then takes the form of a perceived increase in burden but is not accompanied by an increased desire to institutionalize. Triangulating these findings shows that family potentiation is true and effective in the experimental zone. The level of handicap diminishes and informal caregivers feel a corresponding heaviness in their burden, but they don't experience an increased desire to institutionalize their relative. It is understandable that greater involvement would be accompanied by an increased perceived burden. At the same time, the absence of any difference in desire to institutionalize suggests to us that informal caregivers do not respond to this situation too negatively.

General Discussion

Analyses of our study were conducted in the light of "intention to treat"; that is, the presumption is made that all participants have benefited from "the treatment", namely RISPA. Obviously, not all participants had a case manager or used the single entry point (to take two examples). Since this was a population-based effectiveness study, subjects did not all receive the intervention in question (or all of its components), and this dilutes the observable impact. This represents both a limitation of our study and an insurmountable aspect of a population-based study. For that matter, not all participants needed a case manager. An effective RISPA must identify individuals who do require case management and refer them. Difficulties accessing services are present in both experimental and comparison zones and limit leeway in distributing services, which represents yet another challenge to integration (and to measuring its impact).

We must also take into account the fact that implementation had not yet reached 100 %. Rather, over the course of Year 3 of the study, the degree of implementation had reached 80 %. As well, it should not be forgotten that there is a time lapse between an intervention and its observable effects. Thus for example, a case manager who comes into the position will not have an observable impact at the population level right away. Extending this study beyond the first two years made it possible to observe RISPA's effects at a more advanced stage of implementation. The time needed to implement a RISPA should not be underestimated. This is discussed in other chapters of this book, but it is nonetheless important that we indicate its relevance to the impact we observed on elders and those close to them.

Implementation did not take place at the same level across the three experimental zones; nor was it equal for all integration components. This may have produced varying results. As well, integration in the comparison zones was not zero. For example, shared instruments such as the Multiclientele Assessment Tool had been implemented across Quebec as of 2002. Thus, the comparison zone actually was injected with a small dose of integration.

It is impossible for us to determine the individual degree of exposure to RISPA for each participant in the study. For instance, it wasn't possible to determine whether each individual patient had used the single entry point or benefited from any given aspect of coordinated action. We were able to determine the proportion of study participants who had received case management for at least one day over the course of the study, namely 17.8 % of the 751 experimental subjects (14.7 % in Sherbrooke, 16.5 % in Coaticook, 23.9 % in Granit). Supplementary analyses will be conducted relative to these subjects in order to determine the duration of exposure to case management (e.g., coming under case management during Year 1 or Year 3) and its effect on other variables (functional autonomy, death, institutionalization, etc.). For example, while Coaticook subjects came under case management mainly towards the end of the study, might they evidence specific effects as compared with subjects who were not exposed to case management and were paired with them? The supplementary analyses to come will provide answers to these questions.

Despite all the obstacles to determining population-based impact, some positive and significant effects were observed among the elderly. The strength of a population-based study resides precisely in its ability to identify impact not just on active users of the system, but also on those who should be active users. The identification of subjects at risk of functional decline done for this study made it possible to target elders who needed services. The results observed in the experimental cohorts show that RISPA, once implemented, produced observable, significant, and positive effects overall.

Conclusion

The main conclusions regarding RISPA's effects on elders and their close circle are:

- Over four years, no effect on death, institutionalization, and disabilities.
- Significant reduction in handicap levels.
- Functional decline 6.3 % lower in experimental zone during the last two years.
- Incidence of functional decline 14 % lower in experimental zone in Year 4.
- Positive and significant effect on satisfaction levels.
- Positive and significant effect on empowerment levels.
- Increased felt burden by informal caregiver parallel to increased number of hours of assistance to relative, but without effect on caregiver's desire to institutionalize relative.

It can be concluded that RISPA, once implemented, made it possible to identify disabled elders and direct them optimally to required services. The supply of CLSC health services did not significantly increase during the study time in either the experimental or the comparison zones. Nevertheless, we can conclude that existing services were used in a more effective way in the experimental zone, as is evident in positive effects on functional decline and level of handicap. Moreover, elderly people are more satisfied with services in the experimental than in the comparison zone, as well as being more empowered and involved in health-related decisions that concern them. In the experimental zone, the people close to users significantly increased their assistance to their disabled relatives. The main informal caregivers felt an increase in the burden of care, but had no increase in desire to institutionalize their relatives. Supplementary analyses will shed more light on these findings.

Our next chapter (13) presents our findings on the impact of RISPA on health services and their cost and a general conclusion on RISPA's performance. Findings on impact as a whole will be discussed there from the perspective of consistency, under which cost is placed in relationship to observable impact.

References

1. Hébert R, Bravo G, Korner-Bitensky N, Voyer L. Predictive validity of a postal questionnaire for screening community dwelling elderly individuals at risk for functional decline. Age and Ageing 1996; 25:159-67.

2. Hébert R, Guilbeault J, Desrosiers J, Dubuc N. The functional autonomy measurement system (SMAF): a clinical-based instrument for measuring disabilities and handicaps in older people. *Geriatrics Today: J Can Geriatr Soc* 2001; 4: 141-147.

3. Gagnon M, Hébert R, Dubé M, Dubois M-F. Development and Validation of the Health Care Satisfaction Questionnaire (HCSQ) in Elders. Journal of Nursing Measurement 2006; 14(3): 190-204.

4. Gagnon M, Hébert R, Dubé M, Dubois M-F. Development and validation of an instrument measuring individual empowerment in relation to personal health care: The Health Care Empowerment Questionnaire (HCEQ). Am J Health Promot 2006; 20(6):429-35.

5. Zarit SH, Orr NK, Zarit JM. The hidden victims of Alzheimer's disease: Families under stress. New York: New York University Press; 1985.

6. Hébert R, Bravo G, Préville M. Reliability, validity and reference values of the Zarit burden interview for assessing informal caregivers of community-dwelling older persons with dementia. Can J Aging 2000; 19(4): 494-507.

7. Morycz RK. Caregiving strain and the desire to institutionalize family members with Alzheimer's disease. Research on Aging 1985; 7(3), 329-61.

8. Canadian study on health and aging working group. Canadian study on health and aging: Study methods and prevalence of dementia. Can Med Assoc J 1994; 150: 899-913.

9. Hébert R, Spiegelhalter DJ, Brayne C. Setting the minimal metrically detectable change on disability rating scales. Arch Phys Med Rehabil 1997; 78:1305-8.

10. Dubuc N, Hébert R, Desrosiers J, Buteau M, Trottier L. Disability-based classification system for older people in integrated long-term care services: The Iso-SMAF profiles. Arch Gerontol Geriat 2006; 42, 191-206.

11. Leutz WN. Five laws for integrating medical and social services: Lessons from the United States and the United Kingdom. Milbank Quarterly 1999; 77(1):77-110.

12. Tourigny A. Durand P. Bonin L. Hébert R. Rochette L. Quasi-experimental Study of the Effectiveness of an Integrated Service Delivery Network for the Frail Elderly. *Canadian Journal on Aging* 2004; 23(3):231-46.

13. Durand P, Tourigny A, Bonin L, Paradis M, Lemay A, Bergeron P. Mécanisme de coordination des services géronto-gériatriques des Bois-Francs. Rapport final sur les résultats #QC403 remis au Fonds d'adaptation des services de santé, 2001.

14. Béland F, Bergman H, Lebel P, Clarfield AM, Tousignant P, Contandriopoulos AP, Dallaire L. A system of integrated care for older persons with disabilities in Canada: Results from a *randomized controlled trial. Journal of Gerontology: Series A- Biological Sciences and Medical Sciences* 2006; 61(4):367-73.

15. Yordi CL, Waldman J. A consolidated model of long-term care: Service utilization and cost impacts. Gerontologist 1985; 25(4):389-97.

16. Newcomer R, Harringtion C, Friedlob A. Social Health Maintenance Organizations: assessing their initial experience. Health Services Research. 1990; 25(3):425-54.

17. Manton KG, Newcomer R, Lowrimore GR, Vertrees JC, Harrington C. Social/health maintenance organization and fee-for-service health outcomes over time. Health Care Financ. Rev. 1993; 15(2):173-202.

18. Challis D, Darton R, Johnson L, Stone M, Traske K. An evaluation of an alternative to long-stay hospital care for frail elderly patients: II. Costs and effectiveness. Age Ageing. 1991;20(4):245-54.

19. Kodner DL, Kyriacou CK. Fully integrated care for frail elderly: Two American models. International Journal of Integrated Care 2000; (www.ijic.org) 1(November 1):1-24.

20. Johri M, Béland F, Bergman H. International experiments in integrated care for the elderly: A synthesis of the evidence. Int J Geriatr Psychiatry 2003; 18:222-235.

21. Branch LG, Coulam RF, Zimmerman YA. The PACE evaluation: Initial findings. Gerontologist 1995; 35(3):349-59.

22. Branch LG. Evidence-based evaluations of PACE. J Am Geriatr Soc. 1998; 46(1):115-6.

23. Gross DL, Temkin-Greener H, Kunitz S, and Mukamel DB. The growing pains of integrated health care for the elderly: Lessons from the expansion of PACE. Milbank Quarterly. 82(2): 257-82, 2004.

24. Bernabei R, Landi F, Gambassi G, Sgadari A, Zuccala G, Mor V, Rubenstein LZ, Carbonin P. Randomised trial of impact of model of integrated care and case management for older people living in the community. BMJ. 1998;316(7141):1348-51.

25. Landi F, Onder G, Russo A, Tabaccanti S, Rollo R, Federici S, Tua E, Cesari M, Bernabei R. A new model of integrated home care for the elderly: Impact on hospital use. J Clin Epidemiol. 2001;54(9):968-70.

26. Raîche M, Hébert R, Dubois M-F, Grégoire M, Bolduc J, Bureau C, and Veil A. Le repérage des personnes âgées en perte d'autonomie modérée à grave avec le questionnaire PRISMA-7: présentation, implantation et utilisation. *La Revue de Gériatrie* 2007; 32(3): 209-218. This article is reproduced in translation as Chapter 22 of the present book.

27. Hébert R, Robichaud L, Roy PM, Bravo G, and Voyer L. Efficacy of a nurse-led multidimensional preventive programme for older people at risk of functional decline. A randomized controlled trial. Age Ageing 2001; 30: 147-53.

Acknowledgements

We wish to extend warm thanks to all participants in the study and their informal caregivers. Sincere thanks as well to all the individuals who worked on the project over the course of numerous years.

Funding

This project was funded by the Canadian Institutes of Health Research, the Ministère de la Santé et des Services sociaux du Québec (Quebec department of health and social services), and the Agence de la santé et des services sociaux de l'Estrie (the Estrie regional health and social services agency).

Chapter 13
RISPA Overall Performance: Impacts on the Use of Health Services, Their Costs and Efficiency under the PRISMA-Estrie Study

Michel Raîche, Réjean Hébert, Danièle Blanchette, Suzanne Durand, Marie-France Dubois, N'Deye Rokhaya Gueye, and the PRISMA-Estrie group

---

Highlights

- Integrated care brings about an alternative use of services by the elderly; we present detailed findings.
- The cost impacts are examined; we observe no difference in overall costs.
- The overall positive impacts of the RISPA coordination model demonstrate the efficiency of this approach.
- RISPA performance is discussed.

Introduction

Integrated care represents an intervention in the organization of services not only for the benefit of the system's users, but also for the population of a given region. Under the PRISMA-Estrie study, the use of the services by the elderly population and their related costs can be modified by implementing the integrated service delivery network for the elderly (French acronym: RISPA). This chapter describes the impacts of a progressively implemented RISPA on the use of services and on costs in the experimental zone, compared with the comparison zone. The changes over the four years of the study are presented.

This impact study of service use and costs meets a number of objectives. It highlights the transformation in the services offered arising from integration. Through an analysis of economic indicators, we can measure this transformation aggregately, emphasizing a societal perspective.[1] For example, it is difficult to combine consultations with health professionals and days in long-term care facilities (CHSLD). However, the total cost of these two components, like the cost for the range of services, provides an overall view of the RISPA's impacts.

Moreover, by establishing the relationship between the economic impacts of RISPAs for the elderly and their caregivers and their overall impacts, we can draw conclusions about their efficiency. Efficiency refers to the capacity of a RISPA to produce the best results using the resources available. Efficiency can also be defined as the optimal use of resources. In a context of limited resources, this is a priority. It lets us draw conclusions about the range of impacts observed as a function of investments made and resources reallocated to the integrated service delivery network. In short, efficiency is a measurement of the RISPA's overall performance.

Chapter 11 described the general methodology of the PRISMA-Estrie study. At the beginning of this chapter, we elaborate on certain methodological points concerning the collection of data about the use of health services and the determination of their costs. We then present and discuss the findings on the impacts of the RISPAs on service use and costs. The following section covers the entire range of the RISPA's impacts, presenting initial observations on its efficiency. We conclude with a discussion of the overall performance of the RISPA under the PRISMA-Estrie study.

Methodology

Service Use

Since this study is population-based, concern for determining RISPA impacts on the range of health and home-care services (and their costs) was present right from the design phase. Nevertheless, the challenge was daunting. The multifactorial nature of functional decline means that the services required to ensure that the elderly do not find themselves handicapped are extremely diverse. In addition to public services, private services (e.g. those provided by private residences) and those offered by volunteer organizations (e.g. Meals on Wheels) are in very high demand. The sources of information raised a number of concerns from the outset.

There is a mistaken belief that public services are compiled somewhere in comprehensive and reliable databases. This is neither the case for comprehensiveness nor reliability. Hospitalizations are compiled in the MED-ÉCHO databases of the Régie de l'assurance-maladie du Québec (RAMQ). Medical procedures for physicians invoicing on a fee-for-service basis are in another of the RAMQ's databases. Salaried general practitioners employed by Centres locaux de services communautaires (CLSCs) are not stored in these databases. Interventions of professionals and homemakers are compiled in the databases of the *Système d'information clientele* (SIC) of the CLSCs.

Given that the study initially covered seven CLSC regions, an equal number of databases needed to be queried and seven authorization requests needed to be made. The query methods and the reliability of the information obtained from the SIC's databases posed some problems. The experience of the

Montérégie study (see Chapter 19 herein and Chapter 12 in the first PRISMA book[2]) unequivocally demonstrates that this information should only be used following a rigorous cleansing process carried out over a number of years. Initially, we did not have the thorough understanding of this process that we now do, but the procedure had been initiated and we knew enough to make sound decisions in the matter. Moreover, the RAMQ databases appear not to be error-free.

Regarding the data on services to assist with activities of daily living (ADL) and instrumental activities of daily living (IADL) made available in private homes, there is apparently no municipal—let alone regional—database. The same applies to the services offered by volunteer organizations such as Meals on Wheels and support groups.

We rapidly realized that the best and only source of comprehensive information was the elderly patients themselves or their caregivers. For this reason, we decided to maintain regular telephone contact with them and to provide them with a calendar to facilitate information gathering. A previous study carried out by our team[3] demonstrated the feasibility of this method for collecting most of the necessary information on service use. By providing participants with a calendar, acquainting them with its use, and following up with them, this became the only possible method for collecting the full range of required information.

The calendar was provided to study participants at the initial meeting with them, along with written instructions, an explanation of the information we were looking for and how to record it. These instructions were reviewed in detail in the first of the bimonthly telephone calls, as well as throughout the study and during the annual home visits. The calendars for subsequent years were either handed out to them in person at the time of their assessment, when this coincided with the replacement date, or mailed out to them with a signed letter from the interviewer who performed the assessment.

The information gathered from the subjects and caregivers covered, among other things, hospital-related data such as ambulance trips, emergency-room visits, and hospitalizations (duration, department, surgeries). Consultations with health professionals outside of the hospital were recorded (dates, specialty, and travel, where applicable). Lastly, the use of community and health services was monitored. This information covered visits to day hospitals and day-care centers, number of hours of home support for IADL (e.g. housekeeping) or for ADL (e.g. assistance in bathing), number of meals from Meals on Wheels, number of hours of companion sitting, and various volunteer services (e.g. community transportation). The funding sources of all of these services (public, private, volunteer) were recorded.

With a view to efficiency and to minimizing recall bias, subjects were contacted by telephone on a bimonthly basis. We term this method—with its directions, schedule, and regular reminders—"assisted self-reporting." A test–retest and inter-interviewer reliability study was carried out (agreement of information when collected at different times or by different interviewers).[4] A near-perfect agreement was obtained for hospitalizations, day surgeries, medical appointments, housekeeping assistance (IADL), and the use of volunteer services. The agreement was high for emergency-room visits and for personal care support (ADL). For visits to/from nurses or other health professionals, the agreement could be qualified as moderate to high. The fact that no service use variable received anything lower than this level creates a high degree of confidence regarding the findings.

Economic Evaluation

The second element covered in this chapter is cost impact. The cost elements that enter into this economic analysis are accommodations, maintenance, diet, health and social services (e.g. emergency-room visits, hospitalizations, appointments with health professionals, home support), medication use, and the cost of implementation and operation of the RISPA (hereafter, "RISPA cost").

The compilation of service costs, excluding medication and RISPA cost, is calculated using the number of units of each type of service as identified by the participants. These units—hours, visits, and days—are multiplied by the corresponding unit cost. The method for calculating the unit costs of each service type is presented in detail in Chapter 21. Note that the unit costs in question are identical in the experimental and comparison zones. The medication costs were obtained from the RAMQ's pharmaceutical services database for each participant according to the dates they entered and left the study. The RISPA costs were evaluated and are presented in Chapter 10. They are broken down for the experimental zone only. Note, however, that what they represent are the differential costs incurred as a result of RISPA implementation and operation. This category does not reflect the cost of operating an integrated network, but rather the costs over and above those of a non-integrated network.

We take a societal approach, including costs from the public, private and volunteer sectors. However, the costs corresponding to the assessed monetary value of help provided by family and volunteers is not presented in this text. As the book was going to press, these analyses had not been completed. They will be completed and published at a later date.

It is important to note that the costs are compiled **in 2002 dollars** in order to highlight the disparities in use. Accordingly, the cost variations seen in the findings are attributable to variations in service use (expected in an aging sample of participants) and not to inflation. In short, the methodology provides a common foundation with which to measure the RISPA's impact on the use of multiple services over a number of years.

Statistical Analyses

The primary analysis consists of comparing the experimental group with the comparison group. The patterns of change over time are compared and annual comparisons are performed. The change in each group with respect to itself is also examined. A person–year-based weighting was used in order to establish an annual basis for the monitoring periods.

Service use is first examined to determine the proportion with at least one incidence of use per year (e.g. proportion of subjects having visited the emergency room at least once during the year), resulting in a dichotomous variable. Among subjects having used a service at least once, we then examine continuous variables such as the average number of visits or the duration of stay. For the dichotomous variables, the annual comparisons and the patterns of change over time are performed using the GEE (generalized estimating equation) statistical model for dichotomous outcomes. Using the GEE model enables us to account for the interdependence among subjects observed at different times. For the continuous variables, multilevel models of change were used in order to simultaneously take into account intra- and inter-individual changes.

For costs, distributions of the variables are highly asymmetrical. We observe very high costs for certain subjects, while those not having used the service have a cost equivalent of zero. This distribution does not allow us to treat the variables as normally distributed. Therefore, a classification into five categories (zero use, followed by quartiles) was performed for each variable. The annual comparisons and time-change comparisons are performed with GEE analyses using Poisson's model.

Findings and Interpretation

Note that 1,501 subjects were recruited and monitored in both the experimental and comparison zones, (n=728 and n=773, respectively) in cohorts A and B (see Chapters 11 and 12). A maximum of 3,455 person-years are used for the present analysis: 1,779 person-years for the experimental group and 1,676 person-years for the comparison group.

Impacts on Service Use

Below we present the findings for the four years of the study. Note that certain disparities unfavorable to the experimental zone were observed during the first year. The change in health service use must be observed with these disparities in mind. In order to facilitate the presentation of the findings, the same codes—X and C—were used for the experimental group (Estrie) and comparison group (Chaudière-Appalaches) as in the previous chapter. Another similarity in the presentation of the findings is that the three p values close to the curves indicate the outcomes of the three statistical tests for the change over four years. The two initial values concern the change in each group with respect to itself (e.g. if an increase has taken place, is this increase significant?) and the third represents the comparison in the changes in the two groups. A p-value under 0.05 indicates a significant outcome. We also compared the findings for each year, with the significant outcomes appearing above the x-axis. Note that the findings for CHSLD admittance were presented in the previous chapter, since this variable is a component of functional decline. No differences were observed between the experimental and comparison zones for CHSLD admittance.

Emergency-room visits

At least one emergency-room visit

Figure 13.1 shows that the comparison group behaves as expected, i.e., showing a gradual increase in the proportion of subjects using emergency rooms, due to subject aging and the concomitant increase in health problems. Note that the subjects in question were an average of 83 years old when they joined the study. Initially, the proportion visiting the emergency at least once per year was 32 %; by the end, the proportion had increased to 54 %. This increase is statistically significant in the comparison group.

The initial proportion is markedly and significantly higher in the experimental group than in the comparison group, with 46 % of subjects visiting the emergency room at least once a year. After four years, this proportion is 49 %, which is not a significant increase. The difference is significant when the evolutions in each zone are compared.

Figure 13.1
Proportion of subjects with at least one emergency-room visit

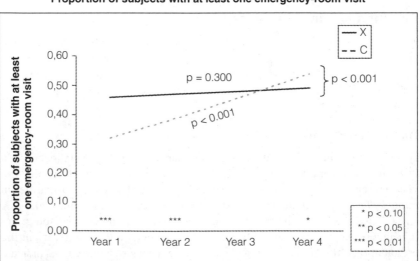

In the case of at least one emergency-room visit

For individuals making at least one emergency-room visit, we also examined the average number of visits, the percentage of visits followed by hospitalization, as well as the rate of return emergency-room visits within ten days. Among the subjects with one emergency-room visit, the average number of visits was initially two per year and remained almost unchanged for both groups throughout the study. No significant disparity was observed between the two groups (p = 0.428).

Regarding emergency-room visits followed by hospitalization, it is not surprising that, since the subjects in the experimental zone used the emergency room more as a point of entry into the system at the beginning of the study, these visits were followed less frequently by a hospitalization. While the difference is significant during the early years of the study, the experimental zone and the comparison zone coincide after four years. In other words, the two zones show reverse trends (p = 0.043), influenced by initial use and its changes over time. Regarding return emergency room visits within ten days without hospitalizations, we observe a stable rate of return visits around 10 % in both groups and no statistical difference (p = 0.300) between them.

Hospitalizations

At least one hospitalization

Figure 13.2 shows that the comparison group behaves as expected; specifically, it shows a gradual and statistically significant increase in the proportion of subjects being hospitalized. The proportion of subjects hospitalized at least once per year went from 28.4 % to 36.1 % in four years. In contrast, the experimental group evidences somewhat of a plateau. The proportion of subjects hospitalized

Figure 13.2
Proportion of subjects with at least one hospitalization

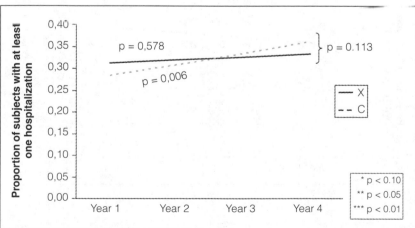

at least once per year in this group went from 31.3 % to 33.3 % in four years, but this slight increase is not significant. Comparing the evolution in the two zones revealed no significant statistical difference.

In the case of at least one hospitalization

Among subjects having been hospitalized at least once, the average number of hospitalizations was initially two per year and remained unchanged for both groups for the study's duration (p = 0.906). The average length of stay is stable and statistically equal (p = 0.200) in the two groups, falling from 10 to 8.7 days in the comparison group and rising from 10.7 to 12 days in the experimental group. The findings on re-hospitalizations in 30 or 90 days or emergency-room visits less than 10 days after hospitalization show no differences.

Public and Private Services for the Elderly Presenting Functional Decline

At least one use of a public service for the elderly presenting functional decline

Looking at the use of public services for the elderly presenting functional decline (CLSC home-care services for ADL or IADL, hospital or day-care center) reveals that the proportion of subjects using these services at least once tends to increase in parallel in the two groups (Figure 13.3). Nevertheless, the increase is not significant over four years. A higher proportion of subjects in the comparison zone used at least one public service; the difference of 6 % is significant and remains constant over the four years.

Figure 13.3
**Proportion of subjects with at least one use of a public service
for the elderly with functional decline**

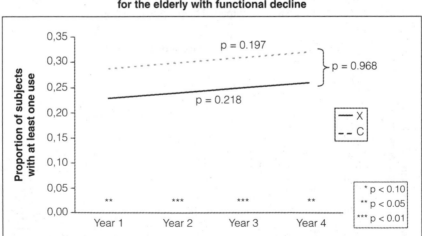

At least one use of a home-care service for ADL and IADL

A closer examination of the use of public and private home-care services for ADL and IADL shows a significant increase in both zones. There is, however, no significant difference in the change between the two zones (Figure 13.4). Over 60 % of participants used public and private services for IADL throughout the study, whereas the proportion varies between 40 % and 50 % for ADL.

Figure 13.4
Proportion of subjects with at least one use of a home-care service for ADL or IADL

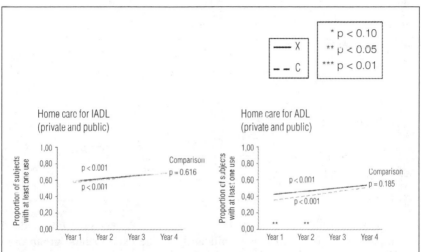

Volunteer Services

At least one use of a volunteer service

Around 12 % of comparison zone participants and 20 % of experimental zone participants made use of a volunteer service each year. These services include meals served in the community or at home (Meals on Wheels), escorts on outings (care-related visits, social outings, shopping), and community transportation. While more participants in the experimental zone made use of these services, the zones show no significant differences in frequency use evolution (p = 0.316).

Consultations with Health Professionals

At least one appointment with a health professional (Figure 13.5)

This category includes consultations in person with health professionals in the office, at outpatient clinics, at CLSCs, or in the patient's home; appointments occurring during a hospitalization or emergency-room visit are not included nor are telephone consultations. Generally speaking, almost all of the subjects in

Figure 13.5
Proportion of subjects with at least one visiit to/by a health professional

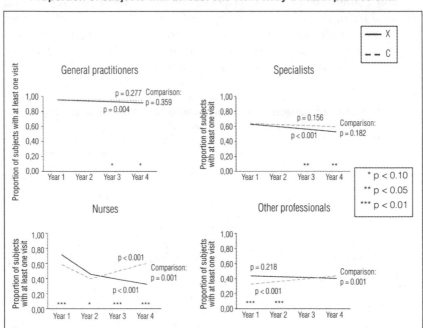

both groups consult a general practitioner at least once per year. For medical specialists, this proportion falls significantly in the experimental group only (p < 0.001), decreasing from 60 % to 50 % over the four years, while the comparison group remains stable at around 60 % over the same period. The change is not significantly different from one group to the other (p = 0.182). The trend in consultations with nurses shows an initial drop between the first and second years followed by an increase in the comparison zone and continued, but less marked decline in the experimental zone. A comparison of the changes yields a significant difference. Regarding consultations with other health professionals (physiotherapists, occupational therapists, social workers, and others), the experimental zone initially showed a significantly higher rate of use (p < 0.01), which remained constant, while the comparison zone increased significantly, reaching the level of the experimental zone by the end of the study. The changes in use are significantly different between the groups.

Findings on Service Use by Subregion (MRC)

We examined the findings by subregion, comparing twin regional county municipalities (MRCs) of Sherbrooke-Lévis, Coaticook-L'Islet, and Granit-Montmagny. Although when doing so, we needed to allow for the fact that comparisons involving smaller subgroups have more limited statistical power for

detecting significant differences. The overwhelming majority of twin comparisons reflect the findings obtained in the overall comparisons of experimental
and comparison zones. In this section, we present only the particular outcomes
where distinct and significant differences were observed.

Regarding hospitalizations, the overall trends observed are magnified
when the analysis is limited to the rural MRCs with a hospital center. While the
proportion of residents in the Granit experimental region with at least one hospitalization annually is quite stable at 35 % over the four years (p = 0.317), it
rises from 29 % to 41 % (p = 0.030) in the Montmagny comparison region.
Therefore, the disparity in change between these two zones is significant over
the four years (p = 0.026).

Economic Impacts

Note that the costs presented below are all calculated in 2002 dollars. This being
the case, all variations observed are due to differences in the use of services and
in no way reflect the influence of inflation. The figures presented in the following section illustrate the average annual costs per person, weighted according to
the number of days of participation of each elderly person. The statistical analyses also take into account intersubject variance (which can be very high for
certain services such as hospitalizations that concern a small segment of the
sample). There may therefore appear to be disagreement between graph and statistical test. Nevertheless, average cost is a valuable index for budget forecast-
ing, and statistical analysis that shows a significant difference must also be held
up to the light of economic reality in order to judge whether or not the difference
is significant from an economic standpoint.

Total Cost

We begin with the total cost, including the public and private components. Note
that the total includes the cost of all accommodations, regardless of type, health
and social services, medications, and the RISPA cost. Overall, annual costs
increase significantly in both zones, but the comparison of the two zones yields
no significant differences between them in the trends or costs for the four years
(Figure 13.6). The RISPA cost, included in the findings for the experimental zone,
seems to have been offset by the savings on services. In four years, the average
total annual costs rise from around $17,000 to $20,000 per elderly person.

Total cost: public share

When we examine total public costs alone, we observe the same overall phenomenon as for combined public and private costs, specifically, a significant
increase in both zones over the four years, with no significant difference in the
comparison of the two zones (Figure 13.7). The increase is attributable to the
aging of the participants, and consequently, their increasing use of public services. The annual average total public costs rise from around $8,000 to around

Figure 13.6
Total annual average cost per person

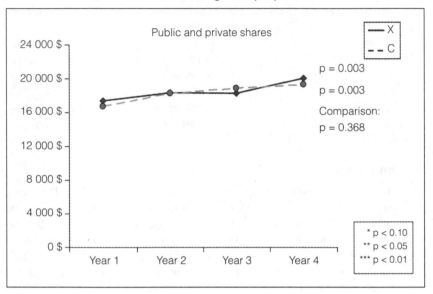

$10,000, equivalent to half of the combined public and private total, illustrated in Figure 13.6.

Total costs: private share

When we examine the total private costs alone, in the experimental zone, we observe a decrease that is significant statistically but not economically, with the average annual cost dropping from $9,300 to $9,200. Annual costs appear to be constant in the comparison zone. The comparison in change in annual costs in the two zones reveals a statistically significant difference (Figure 13.7) of around $600 with respect to the average annual cost over the last two years. The RISPA's effect seems to have been to attenuate private costs assumed by the elderly and their families. What is clearly shown is that the RISPA does not result in a transfer of costs from public to private. This would have meant a savings for the pubic system with an increased burden of private costs shouldered by the elderly.

Cost of Hospital Services

Cost: emergency-room visits

Figure 13.1 shows the proportion of participants who visited the emergency room at least once in a given year, while Figure 13.8 compares the annual cost per participant for emergency-room visits based on an average of all participants (including those who did not visit the emergency room). Note that the

Figure 13.7
Total annual average cost per person

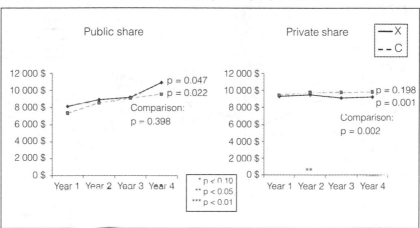

Figure 13.8
Annual average cost per person for emergency-room visits

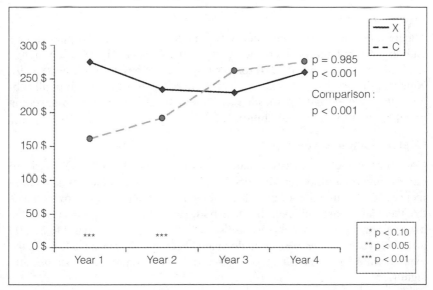

standard cost of an emergency-room visit (see Chapter 21) is $265. The curves representing cost trends for emergency-room visits generally follow the curves of the variable for "at least one emergency-room visit."

Figure 13.9
Annual average cost per person for hospitalizations

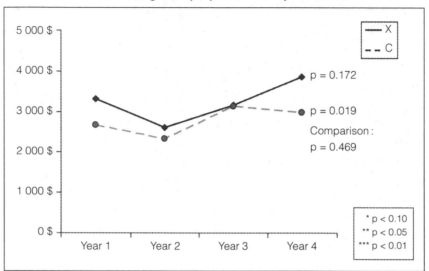

Cost: hospitalizations

The hospitalization costs presented below include costs for all hospitalizations and surgeries but not for emergency-room visits. We do not observe any significant difference between the two zones with respect to cost trends (Figure 13.9). Note that the graphs are based on average costs. For more than half of all subjects, this is zero, and factors such as surgeries and length of hospitalization greatly influence finding variability.

Cost of Home-care Services

Costs for home-care services include assistance with ADL and IADL, visits to day hospitals and day-care centers, and home-care consultations and treatments. Our examination of overall combined public and private costs reveals that there has been significant change in both zones. In the comparison zone, the average annual costs per person rose steadily from $3,800 initially to $5,300 after four years. While these costs fluctuated between $3,500 and $4,000 in the experimental zone, the differences between the two zones are not statistically significant.

ISOLATING THE PUBLIC COMPONENT of home-care costs reveals that both the experimental and comparison zones show significant increases over four years. A comparison of the changes, however, shows no significant differences (Figure 13.10). These findings are consistent with the fact that, during the study, no differential investments were made in the experimental zone over the comparison zone to increase the quantity of home-care services.

Figure 13.10
Total annual average cost per person for home-care services

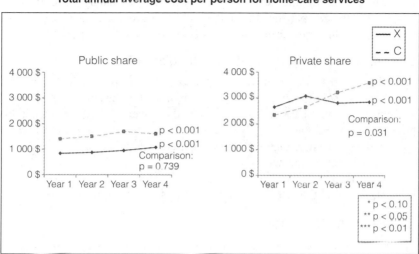

OUR EXAMINATION OF THE PRIVATE COSTS OF HOME-CARE SERVICES reveals a significant difference between the two zones in cost trends (Figure 13.10). The comparison zone shows rising average annual costs, starting at $2,300 and ending at $3,600 after four years. In the experimental zone, which initially showed average annual costs slightly higher than those in the comparison zone, the RISPA seems to have had a stabilizing effect in the last two years, with an average annual cost of $2,900. This explains the significant difference observed between the zones in the comparison of change.

Cost of Consultations with Health Professionals

Analyzing the annual cost for all consultations with health professionals (doctors, nurses, social workers and others), public and private sector combined, including home-care consultations, reveals the same general trends as for home-care services—that is, a relative stabilization in the experimental zone with a steady increase in the comparison zone. We also observe a significant difference between the zones related to trends in average annual costs over four years. The average annual costs in the experimental zone drop from around $850 to around $700, while those in the comparison zone begin at $900 and increase to $1,300 ($p < 0,001$). Considered independently, consultations with nurses also show significant differences in cost changes. Average annual costs in the experimental zone fluctuate between $320 and $360 and those in the comparison zone gradually increase from $360 to $760 ($p < 0.001$).

On the other hand, the costs of consultations with family doctors trend slightly differently. The changes in both zones are still statistically significant, but the average annual costs tend to decline in both zones. This cost is initially $220 (the equivalent of just over 5 visits) for both zones and by the fourth year, it is $200 in the comparison zone and $160 in the experimental zone. The difference is roughly equivalent to one visit fewer per year (p = 0.006).

Outcome of Economic Analysis by Subregion (MRC)

There is no statistically significant difference between twinned MRCs in total annual costs. Obviously, for the examination of the findings by type of service, the reduced sample size entails a decrease in the power to detect significant differences. For the economic analysis by MRC, none of the findings by service type shed any new light on the matter compared with the overall findings when comparing the experimental and comparison zones.

Discussion of Service Use and Costs

Impact on the Use of Health Services

The study did not put forward a hypothesis predicting that any given service would see an increase or decrease in use. The hypothesis was rather that, in general, we would see a *difference* in service use by the subjects in the experimental zone compared with the subjects in the comparison zone as the RISPA was implemented. This difference in use would translate into greater efficiency.

In fact, differences in the trends in service use were observed. Therefore, we can say that the integration of services was responsible. Have we achieved the goal of providing "the right service, at the right time, by the right institution, and at the lowest cost"? There is undoubtedly work to be done, particularly regarding the accessibility of home-care services, but given the desirable outcome on emergency room use and consultations with health professionals, the generally positive impacts on hospitalization (stabilization), together with the demonstrated impacts on satisfaction with services in general (and other impacts discussed in Chapter 12), integration is a step in the right direction. The elderly in the experimental zone use the services differently, are more satisfied with them, and generally experience positive outcomes.

Some remarks are in order regarding the discussion of our study's findings. Few direct comparisons can be carried out with other studies on the same type of service use. Moreover, not only does the structure of the health system differ considerably from one country to another, but also from one information source to another. In our case, the fact that we gathered the data from the participants enabled us to obtain information on private and volunteer services in addition to public ones. By contrast, the Bois-Francs[5-6] and SIPA (système de services intégrés pour personnes âgées en perte d'autonomie)[7-8] studies in Québec made use of administrative databases, much like studies on PACE (*Program of All-inclusive Care for the Elderly*) in the US[9-11] and others in Italy[12-13].

The positive impact on emergency room use is a very interesting finding. Initially, a higher proportion of subjects in the experimental zone used the emergency room as a point of entry into the system. This reading of the situation is confirmed by the fact that this higher proportion of emergency-room visits was followed by a lower rate of hospitalizations compared with the comparison zone. The stabilization in emergency room use in Estrie (no significant increase), and a rate of visits followed by hospitalization that coincides with the level of the comparison zone by the end of the study, indicate a more appropriate emergency room use. The SIPA study found no significant impact on emergency room use,[7-8] while the Bois-Francs study[5-6] found several negative impacts on various indicators (rate of visits, at least one visit per year). It should be noted, however, that the level of use was significantly lower in the experimental zone before the RISPA implementation, and that it is no higher than in the control zone at the end of the study. The study conducted in Italy by Bernabei et al.[12] found a decrease in emergency-room visits in the experimental group. In that study, the explanation cannot be an initially high level of emergency-room consultations, since only 6 % of experimental group subjects used the emergency room over the year of the study, compared with 17 % in the control group. In our study's experimental zone, an initially high level of emergency-room consultations (46 % of subjects over the year) make the RISPA's impacts noticeable and confirm its potential influence. The elderly subjects in Estrie now use the emergency room for "good" reasons more often, for situations where it is called for, and not as a point of entry to the system's services. The single entry point to services implemented under the RISPA seems to have borne fruit. Insofar as our study is concerned, we can credit the RISPA with bringing about a more appropriate use of the emergency room.

We observed a trend toward stabilization in hospitalizations in our experimental zone. Specifically, the proportion of subjects with one hospitalization per year increases insignificantly in the experimental zone, while, in the comparison zone, it increases significantly. The comparison of both evolutions yields insignificant differences ($p = 0.113$), as was the case for this indicator in the Bois-Francs study ($p = 0.11$).[5-6] Note, however, that with our sample size, we were only able to detect a difference of 10 % in hospitalization rates (two-sided alpha level of 0.05, power 80 %). No significant difference was detected in the two studies in the average length of stay and re-hospitalizations. The SIPA study observed no significant difference in hospital use.[7-8] The PACE[9-11] and Italian studies[12-13] showed positive and significant impacts on hospitalizations (number and duration). With no clearly significant impacts observed, the stabilizing effect on hospitalizations in the experimental zone under our study lies halfway between the findings of the other studies in Québec, on the one hand, and the US and Italian studies, on the other.

Findings on the use of public services by the elderly with functional impairment (CLSC home-care services for ADL and IADL, day hospital or day-care center) show a significant difference at the beginning of the study (greater use in the comparison zone). The disparity remains constant, with no significant difference between the trends in the experimental and comparison zones. Both zones showed slight, but insignificant increases in use. At first glance, this is surprising, given the subjects' increasing hardship as evidenced by their significant decline in functional autonomy (see Chapter 12). This seems to reflect the difficulties in accessing CLSC services experienced in both zones, given the relative availability of limited resources. The Bois-Francs study[5-6] found a significant difference between the experimental and control zones in CLSC service use: the former saw a decline in the rate of intervention during the three years out of five for which data are available. This decline in the experimental zone is particularly marked in the CLSC home-care program. By contrast, the SIPA study[7-8] found that the experimental group received 62 % more hours of home health-care services than the control group ($p < 0.05$). The SIPA entailed an increase in home-care services through a specific budgetary allocation.

When we examine the use of home-care services for ADL and IADL from public and private sources, we see a significant increase in both the experimental and comparison zones. The comparison of the two zones reveals no significant difference. The Italian study which examined the use of certain home-care services did not detect any significant difference,[12] whereas the various PACE sites show a wide variation in their findings. For example, the proportion of users of assistance for activities of daily living is anywhere from 16 % to 94 %, depending on the experimental site.[11] An increase in the use of home-care services was found, however, for all experimental sites combined.

We observed no significant difference between the experimental and comparison zones in the trends in use of volunteer services. To our knowledge, this is the first study that evaluates the impacts of an integrated system on a number of these services. Only one other integration study conducted in Italy examined the use of Meals on Wheels, with no significant difference reported. Our study found this to be the most frequently used volunteer service. The use of volunteer services seems to be influenced by their availability in the region; the trends in use do not appear to be influenced by the RISPA.

Regarding consultations with health professionals, in a number of cases—specifically, with general practitioners, medical specialists and nurses—we observed declines in the experimental zone. We observed a significant difference between the experimental and comparison zones in trends in consultations with nurses and other health professionals (e.g. physiotherapists, occupational therapists, social workers), with the comparison zone seeing increased use. Some case managers and administrators in Estrie suggested that the findings may reflect case managers' efforts to "economize" on professional consultations. This explanation is plausible; but were it true, we would expect to see an increase in consultations with other professionals, which is the category that includes consultations with these case managers. But this is not the case. What we actually observe is a stable rate of consultations with other professionals in the experimental zone, an increase in the comparison zone, and a significant difference between the zones. Are these case managers, by means of their regular telephone contact with their clientele, able to "economize" on consultations for every category of health professional? Our data are insufficient to test this explanation and to confirm it with certainty, but it is a possible reflection of the mechanism at work. One Italian study reported a significant decline in visits to general practitioners,[12] but the opposite was observed under the SIPA study.[7-8] A greater number of consultations with health professionals was seen in the experimental groups in the Bois-Francs[5-6] and PACE[9-11] studies.

Emergency-room visits and hospitalizations aside, it is interesting to note that both increases and decreases in service use may be interpreted as positive, depending on the integration study. These differing readings of the trends are probably influenced by the way the original situation was seen to be problematic. A decrease in the use of medical services will be viewed as positive if the services were originally inundated. Integration seems to reshuffle the cards, so to speak.

To summarize our study's highlights, we found that integration brought about a more appropriate use of emergency rooms, a stabilization in hospitalizations in the experimental zone, decreases in consultations with a number of types of health care professionals, no difference in CLSC home-care services, assistance with ADL and IADL, or use of volunteer services.

Economic Impact

Since the total costs in the experimental zone are neither statistically nor economically different from those in the comparison zone, we can draw the preliminary conclusion that service integration does not result in any supplemental costs from the perspective of an entire population. Although one of Lentz's "five laws of integration"[14] holds that integration involves costs before yielding savings, it seems that, in the case of Estrie, the costs were offset relatively quickly by the savings likely stemming from better-adapted services.

The RISPA does not appear to transfer any public costs to the elderly in the form of private services that they incur. On the contrary, we see a slight but statistically significant decline in private costs assumed by the elderly in the experimental zone.

When comparing the PRISMA–Estrie findings with the Bois-Francs[5-6] and SIPA[7-8] studies, it is important to note that the approaches and the costs under consideration vary. The main difference is that in the latter two studies, the costs examined were obtained from participant files and the costs of non-public services could not be considered. On the other hand, these are the actual, inflation-adjusted costs for each participant. For the PRISMA–Estrie study, we used standardized costs (constant 2002 dollars). Both the SIPA and Bois-Francs studies considered the costs of accommodations for CHSLDs alone. In the PRISMA–Estrie study, we considered the accommodation costs regardless of housing—in our view, a better basis of comparison.

Note, however, that neither the Bois-Francs nor the SIPA studies found a significant increase in total costs in the experimental group. The cost break-down was affected by the changes in the types of services used by the group, but with no impact, either positive or negative, on total cost.

Using very different methodologies, the two Italian studies found cost reductions too. Whether or not these reductions are significant is not indicated, however percentage wise, they amount to 23 %[12] and 27 %[13] in one year. In the latter case, the costs involved are exclusively hospital costs, whereas in the former, Bernabei et al.[12] evaluated a range of institutional and home-care costs in a randomized clinical trial with 200 participants. The PACE studies produced contradictory findings: some positive, some insignificant.[9-11] A cost reduction is intrinsically a positive finding, however, in order to evaluate efficiency, cost impacts must be compared with human impacts, which is discussed in the next section.

Preliminary Observations about RISPA Efficiency

A practical approach to examining the findings presented in this chapter and in the chapter on the impacts on the elderly and their caregivers, consists of arrang-ing these impacts in an efficiency table[15] that correlates costs and impacts. They can be rated as higher, lower, or equal to one another (Table 13.1). We can make a claim of efficiency in cases where the impacts in the experimental zone are higher than those in the comparison zone and the costs equal or lower. We can also make this claim if the impacts produced are equivalent and the costs lower (shaded region).

Table 13.1
Efficiency Table: experimental zone vs. to comparison zone

		EFFECT		
		Higher	**Equal**	**Lower**
COST	**Higher**	less efficient	less efficient	to evaluate
	Equal	less efficient	equally efficient	more efficient
	Lower	not efficient	more efficient	more efficient

Our examination of economic impacts shows equivalent costs in both zones. We placed each of the variables we measured into one of three categories according to the impacts observed: lower, equal, or higher (Table 13.2).

Table 13.2
Efficiency results: experimental zone compared to comparison zone

	EFFECT		
	Lower	**Equal**	**Higher**
COST =	Less efficient: Caregiver's Burden?	Equal efficient: Mortality Disabilities Desire to institutionalize	More efficient: Decline Handicaps Satisfaction Empowerment

At first glance, we see that the higher efficiency outweighs lower efficiency, since the impacts are either equal or higher in the experimental zone. This is evidence in support of an increase in efficiency under RISPAs. Future research is needed to flesh out these preliminary analyses on efficiency.

Conclusion on Overall RISPA Performance

Integrated care aims to better coordinate the services offered in a community. As a result of the integration of services for the elderly carried out under the PRISMA-Estrie study, we were able to see trends in the movement of a number of variables over four years. The study confirms that integration leads to flexibility in the use of services. It can bring about adjustments in service use, some of which (e.g. more appropriate use of emergency rooms) would be a great advantage to the system. Integration has proven its capacity to produce different outcomes. It is now patent that we mustn't assume that we cannot achieve more with the same resources.

Since, on the whole, efficiency has been demonstrated, generalized implementation is recommended. Overall, integration of services generates positive impacts for the elderly, on the use of health services, and with no resulting cost difference. Our findings concerning caregivers require more in-depth analysis to be able to draw conclusions about them.

Keep in mind that the largely positive impacts and increased efficiency were observed despite the fact that integration was not absent in the comparison zone. Although most of the integration tools and mechanisms were not implemented in the comparison zone, to a certain extent, common tools were used. The Multiclientele Assessment Tool, for example, became in 2002 the standard in the ministry of health and social services. In the years that followed, it was implemented throughout Québec, including in the Chaudière-Appalaches region. This implies a certain degree of contamination of the comparison zone. Moreover, integration was never 100 % complete in the experimental zone, but rather 78 % complete following the third year of the study. Only 134 experimental subjects out of 751 (17.8 %) had access to case management at least one day during their participation in the study.

The Bois-Francs[5-6] and SIPA[7-8] studies also found overall positive impacts. Considering that these three projects were all carried out in Québec, using different but complementary approaches, we can definitively conclude that integration is beneficial to the health and social services system. The SIPA project was a randomized clinical trial involving the clientele of two CLSCs; the Bois-Francs study was a quasi-experimental study involving the active users of the system; finally, the PRISMA-Estrie study was a quasi-experimental study taking a population-based approach (active users and non-users of the system). Three comprehensive studies all weigh in favor of integration.

Over the years, Québec has become a world center for research on integration, as can be readily seen by attending international symposia or conferences on integration. Moreover, researchers from other countries where integration studies have taken place generally look to Québec's experiences with near admiration. In their view, our health-care system was relatively integrated even before the Bois-Francs, SIPA, and PRISMA-Estrie projects. The mere fact that health services and social services fall under the same government department—part of a publicly funded system with a tradition of interdisciplinary collaboration—is proof that integration exists. The fact that Québec is moving from the "linkage" level to the "coordination" or "full integration" levels, to use Leutz's model,[14] and that we are able to measure the impacts is astounding to some. Highly disjointed health-care systems with shared public and private responsibilities are much the norm in most Western countries. Even in Québec, we often overlook this fact, but observers from elsewhere remind us of it at each gathering. Of course, Québec's health-care system has its own problems to solve, but we can build on certain valuable achievements.

Québec's health-care policy makers would do well to implement RISPAs of this type to take advantage of their benefits. RISPAs are not a panacea, but we now know that *not* integrating services will result in negative impacts. Despite the fact that investments in home care have been modest in recent years ('modest' is actually a generous adjective to describe the experimental zone in Estrie), integration has shown positive impacts. In short, the scarcity of resources is not an excuse to avoid integration. On the contrary, integration will enable us to ensure that the available services will be managed optimally.

The creation of the Centres de santé et de services sociaux (CSSS) in Québec helped to eliminate administrative obstacles facing integration. It is time for clinical integration to take place. The health and social services system is now equipped with a winning blueprint bearing the promise of efficiency with which to face the coming demographic transition.

Bibliography

1. Drummond, M.F., B.J. O'Brien, G.L. Stoddart, and Torrance, G.W. *Méthodes d'évaluation économique des programmes de santé.* Paris: Économica, 1998.

2. Tousignant, M., Hébert, R., Dubuc, N., Coulombe, C. "Public funding of home care services for frail older adults: are the needs being met?," in *Integrated service delivery to ensure person's functional autonomy,* edited by R. Hébert, A. Tourigny, and M. Gagnon, 225-40. Québec: Edisem, 2005.

3. Hébert, R., Robichaud, L., Roy, PM., Bravo, G., and Voyer, L. "Efficacy of a Nurse-Led Multidimensional Preventive Programme for Older People at Risk of Functional Decline: A Randomized Controlled Trial," *Age and Ageing* 2001; 30: 147–53.

4. Dubois, M-F., Raîche, M., Hébert, R., and Gueye, N-R. "Assisted Self-Report of Health-Services Use Showed Excellent Reliability in a Longitudinal Study of Older Adults," *Journal of Clinical Epidemiology,* 2007; 60(10): 1040-45.

5. Tourigny, A., Bonin, L., Hébert, R., and Rochette, L. "Quasi-experimental Study of the Effectiveness of an Integrated Service Delivery Network for the Frail Elderly," *Canadian Journal on Aging* 2004; 23(3): 231-46.

6. Durand, PJ, Lemay, A., Tourigny, A., Bonin, L., and Paradis, M. *Développement et implantation d'un système de prix de revient des soins et des services à domicile dans le cadre du projet de démonstration d'un réseau intégré de services dans les Bois-Francs avec une coordination des services de gestion de cas* (case-management): Rapport QC123. Fonds pour l'adaptation des services de santé, 2001.

7. Béland F., H. Bergman, P. Lebel, A.M. Clarfield, P. Tousignant, A.P. Contandriopoulos, and L. Dallaire. "A system of integrated care for older persons with disabilities in Canada: results from a randomized controlled trial," *Journal of Gerontology: Series A - Biological Sciences and Medical Sciences* 2006; 61(4): 367-73.

8. Béland F., Bergman, H., Dallaire, L., Fletcher, J., Lebel, P., Monette, J., Denis, J-L., Contandriopoulos, A-P., Cimon, A., Bureau, C., Bouvier, L., and Dubois, D. *Évaluation du Système intégré pour personnes âgées fragiles (SIPA): Utilisation et coûts des services sociaux et de santé.* Ottawa: Canadian Health Services Research Foundation: 2004.

9. Kodner D.L., and Kyriacou, C.K. "Fully Integrated Care for Frail Elderly: Two American Models," *International Journal of Integrated Care* 2000; (www.ijic.org) 1(november 1): 1-24.

10. Johri, M., Béland, F., and Bergman, H. "International Experiments in Integrated Care for the Elderly: A Synthesis of the Evidence," *International Journal of Geriatric Psychiatry* 2003; 18: 222-235.

11. Branch, L.G., Coulam, R.F., and Zimmerman, Y.A. "The PACE Evaluation: Initial Findings," *Gerontologist* 1995; 35(3): 349-59.

12. Bernabei R., Landi, F., Gambassi, G., Sgadari, A., Zuccala, G., Mor, V., Rubenstein, L.Z., and Carbonin, P. "Randomised Trial of Impact of Model of Integrated Care and Case Management for Older People Living in the Community," *British Medical Journal* 1998; 316(7141): 1348-51.

13. Landi F., Onder, G., Russo, A., Tabaccanti, S., Rollo, R., Federici, S., Tua, E., Cesari, M., and Bernabei, R. "A New Model of Integrated Home Care for the Elderly: Impact on Hospital Use". *Journal of Clinical Epidemiology* 2001; 54(9): 968-70.

14. Leutz W.N. "Five Laws for Integrating Medical and Social Services: Lessons from the United States and the United Kingdom," *Milbank Quarterly* 1999; 77(1): 77-110.

15. Durand S., Blanchette, D., and Hébert, R. "L'intégration des services pour les personnes âgées et l'efficience," *3ᵉ Journée de recherche du Réseau québécois de recherche sur le vieillissement. Québec*, Québec, 2004.

Acknowledgements

We extend our warmest thanks to all study participants. We also gratefully acknowledge all those who contributed to the project over the years.

Funding

This project was funded by the Canadian Institutes of Health Research (CIHR), the Ministère de la santé et des services sociaux du Québec, and the Agence de la santé et des services sociaux de l'Estrie.

Chapter 14
Evaluation of an Information System within an Integrated Services Network for Frail Seniors: Its Use and User Perception of Usefulness and Impact

Diane Morin, André Tourigny, Line Robichaud, Daniel Pelletier, Lucie Bonin, Aline Vézina, Luc Mathieu, Martin Buteau

Highlights

- The geronto-geriatric information system (SIGG) is innovator because it aims at supporting a long-lasting follow-up by multidisciplinary health professionals working at different levels of care.
- The introduction of SIGG was done in a context: where health professionals had to adapt to an new integrated services delivery network and at the same time to learn how to use a new electronic health record.
- Many technical obstacles were encountered throughout the studied period.
- Despite these technical problems, the users perceive many advantages to the SIGG, especially in primary health care.
- Data from SIGG databases show that information is shared between health professionals from different fields and from different services.
- The SIGG appears to be an effective strategy to support interdisciplinary work in integrated services delivery network.

Keywords: electronic health record, information systems, service quality, interdisciplinarity, integrated services delivery network

Abstract

The geronto-geriatric information system (SIGG) analyzed in this study is an interdisciplinary and interfacility electronic health record designed for information sharing within an integrated services delivery network for frail seniors. This study describes SIGG use and its perceived usefulness and impact. Questionnaires (n=85), group interviews (n=3), patient files (n=5128), inventories of workstations and observation were used to obtain data. Results show that the

SIGG has gained widespread acceptance among health professionals although the pattern of use by workers in primary health care differs from that in secondary care. The SIGG is considered most appropriate in the delivery of services to the frail elderly who use many types of services from different facilities concomitantly. According to users, the SIGG is an effective tool for standardization, coordination and continuity of care, and provides better quality information.

Introduction

SIGG is an acronym for *Système d'information géronto-gériatrique*, a gerontogeriatric information system. It is an interdisciplinary and interfacility information system that includes an electronic health record. It was introduced in 1998 to support information sharing throughout an integrated services delivery network for more than 11,000 frail elderly people living in the Bois-Francs Region (Province of Quebec, Canada)[1-2]. It is a computerized clinical information system shared by health professionals, service providers and managers (nurses, social workers, physicians, pharmacists, physiotherapists, occupational and physical therapists, nutritionists, community groups providing services to elders) from different partnering facilities within the integrated services network (hospitals, local community care centres, day care centres, rehabilitation units, geriatric ambulatory services, long-term nursing homes, physicians' offices). Developed through an interfacility and interdisciplinary collaborative effort, the SIGG currently has 250 users. Between 1998 and 2003 a total of 5128 electronic charts for frail seniors have been entered into the SIGG. In addition to identification, contact and sociodemographic data, the SIGG contains seven other forms: (1) the multiclientele evaluation form (OÉMC), (2) a functional status profile[3-4] (SMAF), (3) a service request form, (4) an intervention plan, (5) an individualized service plan chart, (6) a medication profile and (7) follow-up memos. There is real-time access to all forms throughout all facilities.

The study targeted specific issues raised after several years of SIGG implementation. SIGG users and managers involved were eager to find out how professionals were using the SIGG and if its use led to better outcomes for patients and better care delivery. The study goal was to assess whether the SIGG is an effective tool for improving health care delivery and supporting interdisciplinarity. Specific objectives were to: (1) describe SIGG use, (2) investigate perceived advantages or constraints associated with its use and (3) describe its perceived effects on different aspects of service delivery to frail elderly patients and on interdisciplinarity. The study is part of a larger research program that also investigated how elderly clients and their caregivers view SIGG use.

Figure 14.1

Adapted Model from DeLone & McLean, Seddon & Kurian

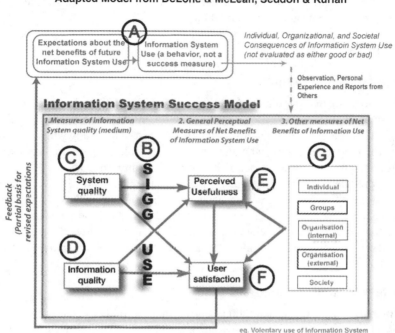

Theoretical model

The theoretical model used is inspired by the DeLone and McLean model[6,7] and takes into account the contributions of Seddon and Kurian[8,9,10] which focuses on six dimensions: (A) user expectations for benefits, (B) system use, (C) system quality, (D) information quality, (E) perceived usefulness, as well as outcomes such as (F) user satisfaction and (G) perceived benefits. This article does not address dimension (A) concerning user expectations since these results have been published previously[11]. They were interpreted taking into account the consistency of health care planning[12], its comprehensiveness and continuity[13], and coordination[14,15], as well as its efficiency, interdisciplinary work, productivity, quality of clinical decisions and the quality of the relationships.

Based on this model, several conditions were set to determine whether SIGG use led to better care and better practices. First, the SIGG had to be used mainly with frail elderly clients. Second, hardware and software had to be suited to the task and flexible enough to avoid hindering health care delivery. Third, users needed to perceive a positive impact on continuity of care, comprehensiveness of care, care coordination, and standardization. Fourth, users needed to perceive that system use improves information quality and helps clinical decision making. Finally, users needed to perceive that system use improves overall productivity and efficiency.

Methods

Population and sampling

The initial targeted population was composed of all SIGG users. At the time of the study, there were 187 users registered in the SIGG security database. They were all considered eligible for the quantitative part of the study which took the form of a survey. For those who were invited to participate in group discussions, three samples were determined using purposive sampling. This type of sampling provides a range of informants based on specific characteristics that are linked to the theoretical concerns. Each of the three groups included six to eight participants (n=21) from different backgrounds (medical, nursing, rehabilitation, nutrition, care management, etc.) as well as from facilities offering different levels of care (medical clinics, home care, day care centres, nursing homes and hospitals).

Data collection and analyses

The study period was from 2000 to 2003. Multiple tools were used to collect data. First, inventories were made of computers and workstations used for SIGG access. At he time of the work station inventories, people were asked about SIGG usage. They were also observed while using the SIGG and asked for facilitating factors, constraints and difficulties associated with their workstation environments. Second, file data was retrieved concerning SIGG forms entered or accessed since 1998. The data provided information on the professions of users and the specific level of care, facility and service in order to facilitate comparison of patterns of use. Third, a 60-minute survey composed of 150 questions for the 6 dimensions was developed[1]. The six dimensions included (1) user perception of computer settings, (2) SIGG use, (3) system quality, (4) information quality, (5) perceived usefulness and perceived benefits, and (6) overall satisfaction. Answers were recorded using a five-point Likert scale, ranging from "Totally agree" (5 pts) to "Totally disagree" (1 pt) or a dichotomic Yes/No scale. The questionnaire had been previously tested for validity and reliability and was sent to the 187 eligible SIGG users. Fourth and last, interview guidelines were drawn up to lead group discussion interviews designed to allow participants to share their views on SIGG use at work and comment on its advantages, disadvantages or constraints, and the changes it might have on relationships with patients and their family, as well as with co-workers, or on workload. They were also asked how they felt the SIGG should be used in the future.

Data from the questionnaire was analyzed quantitatively for frequencies, percentages and basic comparisons (t-test; chi-square). Qualitative material collected during site visits or group interviews was analyzed using a case study approach. Verbatim material was first transcribed and read, and then coded according to dimensions of the DeLone and McLean model[6,7] or according to emerging categories of information. NVivo (v1.3) software facilitated coding which was performed independently by two members of the research team until consensus was reached. In this type of evaluation, data reduction is primarily guided by the need to address the objectives. Coded material was analyzed on the basis of its relation to the central dimensions of the models, as well as on the basis of new and emerging areas of information.

Findings

Users profile

Only 85 of the 187 persons asked to fill out the questionnaire did so. The participation rate was therefore low (45.5 %). Organizational factors prevailing throughout the study and SIGG-related technical problems seem to have influenced participation. We were told that non-participation could have been an indication of dissatisfaction with the lack of corrective measures applied to technical problems. The main characteristics of SIGG user profiles are: 16 % were male, average age was 42.8, 69 % worked in primary care, 31 % worked in secondary care. Most respondents had a full time job (58 % full time, 22 % part time, 20 % other job status). Almost 40 % considered themselves as beginners in computer use and 56 % as intermediate or advanced. Of the 21 persons who participated in the group interviews, 14 % were managers and 86 % were professionals from various disciplines, mainly medicine, nursing, social work and case management.

System Use (B)

Many of the following results are based on data retrieved from the SIGG databases. Data reflects the evolution of the SIGG which was first developed as a set of clinical forms but underwent major revisions and upgrades before and during the study period. System use comprises two major elements: the number of records created in the system and the number of entries made or accessed annually.

Number of elderly people with a SIGG record

In Figure 14.2, a general increase can be observed in newly created or in active files between January 1998 and December 2002. In fact, in December 2002, there were 2854 active records in comparison with 775 in 1998. In 2000-2001, among all seniors aged 65 and over living in the Bois-Francs region, 26 % had

Figure 14.2
Number of active SIGG records from 1998 to 2003

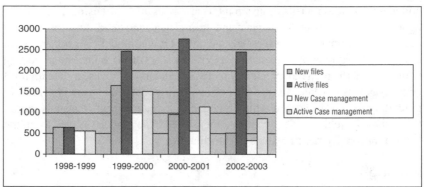

a SIGG record. Among those aged 65 to 74, only about 14 % did. This percentage rises to 34 % for those 75 to 84, and to 64 % for those 85 and over. During that period, the percentage of elderly people with an active record specifically in case management also increased with age, varying from 6 % for those 65 to 74, to 15 % for those 75 to 84, and 31 % for those 85 and over. Overall, 11 % of those aged 65 and over have an active SIGG record in case management for that period.

Use of forms

As previously indicated, the SIGG has seven forms. Figure 14.3 shows there was an increase in use over time for the five most commonly used.

In depth analysis shows that in 2002-2003 in terms of the OEMC multi-clientele evaluation form, the percentage of people aged 65 and over with an active file containing at least one fully completed form did not increase and

Figure 14.3
Number of Main SIGG Forms Use from 1998 to 2003

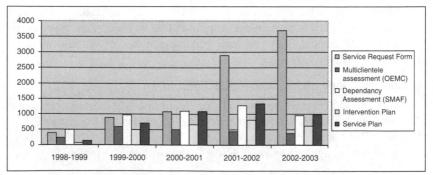

stayed relatively low at 12 %. For active case management records, this percentage rose to 24 %. From 1998 to 2002 the overall number of fully completed SMAF forms also increased. About 20 % of all files retrieved have at least one annually updated or partial SMAF. SMAF forms are found in 50 % of case management files but only 35 % of those are completely filled out. The proportion of active SIGG records with at least one intervention plan in a given year is increasing but still remains very low at 16 %. The use of service plan forms has nevertheless increased regularly over time, rising to 1,325 in 2001-2002.

Because service plan forms are mainly used in case management, analysis of the study period shows that the percentage of active case management files with at least one completed form increased from 18 % to 46 %.

SIGG data entry and use

We observed that the average number of times that SIGG forms were consulted or data was entered increased in relation to client age. Each active file was accessed an average of 39 times in 2001-2002 for patients 65 to 74, and 43 times for those 75 and over. On average, 16 data entries per active file were made in 2001-2002 for patients 65 to 74, and 18 for those 75 and over. Average data entries and consultations also increased when the SIGG file included a SMAF. Averages also rose with higher SMAF scores, showing that SIGG use increases for seniors showing a lower level of autonomy.

The frequency of access is certainly a good indicator of how information is shared between users from different professional backgrounds, different levels of care and different types of facilities. For example, we examined the extent to which electronic entries in the follow-up memos made by case managers were read by health care professionals from primary and second levels of care within

Figure 14.4
Proportion of interdisciplinary follow-up Memos (%)

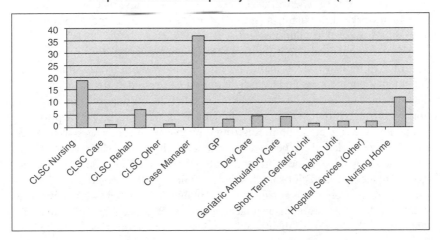

a 30-day period. The breakdown for 765 occurrences of data access over a 30-day period was 37.5 % by other case managers, 19.3 % by residential care staff, 7.5 % by rehabilitation unit staff, 4.6 % by geriatric ambulatory service staff and 2.7 % by intensive geriatric rehabilitation unit staff. This illustrates that primary health care workers are more proactive in using electronic records than are secondary health care workers. We will explore this difference in a subsequent section.

System quality

Desktop models make up 64.6 % of the 110 computers in the network and laptops the other 35.4 %. The range of processors in the computers reflects what was available on the market in the years covered by the study. The network architecture is based on Lotus Notes (v5) and includes servers in five facilities. It ensures file replication every fifteen minutes. Some computers are clearly out of date. Users often complained about poor system performance, but most often the network was at fault. Server network cards were upgraded to solve the problem and, as previously mentioned, the SIGG underwent two major upgrades. Nevertheless, technical problems and disruptions influenced user perception of system quality.

According to the questionnaire, even if only 59 % of the respondents consider the technology to be generally reliable, 80 % are satisfied with how they work and with workstation availability. Workstation ergonomics are generally viewed as acceptable but open to improvement. At the time of observation, workstations were often encumbered with wires, mouse, keyboards and monitors, leaving little room for workspace. Workstation furniture was not always adjusted for maximum user comfort. From a workflow perspective, 38 % of respondents say that they sometimes have to devise alternative solutions to deal with computer or network disruptions. Most users have their own computer, but some share hardware. The work schedule is often the cause of work overload at the end of work shifts, but during group interviews it was said that everyone gets by and finds workable solutions.

Users complained about the fact that computerization does not cover or integrate all their workload mainly because it is required by law that written documents, photocopies and transcriptions must be signed for at the archives department. This remains a daily task. Computerization requires that information be processed quickly on a constant basis in order to be kept up-to-date throughout the care continuum. Entering data into what is expected to be a fast and effective work tool can be cumbersome when the system slows down. Users stated that they depend more and more heavily on computers on an every day basis. Breakdowns and clumsily designed features produce frustration. Technical support for problems is considered acceptable. While 25 % say that the time it takes to deal with problems is unacceptable, 81 % agree that technical assistance regularly does solve their problems. Users want to be consulted on SIGG improvements and development so that answers to their needs are suitable and realistic.

Training delivered covered only the first versions of SIGG. For version 3, some assistance was provided by co-workers but no formal training sessions were offered. The average training time was 18.1 hours, of which 16.6 were said to be received on the job. Almost 80 % of respondents agree that training gave them enough knowledge to work adequately with the computers and the SIGG. Comments are generally positive but point to a need for post-training support. Assistance from colleagues is seen as appropriate but is not viewed as the only suitable solution to improve skills. In fact, 70 % of respondents favour technical support and formal training.

Information quality (D)

Most comments on the quality of information provided by the SIGG are positive. Specifically, a majority of respondents agree that the SIGG gives them more accurate and more accessible information. Complaints mainly concern improving the SIGG's application and customizing it to specific needs, such as adding features that would provide automatically-generated profiles or summaries.

Perceived Usefulness (E)

Perceived efficiency

SIGG users insist that system slowdowns and malfunctions should be corrected to ensure greater performance and increased system reliability. Users recommend keeping the user-friendly interfaces already available in the SIGG's latest version. SIGG users see usefulness as a balance between costs and benefits; between effort put into learning and paybacks in terms of work achievement, better coordination in services and ultimately better care. The following benefits were mentioned by users. First, it saves time resulting in fewer trips to archives, faster interaction, shorter delays, fewer phone calls and reduced clerical tasks. Second, it improves direct access to information offering easier interaction, rapid identification of case managers, caregivers and other services providers. Third, it lowers the need for duplication and repetition for patients in terms of gathering information and managing files at different facilities. Fourth, the SIGG provides improved information security over paper files because there are fewer documents borrowed from the archives and there is greater file traceability on access and services provided. Fifth, it lowers the risk of error in file duplication, errors in patient names and address and provides better legibility. Sixth, it eases care supervision and management in terms of access to a professional health care worker's caseload, services provided according to objectives (IP and ISP forms), follow-up and referrals and caregiver replacements. Last, it eases manager workload and automates consent renewal and other routine tasks.

SIGG efficiency is viewed differently by users at different stages in the intervention process. For respondents involved in secondary health care, SIGG data must be updated quickly if it is to be useful. So these respondents prefer to talk to case managers and family members because they consider that these informants have information that is more up-to-date than the SIGG. On the other hand, users involved in primary care see the SIGG as indispensable for follow-up, case management and reassessment. They feel that the SIGG provides a broader perspective leading to better plan care and services. Informants from different levels of care have different perceptions of SIGG effectiveness.

User Satisfaction (F) and other measures of benefits (G)

The differences in perceived utility according to level of care affect overall user satisfaction. As one respondent said: "...*even if I know nothing about data processing, the SIGG is an extraordinary tool for follow-up, information, communication with caregivers, [...] at every level*". "*It is pitiful [...] because sometimes, I think we are the only ones to use the SIGG on a large scale. Anyone, at any moment, can obtain information on our patients, visits, treatment and services provided. If I want information on a client seen last week by one of my colleagues in primary care, I can get it by looking in the SIGG. But if I want to know what happened in other secondary care units, like the UCDG (hospital) well...it's often missing.*"

The difference in patterns of use and in data entry is also a factor that seems to be highly important. Comments in user group discussions, as well as results from the questionnaire, show a difference in views between professionals from primary and secondary levels of care. The latter view fewer benefits, but also use the system less often and in a less comprehensive way.

Even the system's flaws are viewed as being surmountable and do not affect satisfaction as much as we expected. SIGG users report that, despite problems, they were willing to adapt. They said that they learned how to use the software, safety protocols and passwords quickly. They learned how to navigate within and between different forms, they got used to different settings, and often had to deal with a lack of desktop space. All these adaptive skills were acquired in a short period of time. The SIGG was integrated into the workflow quickly and is greatly appreciated as long as it eases the workload.

Using the SIGG is seen as quite different from paperwork. Users have to take over some clerical work formerly done by other types of personnel (for example, access and manage their records through the SIGG instead of relying on archives personnel). Users would nevertheless like to have even more features integrated into the SIGG, and they would appreciate having it customized to fit more of their needs. Users said they easily became familiar with computers. They say they often use their own time to get better acquainted with new software.

Figure 14.5
Main score (0-5) Results on Perceived Benefits

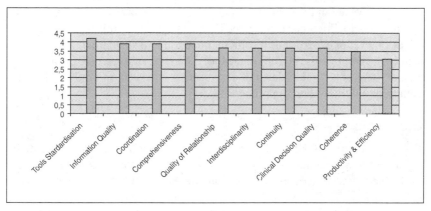

The following figure presents the questionnaire scores on six dimensions of benefits related to clinical work and services. As previously indicated, answers were rated on a five-point Likerttype scale where responses range from 5 "Totally agree", to 1 "Totally disagree".

As seen in Figure 14.5, the mean scores attributed to the dimensions were all relatively high considering the 5-point scale. Ranked by level on agreement on perceived benefits, respondents think the SIGG helps in: (1) tool standardization; (2) coordination, comprehensiveness of care and information quality; (3) continuity of care, quality of the relationship with clients, clinical decision quality and interdisciplinary work; (4) coherence of care. Finally, they rate (5) productivity and efficiency as the lowest dimension.

During group interviews, some professionals expressed reservations about using computers in front of their clients. They think that the computer might hinder the relationship, coming between themselves and their clients. Their comments do not state if this embarrassment is based on their skilfulness with computers or rather linked to the intervention process itself. Nurses added that the use of a laptop at an elder's home is often problematic. They state that they already have a lot of material to carry and the additional weight of the laptop makes it less attractive. Laptop launch and safety procedures are seen as time consuming when time in the home is already limited and too short.

The highest proportions of "do not know" relate to interdisciplinary work. For example, the question asking whether the SIGG favours recognition of colleagues' competence was not answered by 27 % of respondents. A question related to the fact that the SIGG makes clinical leadership more difficult was not answered by 35 % of the respondents. Further analysis also reveals that case managers and social workers perceive significantly more positive effects than their colleagues on different dimensions such as coordination (4.3 vs 3.7), quality of relationship (4.1 vs 3.4), quality of clinical decisions (4.5 vs 3.4) and comprehensive care (4.5 vs 3.7). Intermediate or advanced computer users are also more positive about the benefits of the SIGG than their novice colleagues (4.0 versus 3.7). No difference is observed based on age, sex, work experience, work status or level of expertise as a computer user on tool standardization and continuity of care. Finally, no difference based on level of expertise, profession or primary versus secondary level of care user, is observed on productivity, efficiency, or interdisciplinary work.

Discussion

Before concluding if the SIGG is really an effective tool to improve care delivery and support interdisciplinary work, results have to be discussed in the light of the literature, the theoretical model and its set of conditions, as well as study limitations.

Results show SIGG use is increasing, mainly for people showing lower autonomy as measured by scores on the SMAF. Also, the older a person gets, the greater the chance that they have an active SIGG record. The SIGG is also used more often for persons with multiple problems or requiring more services from different facilities. This is consistent with literature demonstrating greater usefulness for the more frail elderly population[15,16]. Therefore, the first condition, stating that before concluding that it has added value, the SIGG had to be used more often for frail elderly clients, has been met.

The level of shared information and the level of use of the SIGG seem to vary according to different characteristics. There is a difference between intermediary or advanced users and beginners. A difference has been observed between health care providers in primary care and secondary levels of care. Concerning benefits that are perceived, primary care users agree that there are more benefits for coordination, quality of relationship, clinical decisions and comprehensive care. Group interviews highlighted that participants from secondary care felt they needed more up–to-date information, which they claimed was unavailable in the SIGG. For them, the main sources of information are still the patients, their caregivers, hospital records and the case manager. The presence of a case manager is viewed as a shortcut to a more reliable and easily accessible source of information. These results are consistent with the DeLone & McLean Model[6,7], which postulates that user characteristics and information needs directly influence use and satisfaction with an information system. Also according to the model, satisfaction is linked to the variability in the system quality and use[6,7,17]. This study shows that people who agree with benefits are more acquainted with the system and use it more often. Hardware and technical problems, lack of user-friendliness in some features and forms, plus certain upgrades in the last version, all hindered ease of use, but are all considered as modifiable factors. Users suggest improvements. Problems with computers limit their use. Training and technical and professional support are found to be satisfactory but need to be increased. Most users agreed that they can adapt to the computer system's features and do not question the use of the SIGG, but they pointed out that reliability is a minimum requirement for use.

Only a few professionals use the SIGG at a client's home. In the literature, computer or laptop use during visits is still under debate[18]. For some health professionals, it could greatly change the way they interact with their clients. For homecare nurses, the use of a laptop on visits adds to their task. Most professionals are faced with a double challenge: learning how to use the forms and how to use the computer technology supporting it. The secondary care service providers seem to depend on the SIGG's content but would like to have it adapted to specific needs. Even if the SIGG use is viewed as a clear trend[19], improvement in performance and customization could increase its use, probably even in home care. The literature also indicates that professionals are resistant to the use of a laptop, a computer or even a handheld[15]. Nevertheless, most of these factors are or will be modifiable with technological advances. Reviews[20] regarding information systems are consistent with findings by this study confirming that most users would not like to go back to paper and pencil. They expect more and more from computerization. Therefore, the second condition stating that hardware and software characteristics should be seen as generally suitable and adaptable enough in order not to hamper care provision has been met.

Questionnaires, group interviews and system data analyses show that information is indeed shared between caregivers, between levels of care and between facilities thereby supporting collaboration and interdisciplinary work. The SIGG is also seen to enhance care in various ways such as tools standardization, coordination, comprehensiveness of care and information quality. This was also observed in the literature[21,22]. Users are less convinced that the SIGG enhances productivity and efficiency due to repeated technical difficulties experienced with the system. The literature also generated contradictory findings as regards correlation between the use of electronic health records and improvement in productivity and efficiency[23,24,25,26,27,28]. Nevertheless, our third and fourth conditions are met because users generally perceive positive effects of system use on continuity of care, comprehensiveness of care, care coordination, and standardization and also feel that the use of the system improves information quality and helps clinical decision making.

Several efforts were made to minimize selection bias to ensure internal validity. The questionnaire was sent to all SIGG users. The response rate was low (45.5 %) despite two recalls. However, data analyses showed that there was no difference in the number of entries made and accessed by respondents and non-respondents. Nevertheless, it is impossible to evaluate if answers would have been more or less favourable than they actually were. As for information bias which is usually due to systematic errors on answers, encoding or classification, since the interviews and analysis were based on a theoretical framework, and since interview guidelines and questionnaires were validated by a multidisciplinary research team and field work, this bias should be limited. Moreover, triangulation of qualitative and quantitative data analyses revealed quite a high degree of homogeneity among users' perceptions.

Therefore, the observed results show that a SIGG such as the one evaluated in this study can be viewed as an efficient tool to support care and interdisciplinary work.

Conclusion

This study is one of the few examining the impact of an information system on clinical practices, taking into account the viewpoints of users coming from different levels of care, different backgrounds and different facilities. Results from this study show that SIGG use is being increasingly accepted. Its use increases over time, specifically for those who perceive positive benefits for themselves as well as for patients. The SIGG also provides a secure way to access and exchange information rapidly dealing with the needs of a growing elderly clientele. Even with occasional technical flaws, the SIGG is viewed as improving clinical information exchange. Most users generally see many benefits to its use, especially in primary care services. Most of them would not go back to pen and paper files. The perceived usefulness and the satisfaction might even have been higher if the information system had not experienced technical difficulties during the study period. It is therefore possible to state that use of information systems such as the SIGG can be encouraged in an integrated services delivery network for frail seniors.

Acknowledgements

This study was carried out with the support of grants from the Canadian Institutes of Health Research (CIHR), the *Fonds de recherche en santé du Québec* (FRSQ) and from the former National Health Research Development Program (NHRDP).

References

1. Tourigny A, Bonin L, Morin D, Buteau M, Mathieu L, Robichaud L, V.ézina A, Hébert R, Durand P, Pelletier D. *Système d'information géronto-gériatrique, interdisciplinaire et interétablissements: Utilité perçue et utilisation en temps réel - Rapport de recherche*. Québec: Centre de recherche Centre hospitalier St-Sacrement, Unité de recherche en gériatrie de l'Université Laval. 135 p. 2003.

2. Tourigny A, Durand PJ, Bonin L, Hébert R, & Rochette L. Quasi-experimental Study of the Effectiveness of an Integrated Service Delivery Network for the Frail Elderly. *Canadian Journal on Aging* 2004; 23(3): 231-246.

3.   Hébert R, Carrier R, Bilodeau A. The Functional Autonomy Measurement System (SMAF): Description and Validation of an Instrument for the Measurement of Handicaps. *Age and Ageing* 1998; 17(5): 293-302.

4.   Hébert R, Guilbeault J, Desrosiers J, Dubuc N. The Functional Autonomy Measurement System (SMAF): A Clinical-based Instrument for Measuring Disabilities and Handicaps in Older People. *Journal of the Canadian Geriatrics Society* 2001; 4: 141-147.

5.   Hébert R, Durand PJ, Dubuc N, Tourigny A and the PRISMA Group. PRISMA: A New Model of Integrated Service Delivery for the Frail Older People in Canada. *International Journal of Integrated Care* 2003; 3 (March)

6.   DeLone WH, McLean ER. Information Systems Success: The Quest for the Dependent Variable. *Information Systems Research* 1992; 3(1): 60-95.

7.   DeLone WH, McLean ER. The Delone and McLean Model of Information Systems Success: A ten-year Update. *Journal of Management Information Systems* 2003; 19(4): 9-30.

8.   Seddon PB, Kiew MY. *A Partial Test and Development of DeLone and McLean's Model of IS Success*, International Conference on Information Systems (ICIS) Conference Proceedings, Vancouver, 1994, pp.99-110

9.   Kurian D, Galupe RB, Diaz J. Taking Stock: *Measuring Information Systems Success*. Paper presented at the ASAC-IFSAM-2000 Conference, Montréal, Canada. 2000

10. Seddon PB. A Re-specification and Extension of the Delone and McLean Model of IS success. *Information Systems Research* 1997; 8(3): 240-253.

11. Morin D, Tourigny A, Pelletier D, Robichaud L, Mathieu L, Vézina A, Bonin L, Buteau M. Seniors' Views on the Use of Electronic Health Records. *Informatics in Primary care* 2005; 13(2): 125-134

12. Reid Ponte P, Kruger N, DeMarco R, Hanley D, Conlin G. Reshaping the Practice Environment: The Importance of Coherence. *Journal of Nursing Administration* 2004; 34(4): 173-179.

13. Haggerty JL, Reid RJ, Freeman GK, Starfield BH, Adair CE, McKendry R. Continuity of Care: A Multidisciplinary Review. *British Medical Journal* 2003; 327(7425): 1219-1221

14. Aliotta S. Coordination of care: The Council for Case Management Accountability's Third State of the Science Paper. *Case Manager* 2003; 14(2): 49-52

15. Fisher HM, Raphael TG. Managed Long-term Care: Care Integration through Care Coordination. *Journal of Aging and Health* 2003; 15(1): 223-245.

16. Sands D, Rind D, Safran C. Dissemination of Electronic Patient Records Using Primary Care Referrals as a Vector for Change. *Medinfo* 2001; 10: 685-689.

17. Myers BL, Kappelman LA, Prybutok VR. A Comprehensive Model for Assessing the Quality and Productivity of the Information Systems Function: Toward a Fheory for Information Systems Assessment. In E. J. Garrity & G. L. Sanders (Eds.), *Information Systems Success Measurement* (pp. 94–121). Hershey, PA: Idea Group. 1998

18. Ammenwerth E, Iller C, Mansmann U. Acceptance of Information Technology in a Clinical Environment - Results of Quantitative and Qualitative Analysis. In: Brown A, Remenyi D, editors. *Proceedings of the 9th European Conference on Information Technology Evaluation (ECITE)* Paris. pp. 39 - 44. 2002

19. Lenhart J, Honess K, Covington D, Johnson K. An Analysis of Trends, Perceptions, and Use Patterns of Electronic Medical Records among US Family Practice Residency Programs. *Family Medicine* 2000; 32(2): 109-114.

20. Delpierre C, Cuzin L, Fillaux J, Alvarez M, Massip P, Lang T. A Systematic Review of Computer-based Patient Record Systems and Quality of Care: More Randomized Clinical Trials or a Broader Approach? *International Journal for Quality in Health Care* 2004; 16(5): 407-416.

21. Garrison G, Bernard M, Rasmussen N. 21st-Century Health-care: The Effect of Computer Use by Physicians on Patient Satisfaction at a Family Medicine Clinic. *Family Medicine* 2002; 34(5): 362-368.

22. Garrity EJ, Sanders GL. Dimensions of Information Systems Success. In E. J. Garrity & G. L. Sanders (Eds.), *Information Systems Success Measurement* (pp. 13-45). Hershey: Idea Group Publishing. 1998

23. Axford RL, Carter BE. Impact of Clinical Information Systems on Nursing Practice. Nurses' perspectives. *Computers in Nursing* 1996; 14(3): 156-163.

24. Baldwin D. Implementation of Computerized Clinical Documentation. *Home Health Care Management and Practice* 1998; 10: 43-51.

25. Gilbert J. Physician Data Entry: Providing Options is Essential. *Health Data Management* 1998; 6(9): 84-86, 88, 90-82.

26. Kalra L, Fowle A. An Integrated System for Multidisciplinary Assessments in Stroke Rehabilitation. *Stroke* 1994; 25(11): 2210-2214.

27. Sleutel M., Guinn M. As good as it gets? Going Online with a Clinical Information System. *Computers in Nursing* 1999; 17(4): 181-185.

28. Smith D, Rogers S, Hood E, Philips D. Overtime Reduction with the Press of a Button an Unexpected Outcome of Computerized Documentation. *Nursing Case Management* 1998; 3(6): 266-270.

Chapter 15
Seniors' Views on the Use of an Electronic Health Record[*]

Diane Morin, André Tourigny, Daniel Pelletier,
Line Robichaud, Luc Mathieu, Aline Vézina,
Lucie Bonin, Martin Buteau.

Abstract

In the Mauricie and Centre-du-Québec region of the province of Quebec, Canada, an integrated services network has been implemented for frail seniors. It combines three of the best practices in the field of integrated services, namely: single-entry point, case management and personalized care plan. A shared interdisciplinary electronic health record (EHR) system was set up in 1998. A consensus on the relevance of using EHRs is growing in Quebec, in Canada and around the world. However, technology has outpaced interest in the notions of confidentiality, informed consent, and the impact perceived by the clientele. This study specifically examines how seniors who are frail perceive these issues. The conceptual framework is inspired by the DeLone & McLean model whose main attributes are: system quality, data quality, utilization modes and the impact on organizations and individuals. This last attribute is the focus of this study, which is a mixed specifications descriptive investigation with both a quantitative and a qualitative component. Thirty seniors were surveyed. Positive information they provided falls under three headings: (i) being better informed, (ii) trust and consideration for professionals and (iii) appreciation of innovation. The opinions of the seniors are generally favourable regarding the use of computers and the EHR in their presence. Improvements in EHR systems for seniors can be encouraged.

---

[*] This chapter is reprinted with the kind permission of *Informatics in Primary Care*, where it appeared as: Morin D, Tourigny A, Pelletier D, Robichaud L, Mathieu L, Vezina A, Bonin L, Buteau M. «Seniors' views on the use of electronic health records», 2005; 13(2):125-33.

Background

In February 1997, an integrated services network for frail seniors was set up in the Bois-Francs Area within the Mauricie and Centre-du-Québec Region in the Province of Quebec, Canada[1, 2]. It was designed to correct several deficiencies related to coordination of health care and services for frail seniors[3-10]. It combines what are considered as three of the best practices in the field of integrated care[11], namely: single-entry point, case management and individualised service plans. Within this network, coordination is a central component. It relies on a team of case managers who are responsible for triage, information, orientation, follow-up and evaluation. Their duties involve: (i) developing individualised-service plans with frail seniors and their family support networks, (ii) negotiating and coordinating the planned services with providers, (iii) ensuring that these services are in fact delivered at the proper time, (iv) ensuring that services are adjusted to any changes in the health profile or in the family support network and (v) ensuring that services are evaluated. Within this model of integrated care, interactions among professionals and between care facilities are more frequent than in usual care and this is mainly due to a greater need for consensus and follow-up in the individualised-services plans. To support interactions between professionals and facilities, a shared interdisciplinary electronic health record (EHR) was set up in 1998[12]. It contains: (i) identification and consent management, (ii) security and confidentiality measures, (iii) health profile, (iv) medications profile, (v) change in functional status, (v) individualised-services plan and its revision system, (vi) follow-up memos, (viii) requests for services and finally, (ix) data extractor. At the end of 2004, the EHR was used by 250 professionals to support services provided to more than 5,000 frail seniors. With the rapid development in the field of EHR, a certain number of questions must be raised. Among them, one of the most significant is how to make sure that the point of view of frail seniors is taken into consideration regarding issues such as sharing computerised health data, confidentiality and informed consent. These issues are rarely raised in the literature but are specifically addressed in the present study which is embedded in a larger research programme aimed at evaluating several facets of an interdisciplinary information system for frail seniors that includes EHRs[13].

Literature review

Electronic Health Record to Support Professional Practice

Many articles are available on EHRs in international literature. In these studies, EHRs are for the most part used within the same health care unit or within the same facility such as hospital. The rare studies in which an EHR is used in an interdisciplinary context, deal with a single type of clientele[14-16]. Only a few studies address computerisation of data within integrated health care systems such as for seniors, cardiac patients or other chronic illnesses[17-19].

Seniors' Views on Sharing Information, Confidentiality, and Consent

Few studies deal with what frail seniors or their families know about EHRs or with their concerns about computerisation. Among those, there is no consensus regarding patients' degree of knowledge. Some studies indicate that patients do have a good understanding of EHRs, while others show they don't[20-22]. Risdale and Hudd[21] conclude that an EHR must be sufficiently user-friendly in order for patients to feel it can be easily used, to see the data and be reassured that it remains confidential. They note that very old patients would accept the EHR even when on-screen data is complex. These authors suggest that the most important factor of all is patients' trust in their physician. A recent study concludes in the same way after examining how patients suffering from chronic heart failure, access their EHR and how they feel this affects their relationship with the professionals caring for them. Overall, the patients are satisfied with the information they find in their EHR and this has a positive impact on their acceptance of the planned therapy[17].

In studies where professionals used laptop computers for home visits, patients stated that they were better informed of their care plan and had better interaction with health care providers[23, 24]. In other studies, seniors felt that the professionals were more involved with the computer than with them as patients[25]. For medical practice, many studies have shown that introducing an EHR does not decrease patient satisfaction[12, 20, 21, 26-28]. There are nevertheless very few studies that deal specifically with confidentiality and consent. In these studies, results conclude that seniors have little concern for confidentiality, and even when they are concerned, they allow data to be made available on the condition that their physician gives consent[21, 22, 29-31]. The literature is so rare on this point that Barber[32] says that "... *the need is for a clear policy about the use of patient data ... providing openness, transparency and security for patients and healthcare professionals...* (p.21)" Layman[33] also suggests that "*A multi-pronged solution that incorporates adherence to regulations and standards, promotion of codes of conduct and ethics, and creation of a culture of info-ethics is recommended.* (p.12)"

In Brief

There is wide consensus on the relevance of using an EHR when caring for frail seniors. The EHR used in the Mauricie and Centre-du-Québec region certainly differs from others due to its interdisciplinary character and especially its deployment across several levels and types of facilities. There are numerous factors encouraging or constraining the use of an EHR, but in general, good knowledge of the system by the professionals and patients' trust in the professionals, increase EHR acceptability and use. Frail senior patients can be interested in and easily accept this type of innovation. However, technology has outpaced interest in the notions of confidentiality, informed consent, and the impact perceived by the clientele. This study specifically deals with how these issues are perceived by frail seniors.

Conceptual framework

The conceptual framework selected for this study is inspired by the DeLone & McLean[34] model. It often has been used in studies evaluating the introduction and impact of computerisation[35-37]. The central concepts of the model may be summarised as follows: system quality, data quality, utilization modes and the impact on organizations and on individuals. The central concept of impact on individuals is composed of two main attributes, which are the effect of the system on the professionals and the effect of the system on the clientele. This study addresses the latter.

Methods

Population and sampling

This is a descriptive study using a mix design including qualitative and quantitative approaches. In 2001, a sample of elderly people was selected among a population of 2,500, according to three main criteria. The primary criterion was the fact of having an active EHR. The second criterion was related to having had a case management episode during the prior six months. The third criterion was the fact of having a fully-completed measure of functional status using the *Système de mesure de l'autonomie fonctionelle* (SMAF), a negatively-scored standardised instrument, widely validated in comparable environments[38, 39]. The sample of seniors was then stratified in relation to level of functional status measured by the SMAF (SMAF ≤-30 or SMAF >-30), and in relation to living arrangements (own home or private facility). These stratifications produced a subset of 206 eligible individuals who were all personally contacted to determine if they considered they had an experience with their EHR. A total of 56 seniors stated they had previous experience with the HER and among them, 30 accepted to be interviewed. The 26 seniors who refused stated they were too weak or too ill to participate in an hour-long interview. They were also those with the lowest SMAF scores (SMAF ≤-30).

Instruments and Procedures

The interviews were conducted at the seniors' homes and lasted an average of 50 minutes. The three main topics addressed were: (1) free and informed consent regarding data transmission via the EHR, (2) general reactions to computer use and the EHR, and (3) perceived advantages, disadvantages and impact of computer use and the EHR. The interviews were conducted in two parts. First, a questionnaire comprising 20 closed-ended questions was administered. The questionnaire was previously tested. Answers were either on a 4-point (ranging from Strongly Agree to Strongly Disagree) or on a Yes/No scale. An additional choice of "I do not know" was possible when the 4-point scale was used. The following are three examples of statements or questions included in the closed-ended questionnaire regarding consent and confidentiality: "When my permission was requested, I felt free to accept or refuse"; "I am confident that only authorised persons will have access to my records" and finally, "When professionals use a computer during the home or office visit, where you interested to look at the screen? " Answers were analysed using the statistical software SAS-V8. After completion of the questionnaire, six open-ended questions were asked. These had been pre-tested. An example of a question is: "Are you concerned by the fact that data on your health could be shared over the network? " Answers were analysed by two independent researchers using the software NVivo-V2.0.

Results

Participants' profile

As shown in Table 15.1, the mean age of the participants was 78. Women formed the majority. Approximately one quarter was married. Most seniors lived in their own homes and were retired. As could be expected, since participants were frail seniors, the large majority of them considered their health to be poor or only acceptable.

Table 15.1
Participants' profile

Characteristics	Men n=10	Women n=20	Total
Age (mean)	78.0	78.2	78.1
Civil status	%	%	%
Single	10.0	13.3	23.3
Married	16.7	10.0	26.7
Divored/Separated	3.3	10.0	23.3
Widow	3.3	23.3	26.7
Education	%	%	%
Primary	26.7	43.3	70.0
Secondary	3.3	10.0	13.3
College/University	3.3	13.3	16.7
Living arrangements	%	%	%
Personal home	16.7	60.0	76.7
Family home	3.3	0	3,3
Private seniors' home	13.3	6.7	20.0
Work	%	%	%
At work	0	3.3	3.3
At home	0	33.3	33.3
Retired	33.3	30.0	63.3
Perceived quality of health	%	%	%
Excellent	0	3.3	3.3
Good	13.3	13.3	26.7
Poor	10.0	46.7	56.7
Bad	10.0	3.3	13.3

Table 15.2
Participants' Views – Quantitative Section

STATEMENTS	Completely or Partially Disagree (%)	Completely or Partially Agree (%)	Don't know (%)
Consent			
1. When my permission was requested, I felt free to consent or refuse	0	100	0
3. I was well informed	5.6	88.8	5.
4. Explanations were clear	11.1	84.3	5.6
5. I was informed I could withdraw my consent at anytime	27.8	61.8	11.1
6. I had sufficient time to decide	10	84.4	5.6
Information			
7. I knew what it was all about	11.1	83.3	5.6
8. I was informed I could access my file	38.9	38.9	22.2
9. I feel confident that only authorised persons will have access to my records	0	88.9	11.1
Practice			
10. I felt the professional had to stop talking to me when working in my file	53.4	43.3	3.3
11. I felt this file was a nuisance	93.3	6.7	0
12. I felt the professional was not listening to me when working with the file	96.7	0	3.3
13. I felt less satisfied because of the file	93.3	3.3	3.3
14. I don't like it when the professional uses the file when I'm there	100	0	0
General Questions	Yes (%)	No (%)	
15. Occasionally, do professionals use a computer during the home or office visit?	100	0	
16. When professionals use a computer during the home or office visit, where you interested to look at the screen?	41.4	58.6	
17. Were you offered to look at the screen?	17.3	82.7	
18. Did you look at the screen?	31.0	69.0	
19. Were you interested to know or see more	33.3	66.7	
20. Were you offered to see more of the file?	6.9	93.1	
21. Did you read the information in your file?	15.4	84.6	

Participants' Views

Results from the Closed-ended Questions

As presented in Table 15.2, the results show that a majority of seniors were in agreement with the fact that they felt free to consent to the use of the EHR. The majority considered themselves fairly well informed. Nonetheless, 40 % stated either they did not remember being informed that they could withdraw consent at any time and have access to their EHR or that they did not know.

The majority of seniors stated that they were not invited to look at the screen or at their EHR contents but for those who said they were, they said they had no interest in looking at or consulting the EHR.

Results from the Open-ended Questions

Information available and follow-up

The participating seniors feel that the information is quickly available and is complete. They feel that the professionals possess a great amount of data on their health and lifestyle. They state: *"They know my whole life story!"*; *"It's all there."* These expressions briefly summarize comments made concerning the information contained in the EHR. Seniors feel that the EHR gives professionals better information about their health and life situations in general. They consistently note that the EHR appears to make work easier for the health care workers. They say that information is exchanged more quickly between professionals and between health care facilities. They appreciate that the data is available; especially for those professionals directly involved in the health care or services they receive. They express this as follows: *"Health care workers are better informed and more knowledgeable about what I might need."*

Some of them feel that computerisation is unavoidable and that it will not have a negative impact on the quality of data. *"I felt important. I prefer the computer. We need to keep up with progress. I am pleased my record is computerised."* Among those interviewed, some did mention that there might be fewer errors with an EHR. However, one or two respondents did mention the possibility that errors could slip in during data collection. *"In my opinion, there are only advantages as long as the data is not lost."*

Finally, some individuals pointed out that their follow-up care seemed more systematic. They seem to get an impression of professionalism and effectiveness from the use of modern tools. They say: *"They know what they are doing ... They have all the information ... Everything is there."* These statements illustrate and summarise the comments made about the information contained in the EHR.

Rapidity and accessibility

Other comments were made regarding the fact that the information is quickly available and that this saves time. An overall impression of effectiveness is the result for many, *"The health care workers know what they are doing."* The participating seniors believe that the EHR reduces the risk of error and ensures better coordination during follow-up. Some explained that using this technology gives the impression of being clear, correct and effective. However, they do often emphasize that this technology is mainly a tool for the professionals. They have difficulty in saying what advantages it has for them. They do specify that they are not the best to judge the issue noting, "*I do not know the advantages, but I am sure there are many.*" Some of the elderly mention the fact that they are not obliged to repeat themselves thanks to the EHR. Others however do not find that there is less repetition. Seniors perceive that it may be more rapid and effective and generally emphasize that they do not see any change or any reason not to use the computerised system. However, they get a general impression of effectiveness, accuracy and better communication and cooperation among health care workers. For the seniors, this aspect is seen both as reassuring and encouraging since they feel health care workers are using the best tools available to provide care.

Confidentiality and security

Seniors feel that their data is safe in an EHR: "*I have a computer myself and I know how it works. You need a password to do anything. So I am not concerned if someone attempts to break in.*" "*I am sure the records are well protected at the facility (sic).*" Several mentioned, "*I can trust the professionals.*"

Among those interviewed, some specified that they felt safe with all the measures taken to ensure the security of personal information. Some did express concern over possible errors and some with confidentiality. "*Well, I believe that some individuals with bad intentions could look at my record but that is not really disturbing since there is nothing in it that is revealing.*" "*I am fairly confident, there are curious people everywhere.*"

Convergence among the sources of information

It can be concluded that the results stemming from the closed-ended questions converge with open-ended ones. Both conclude that seniors are relatively favourable to EHRs. They see no major disadvantage to its use. They feel that the data contained in an EHR is useful and accessible more quickly to the professionals who are caring for them or providing services. The question of consent is less clear. The responses obtained to questions dealing with access to the records and the right to withdraw consent reveal in fact that this information, while apparently presented and stated in the documents given to the individuals, escapes many. Some seniors feel that when they accept services they accept as a matter of course that their information is made available. Most of them feel that their consent to health care and the fact that information circulates electronically may be revoked at any time but for a large proportion, consent procedure is still unclear. They nevertheless have confidence in the professionals who are involved in their health care and services.

Discussion

The central concept explored in this study was the impact on the individual caused by an innovation such as the EHR. More specifically, the intent was to determine how the seniors who had already used it view this new type of information system. Positive comments made by the seniors fall into three categories: (1) being better informed, (2) trust for professionals and (3) appreciation of innovation.

Regarding the first point, the majority of seniors stated that the EHR improved the quality of the information. They felt that all the information was available and as a result, the health care and services they receive will be increasingly appropriate. Some individuals did say that they did not remember that they had access to the contents of their record or that they could withdraw consent if they so wanted. Even when this information appears in writing in the documents given to the individuals, it would be advisable to review the format and the contents of information exchanged between health care workers and the individual patients when consent is initially obtained or when it is renewed. Very few expressed concern to the effect that the information would not remain confidential. Available literature does also mention that individuals using an EHR have little concern for confidentiality and accept that their data is made available on the condition that their physician gives consent and that adequate security is ensured[21, 22, 29-31]. This does illustrate the importance of providing more information to seniors and their families regarding their rights and the measures taken to ensure the confidentiality of the information.

Concerning the second point, it is very apparent that seniors place their confidence in the professionals providing their health care and services. The EHR seems to have made this confidence explicit in a context where seniors may have a limited view of the technology. This dimension is less explicit in the literature[17, 18, 40]. The results of this study are therefore innovative in this regard. Nonetheless there is a need to develop a true partnership with seniors so that the model, which supports clinical practices, also includes empowerment and the development of self-care management.

Finally, the third point involves appreciation of innovation. This impact was rather unexpected since current literature does not mention it. On the contrary, several studies have observed that the older the individual (including health care workers), the more reluctant they were to innovation[41-43]. This finding strengthens interest in other studies involving frail seniors and their families regarding the perception of and the integration of technological innovation.

This study does have certain limitations. In fact, it was conducted as part of a research programme that examined several aspects of professional practice within a network of integrated services. Participating seniors therefore knew that various types of innovation would be introduced into their care delivery system in which EHR was one facet. It is possible that individuals who accepted to participate were more open than others to accepting innovation of various kinds. In this sense, they may have provided us with a more optimistic view than anticipated. The specific social and geographic foundations of this study may mean that its potential for generalization is relatively limited. Nevertheless many of the results observed do agree with available literature and reinforce evidence that the EHR is deemed acceptable, although it must be used in a transparent manner and in a way that empowers individuals to remain vigilant and well informed.

Conclusion

The goal of this study was to understand how seniors perceive the EHR in terms of consent and confidentiality and what are the advantages that its use offers. It is important to remember that the EHR in this study was implemented to meet new requirements for data exchange generated by the initial network of integrated services for frail seniors. Nowhere else in Quebec is there an EHR simultaneously linking so many professionals, services, levels of care and types of facilities. The professionals were faced with the dual challenge of mastering the implementation of an integrated services network with the new methods it involved, while at the same time learning computer skills as well as EHR content and techniques.

For seniors, this innovation was perceived as quite positive. Overall, their comments were favourable concerning use of the EHR as well as concerning the use of a computer in their presence. Seniors in the Mauricie and Centre-du-Québec region feel that their health information circulates faster between professionals and health facilities. Continuous improvement of EHR for seniors should therefore be encouraged.

References

1. Hébert R, Tourigny A, Durand PJ, Group TP. Frail elderly patients – New model for integrated service delivery. Canadian Family Physician 2003;49: 992-997.

2. Tourigny A, Durand PJ, Bonin L, Hébert R, Rochette L. Quasi-experimental study of the effectiveness of an integrated service delivery network for the frail elderly. Canadian Journal on Aging 2004;23(3):231-246.

3. Hébert R, Bravo G, Voyer L. Répertoire des instruments de mesure en langue française pour la recherche gérontologique et gériatrique. Sherbrooke: Centre de recherche en gérontologie et gériatrie; 1993.

4. Paradis M, Bonin L, Tourigny A, Durand PJ, Bussière A, Roy H-A, et al. Réseau de services iintégrés aux aînés des Bois-Francs: mécanisme de coordination des services géronto-gériatriques – Rapport de l'évaluation d'implantation et de processus. Québec: Unité de recherche en gériatrie de l'Université Laval – Centre de recherche du Centre hospitalier affilié universitaire de Québec – Université Laval; 2001.

5. Bolduc M, Trahan L. Programme d'évaluation portant sur le processus de réponse aux besoins de longue durée des personnes âgées ayant des limitations fonctionnelles. Québec: Ministère de la santé et des services sociaux, Direction de l'évaluation; 1988.

6. Trahan L. Les facteurs associés à l'orientation des personnes âgées dans des établissements d'hébergement: une revue de littérature. Québec: Service de l'évaluation, Réadaptation et Services de longue durée, MSSS; 1989.

7. Garant L. Synthèse d'un programme d'évaluation sur la réponse aux besoins de longue durée des personnes âgées ayant des limitations fonctionnelles. Québec: Gouvernement du Québec; 1994. Report No.: 20.

8. Joubert P, Laberge A, Fortin JP, Paradis M, Desbiens F. Évaluation du programme québécois de services intensifs de maintien à domicile (SIMAD). Québec: Unité de recherche en santé communautaire, Centre hospitalier de l'université Laval; 1991.

9. Tourigny A, Côté L, Laberge A, Paradis M, Joubert P. Évaluation du programme québécois des centres de jour. Québec: Unité de recherche en santé communautaire, Centre hospitalier de l'Université Laval (CHUL), Centre de santé publique de Québec; 1993.

10. Tourigny A, Gagnon C, Miller-Stryckman J, Bergeron P, Paradis M, Thomassin L. L'allocation directe au Québec: Des modes de fonctionnement variés à découvrir, des points de vue à faire connaître. Québec: Ministère de la Santé et des Services sociaux, Direction générale de la planification et de l'évaluation & Centre de santé publique de Québec; 1996.

11. Angus DC. Pour un système de soins de santé viable au Canada. Ottawa: Université d'Ottawa; 1995.

12. Legler JD, Oates R. Patients' reactions to physician use of a computerized medical record system during clinical encounters. J Fam Pract. 1993;37 (3):241-244.

13. Tourigny A, Bonin L, Morin D, Buteau M, Mathieu L, Robichaud L, et al. Système d'information géronto-gériatrique interdisciplinaire et inter-établissements: utilité perçue et utilisation en temps réel. Rapport de recherche. Québec: Unité de recherche en gériatrie de l'Université Laval; 2003.

14. Fretschner S, Bleicher W, Heininger A, Unertl K. Patient Data Management Systems in Critical Care. Journal of the American Society of Nephrology 2001;12(Suppl. 17):S-83-S-86.

15. Nielsen LH, Dinesen B, Binder C. Integrating a multipurpose clinical workstation in ambulatory care. In: Toward and Electronic Patient Record '97; 1997; Nashville, Tennessee: Newton, MA; 1997. p. 121-126.

16. Tiessen B, Doan K, Benoit L. Electronic Documentation on a Psychiatric Unit. Canadian Nurse 2001;97(10):27-29.

17. Ross SE, Moore LA, Earnest MA, Wittevrongel L, Lin C-T. Providing a Web-based Online Medical Record with Electronic Communication Capabilities to Patients With Congestive Heart Failure: Randomized Trial. Journal of Medical Internet Research 2004;6(2):electronic #12.

18. Ralston JD, Revere D, Robins LS, Goldberg HI. Patients' experience with a diabetes support programme based on an interactive electronic medical record: qualitative study. British Medical Journal 2004;328:1-4.

19. McCoy HV, Kibort Vila C. Tech Knowledge: Introducing Computers for Coordinated Care. Health & Social Work 2002;27(1):71-74.

20. Ornstein SM. Patient perspectives on computer-based medical records. J Fam Pract. 1994;38(6):606-610.

21. Ridsdale L, Hudd S. What do patients want and not want to see about themselves on the computer screen: a qualitative study. Scand J Prim Health Care 1997;15(4):180-183.

22. Ridsdale L, Hudd S. Computers in the consultation: the patient's view. British Journal of General Practice 1994;44:367-369.

23. Baldwin DR. Implementation of computerized clinical documentation. Home Health Care Manage Prac 1998;10:43-51.

24. Mc Neil-Mc Donald C. Building the Case for Web-based Solutions. Caring 2001;20(9):40-42.

25. Malone N, Loader S, Poulter J. Evaluating the benefits realized from a nurse management information system. J Nurs Manag 1997;5(1):5-9.

26. Als AB. The desk-top computer as a magic box: patterns of behaviour connected with the desk-top computer; GPs' and patients' perceptions. Fam Pract 1997;14(1):17-23.

27. Solomon GL. Are patients pleased with computer use in the examination room? J Fam Pract. 1995;41(3):241-244.

28. Brownbridge G, Herzmark GA, Wall TD. Patient reactions to doctors' computer use in general practice consultations. Soc Sci Med 1985;20:47-52.

29. Bates DW, Ebell M, Gotlieb E, Zapp J, Mullins HC. A proposal for electronic medical records in U.S. primary care. Journal of the American Medical Informatics Association 2003;10(1):1-10.

30. Berg M, Langenberg C, Berg I, Kwakkernaat J. Experiences with an electronic patient record in a clinical context: considerations for design. Medical Informatics Europe'97 1997:811-815.

31. Bomba D, de Silva A. An Australian case study of patient attitudes towards the use of computerised medical records and unique identifiers. Medinfo 2001;10(Pt 2):1430-1434.

32. Barber B. Protecting privacy: transparency, openness and data security – even in transborder applications. British Journal of Healthcare Computing and Information Management 2001;18(1):21-22.

33. Layman E. Health informatics: ethical issues. Health Care Manager 2003;22(1):2-15.

34. DeLone WH, McLean ER. The DeLone and Mclean Model of information systems success: a ten-year update. Journal of Management Information Systems 2003;19(4):9-30.

35. Seddon PB. A respecification and Extension of the DeLone and McLean model of IS success. Information Systems Research 1997;8(3):240-252.

36. Seddon P, Kiew M-Y. A partial test and development of the DeLone and McLean model of IS success. In: internationalconference on information system; 1994; Vancouver, Canada; 1994.

37. Kurian D, Galupe RB, Diaz J. Taking stock: Measuring Information Systems Success. In: ASAC-IFSAM Y200 Conference; 2000; Montréal, Canada: ASAC-IFSAM; 2000. p. 77-90.

38. Hébert R, Carrier R, Bilodeau A. Le système de mesure de l'autonomie fonctionnelle. Revue de gériatrie 1988;13(4):161-167.

39. Hébert R, Carrier R, Bilodeau A. The functional autonomy measurement system (SMAF): description and validation of an instrument for the measurement of handicaps. Age and Ageing 1988;17(5):293-302.

40. Patel VL, Arocha JF, Kushniruk AW. Patients' and physicians' understanding of health and biomedical concepts: relationship to the desing of EMR systems. Journal of Biomedical Informatics 2002;35(1):8-16.

41. Brown RT. Computerized Patient Records (CPR) in primary care: "five years chartless" a Canadian experience. In: Toward an Electronic Patient Record '98; 1998; San Antonio, Texas: Newton, MA: MRI, 1998; 1998. p. 311-314.

42. Dansky KH, Gamm LD, Vascy JJ, Barsukiewicz CK. Electronic medical records: Are physicians ready? /Practitioner application. Journal of Health care Management 1999;44(6):440-455.

43. McConnell EA, O'Shea SS, Kirchhoff K. RN attitudes towards computers. Nursing Management 1989;7:36-40.

Chapter 16
Measuring and Improving the Quality and Continuity of Health Care and Services Delivered to Vulnerable Elders: Pilot Project for People with Cognitive Impairments or Dementia

André Tourigny, Diane Morin, Marie-Jeanne Kergoat,
Nicole Dubuc, Line Robichaud, Jacques Morin,
Lise Côté, Paule Lebel, René Verreault,
Edeltraut Kröger, Zohra Benounissa, and Solange Proulx

Highlights

1. The implementation of measures to continuously improve quality for the elderly is relevant, given the involvement of primary- and secondary-care providers who act in cooperation with partners or other resources working with this target population.
2. The pilot project aims at identifying potential data sources to measure indicators and assess feasibility as well as to measure inter-observer reliability.
3. The process indicators were selected because they already point to the source where action is required and help accurately target efforts to improve quality.
4. Indicators were sought by reviewing copies of clinical and medical files of 29 clients of the home-care services in a health and social services center who have cognitive impairments or dementia. Telephone interviews to survey satisfaction were carried out with 40 people from the sample to complete the review of quality indicators (QIs).

5. The results indicate that the files and interviews are appropriate as data sources. The wording on the consent forms should be clear enough to obviate the need to anonymize the file copies. Out of 68 initial indicators, 61 were assessed by both nurses, but the others were never found, suggesting that, in future projects, either the number of files reviewed should be substantially increased or the number of indicators be reduced. Improving the tools and training for research nurses would be significant advantages in a project of larger scope.

Introduction

Quality of care is an important concern for health agencies in a variety of countries[1, 2, 3, 4]. Despite this interest in quality, the care delivered to the elderly is frequently inadequate, particularly as regards certain geriatric conditions such as dementia, malnutrition, incontinence, and falls[5-8]. Some authors have also pointed out that the level of care for the vulnerable elderly falls well short of acceptable for large variety of geriatric conditions[6]. Other reports about the quality of care[7, 9, 10] support these observations and emphasize that quality assessment studies are rarely carried out for geriatric care[7].

Moreover, it is important that particular attention be paid to geriatric conditions[11] and to the necessity of improving quality in the continuum of care for the elderly, whether in the home,[6, 12] in hospitals,[7, 13] or in placement settings[12, 14, 15]. Specifically in Quebec, the presence of family practice units, the implementation of interdisciplinary family medicine groups, and the creation of local service networks bringing together primary and secondary care promote the identification and implementation of continuous quality improvement measures because of the roles that they play with the vulnerable elderly and their cooperation with the various partners and resources involved with this target group. The relevance of assessing quality logically flows from the position that there must be means for accurately measuring the quality of care in order to determine if it has been improved. Measuring quality contributes to the improvement process improvement,[16-18] while fostering greater efficacy in care organization[16, 17] and promoting the expected changes[17, 18]. Furthermore, measuring quality yields a better understanding of care delivery and relevance, making it possible to improve care, which impacts on the observed results. Consequently, a link has been reported between higher quality of care and the survival rate of the vulnerable elderly living in the community[19].

Objectives

The pilot project is part of a broader quality assessment and improvement process, of which several steps have been completed. The medium-term objective is to develop, implement, and assess a continuous quality improvement process.

This type of process must be appropriate for the clinical and organizational context for the territory of a local network delivering primary and secondary care services to a population of the vulnerable elderly. To help achieve this goal, the pilot project has a general objective of selecting reliable and measurable quality indicators. It also aims at (1) identifying potential data sources for measuring each of the selected indicators and to assess the feasibility of using them in an actual context of delivering primary and secondary care and services; and (2) measuring interobserver reliability.

Reminder of the Steps Completed for the Pilot Project

Definition of Quality

A study on quality has the initial premise that there is consensus about the definition of the concept of quality and that it clearly reflects the issues that the research project aims at dealing with. For the purposes of this pilot project, the definition of quality of the Institute of Medicine (IOM) was used, namely: "The degree to which health services for individuals and populations increase the likelihood of desired health outcomes and are consistent with current professional knowledge[2]." This definition has the merit of considering quality on the individual and population in terms of care processes and health outcomes,[16, 20]while taking into account patient values and expectations as well as keeping pace with changes in knowledge[21].

Conceptual Framework

With the acceptance of this definition, it was possible to move forward with project development by adapting the IOM conceptual framework. It comprises the following quality dimensions: safety, efficacy, care centered on the elderly person and the community, and access. Moreover, equity and continuity bridge these four dimensions. They are compared with the outcomes desired by the elderly and their caregivers, whether they involve staying healthy, getting better, living with disease, or facing the end of life. These two elements are especially important in the context of integrated services networks for the elderly, which are developing in Quebec and everywhere else[22–26]. It should be remembered that safety corresponds to the way in which care and services are provided and that the negative effects on the elderly person and his or her family are kept to a minimum[27]. Efficacy refers to appropriate care or services based on scientific evidence. Care centered on the elderly person and the community fits directly into a partnership approach between the individual and health-care professionals. Rapidly obtaining care at the right place and the right time constitutes the central element of access. Equity presupposes care for all with no discrimination, whereas continuity implies consistency and well coordinated care[2]. The steps leading to the definition of quality and the choice of the conceptual framework are detailed in Chapter 16 of the first book on PRISMA[28].

Measuring Quality

The assessment of quality in this project is based on process indicators rather than on outcome indicators. The latter case requires recourse to complex adjustments, especially to take into account the seriousness of the disease and the associated conditions, which often are topics of discussion[6, 19, 29, 30]. There are other grounds for opting for process indicators: the current trend towards evidence-based practice, the development of practice guides promoting identification of indicators, and a greater capacity for establishing comparisons between regions over time. Typically, process measurement assesses the proportion of eligible patients who receive the recommended care. Process indicators already point to the source requiring action and give direction to efforts to improve quality—that is, the care given—in order to correct the quality issue[9, 29]. Process assessment, particularly in cases of pharmacological treatment of the vulnerable elderly, is especially appropriate in examining the ordering of medication, medication management, patient information and education, and pharmacological follow-up[31].

Conditions Selected

The research team decided on dementia and cognitive disorders, which stand out as public-health priorities[32] because of their significant impact on the individual, family, caregivers, and the entire health-care system. Dealing with this issue requires the involvement of several disciplines; the quality indicators had been the topic of much research, including that of ACOVE (Assessing Care of Vulnerable Elders),[33] which was the main reference for our work. Specifics about the issues selected can be found in Chapter 16 of the first PRISMA book[28].

Validation of Quality Indicators

In order to take into account the integrated care model, professionals from a variety of disciplines were brought together for a number of reasons, including to determine the relevance of the indicators in Quebec's clinical-practice context and their relationship to quality. A total of 33 experts from different fields (medicine, geriatrics, nursing, pharmacy, rehabilitation, nutrition, psychology, neuropsychology, and social work) and different settings (Québec, Montréal, and Sherbrooke) examined some or all of the indicators submitted. A Delphi panel, based on the RAND/UCLA appropriateness method, was used for validation purposes. The indicators were rated in a first round; a second round was conducted when there were significant discrepancies between expert ratings. The outcome was 82 quality indicators, most of which (75 %) inventoried from the ACOVE project, being submitted to panel members, who had to indicate if they agreed with QI validity and determine if the indicators were "appropriate, inappropriate, or uncertain." In the second round, 72 indicators (92 % from ACOVE) were deemed valid by the experts. See Chapter 17 herein for Edeltraut Kröger's text "Indicators Validated for People with Cognitive Impairments or Dementia" for more information on the topic of validation.

Methodology

Collaborating Institution

The project was carried out in the urban area of Québec, in cooperation with the Centre de santé et de services sociaux de la Vieille-Capitale (CSSS/VC). The CSSS/VC is a multivocational institution resulting from the merger of the local community service centers (CLSCs) and residential and long-term care centers (CHSLDs). The CSSS/VC's territory takes in part of the city of Québec and the municipalities of Ancienne-Lorette and St-Augustin-de-Desmaures[34]. The CSSS/VC's coordinator of home-care services (HCS) and ten social workers took part in the pilot project.

Study Population

The eligible individuals were age 75 and older registered with the CSSS/VC's home-care services presenting one or more diagnoses identified with codes in the SIC Plus information system available to CLSCs:[*] Alzheimer's disease, cognitive disorders, delirium, dementia (vascular dementia), and amnesic disorder (N=306). Two random draws were carried out, 193 out of 306 eligible candidates being selected. The social workers with at least five cases included among these 193 subjects made the initial contact. Figure 16.1 illustrates the steps in selecting the sample population.

Between October 7, 2005 and April 15, 2006, ten HCS social workers contacted 131 subjects. A total of 70 records were deemed ineligible (diagnostic coding error, death, placement in a private home for the elderly or CHSLD for more than three months, no active CLSC services, record closed) and 21 individuals declined to participate in the project. The final number of subjects in the study was 40. The 40 subjects were interviewed on the telephone to determine their satisfaction; the records of 29 of the subjects were reviewed.

---

[*] SIC Plus CLSC (client information system) – Selected diagnostic codes: 1507: Alzheimer's disease; 2499: cognitive disorders; 5100: Delirium, dementia, amnesic disorder; 5101: delirium; 5102: dementia (vascular dementia); 5103: amnesic disorder; 5104: other cognitive disorders

Figure 16.1
Selecting the study sample

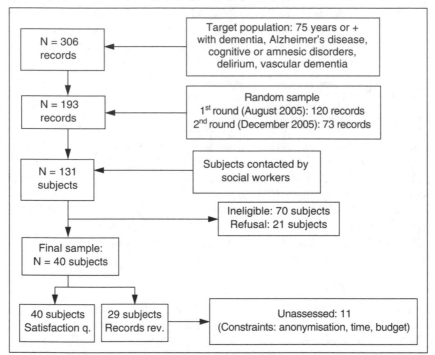

Data Sources

The data sources selected to rate quality indicators were clinical or medical records (CSSS/VC; hospital—complete chart for hospitalization of two days or more; residential and long-term care, specialized geriatric services, records from the attending physician's office) for the preceding two years, that is, from January 1, 2004 to December 31, 2005. The elderly persons themselves (caregiver or legal representative) were also asked to agree to a telephone interview about satisfaction. Lastly, administrative databases were consulted, as necessary.

Data Collection and Procedure: Quality Indicators

The main challenge in this pilot project was gaining access to hospital and medical records, collecting them, and reviewing their contents.

Information sheets (see a sample sheet in the appendix) used in data collection were developed by team members for the 68** quality indicators that were

---

** The team members agreed, after subsequently examining the 72 quality indicators selected, that four indicators were either difficult to find in the records or not recorded. The team removed these four items, replacing them with an equal number from the satisfaction survey used for telephone interviews.

validated by experts in the two Delphi panel rounds. The sheets dealt with pre-established areas, namely, assessment, treatment, follow-up, and continuity. Team members, assisted by a records archivist, provided three days of training to the two research nurses. Two entire records were reviewed as a group. After analyzing five records, an additional day was dedicated to summing up and making any necessary adjustments. Working on their own, the nurses filled out the sheets for the quality indicators in the records. They were also able to enter their own comments, if necessary. The review work began in March 2006 and ran until June 2006.

Photocopies of the records for 38 subjects selected from the initial 40 were requested from institutional authorities or physicians in private practice. Copies of the other two files were not requested due to time and budget constraints. The records were photocopied, instead of consulted at the site, for a number of reasons. Indeed, should a broader project being contemplated, it would be difficult and expensive to conduct the record review at the site. If further details or checking were required, it would entail submitting a new request to the archives department for access to the record as well as additional visits to the institution or the physician's office.

All requests for access to records were accompanied by a consent form duly signed by the elderly person, caregiver, or legal representative. The directors of professional services at the health-care institutions in the Québec area authorized archives department to release the required documents to the research team. Two approaches were used when submitting requests to family physicians. In the first approach, the person in charge of the study telephoned the physicians in question in order to describe the project and request access to the records of the patients participating in the study. This was followed up by a letter to the physicians. In the second approach, the physicians were not called; they were simply sent letters stating the reasons for the request. In both cases, the full contents of the records were requested for the patients taking part in the study, including test and analysis results as well as consultation notes.

The project defrayed the costs for photocopying the records and the time spent by the staff of the institution or physician's office. The project also paid for postal or courier charges for sending and returning the consent forms.

The research ethics committees of the CHA, the CSSS/VC, and Université Laval approved the pilot project, the contents of the consent form, and access to the information in the various records. Commitments to preserve confidentiality and measures to protect the information collected were put into practice throughout the term of the pilot project.

The project coordinator maintained a log throughout the term of the study in order to document any problems or important events. It was also used to note requests for records made to the institutions and family physicians, the number of records received and reviewed, the hours worked by the research nurses, and any difficulties that they may have encountered in performing their jobs.

Data Collection and Procedure: Satisfaction

The HCS social workers made the first contact with the elderly, their caregivers, or their legal representatives for permission to pass on their contact information so that the research team could get in touch with them. When permission was granted, the project coordinator called them to provide details about the research project, specify the type of cooperation expected, inform them about the legal obligation to obtain consent to have access to their records, and determine the procedure for the subsequent telephone interview. Two copies of the appropriate consent form were mailed to the candidates. The coordinator could conduct the telephone interview once the duly signed consent form was received.

The decision was made to opt for telephone interviews instead of face-to-face encounters during this pilot project. Given the eventuality that a broader project could be undertaken, it would indeed be more difficult and expensive to conduct the interviews in person.

The questionnaire was one developed by the PRISMA team [35] on satisfaction with services, to which were added four elements related to quality indicators that were either not in or not found in the hospital or medical records. These questions dealt with waiting time for an appointment with a physician specialist, cooperation and opinion asked for about the overall services delivered; ease in getting an appointment with a physician, if necessary; and advice or referrals about smoking cessation.

The original version of the PRISMA questionnaire contained 34 questions with two components: perception of care and services received, and the importance placed on them. This version was used for the first ten interviews. In December 2005, it was decided to use an abridged version (26 questions) for subsequent interviews. The PRISMA researcher who developed this questionnaire made it available to us. The ethics committees were advised and approved the questionnaire's modification.

The elderly person, caregiver, or legal representative was asked about the use of services, especially hospitalization for two days or more and visits to the generalist physician over the preceding two years.

Statistical Analysis

First of all, the number and proportion of indicators deemed applicable and evaluated in the records reviewed by the nurses were assessed. Decision-rule algorithms were established for each indicator in order to determine if the information about the quality indicators assessed in the records was sufficient to warrant deeming the indicator as met or not. The Kappa coefficient was selected to rate interobserver agreement between the two research nurses, to determine whether a quality indicator a) was applicable to a given patient and b) whether it was met based on record analysis. The average cost and time invested in each record was calculated. As for the satisfaction survey, the team analyzed all the completed questionnaires, the proportion of third-party respondents, and the comments or additional explanations provided by third-party respondents.

Results

Objective 1: Data sources

In validating the content of quality indicators (see Chapter 17, E. Kröger et al.), it was determined whether the information for a specific indicator should have to appear in the clinical record. Indeed, the data sources used were clinical and medical records as well as interviews with the elderly person, caregiver, or legal representative. Consulting administrative databases was not necessary since the type of information collected was already in the records.

Of the 40 people comprising the sample, the records of 38 were applied for and obtained by the CSSS/VC. The records for each of the 38 people were requested, regardless of where they had received care in the preceding two years. As a result, hospital records were requested for 20 people and general physicians provided files for 32 individuals. Thirty-eight records from the CSSS/VC were also received. The time and budget constraints inherent in carrying out the pilot project resulted in the records for 29 people (out of 38) being reviewed.

Objective 2: Feasibility

The research team was confronted by a major ethics issue, namely, anonymizing records. From the outset of field data collection, the heads of archives at certain institutions considered that the wording of the consent form required copies to be anonymized. This procedure is long and expensive, especially in the case of social records, in which names and other information identifying the elderly person, caregiver, or legal representative appear often and regularly.

The anonymization procedure caused delays and costs that were not initially planned for. This soon came to light in applying this procedure to the first eight CSSS/VC records. Continuing along the same lines would have compromised the project due to delays and significant costs. Steps were then taken with the CHA ethics committee to clarify and validate the relevance of not anonymizing the copies. The CHA research ethics committee confirmed the research team's action, considering that all reasonable measures had been taken to safeguard confidentiality. The archives departments were advised of this decision and agreed to continue the photocopying operation without anonymizing the records.

The research team had to face another constraint: having to submit the pilot project and all the modifications that might occur along the way to several ethics committees. Applying the same requirements to a larger project would result in delays and could complicate its execution.

The complete records of 29 people were reviewed. The nurses independently extracted information from patient records. When examining each record, the nurses indicated on the data sheet the presence or absence of the various constituents for each quality indicator. The estimated cost for a nurse to review all the records for a single subject averaged $135, rising to $184 per subject when the satisfaction questionnaire is included. The length and complexity of certain records affected the time required for review. The average time for reviewing a file was five hours. Each nurse invested a total of nearly 150 hours to review the complete records of 29 people.

The telephone interviews about satisfaction took place between October 31, 2005 and May 12, 2006 for all subject in the final constituted sample (N=40). In 75 % of cases, the caregivers primarily responded to the questionnaire and provided information about the use of services. The other interviews were carried out with the legal representatives (17 %) or the elderly individuals themselves (8 %). Respondents easily and successfully responded to the questionnaire. The average interview length was 15 minutes. While telephone interviews suited most of the subjects, three individuals had face-to-face interviews because of their specific situations. Comments made by third-party respondents were recorded at the time of the interview. In many cases, we observed that the third-party respondents were unable to answer questions about help with activities of daily life and personal care since they did not live with the elderly person.

Objective 3: Interobserver reliability

Of the 68 quality indicators that could be applied to the same person, 65 were assessed by at least one nurse for at least one patient and 61 by both nurses for at least one patient. Only 22 quality indicators, however, were assessed by both nurses in 10 or more subjects (Table 16.1).

Table 16.1

Number of quality indicators (QIs) assessed for the 29 subjects in the study

QI assessed for:	QI assessed by Nurse # 1	QI assessed by Nurse # 2	QI for the patient assessed by both nurses	Total number of QIs assessed by the 2 nurses in more than 10 patients
Assessment				
• 1 to 9 subjects	11	15	16	
• 10 subjects or +	18	13	11	11
Treatment				
• 1 to 9 subjects	7	9	9	
• 10 subjects or +	9	7	7	7
Follow-up				
• 1 to 9 subjects	10	13	14	
• 10 subjects or +	10	6	4	4
Total number (% of 68 QIs studied)	65 (95.6)	63 (92.6)	61 (89.7)	22 (32.4)

Interobserver agreement was calculated for two situations:

a) If both nurses deemed that an indicator was applicable to a patient, there was agreement. If both nurses deemed that an indicator was not applicable to a patient, there was also agreement. If the nurses did not concur in their assessments, then there was disagreement. The kappa value for this type of agreement for the 65 indicators assessed in 29 subjects was 0.53 or moderate (Table 16.2).

b) The judgment agreement was calculated for all the indicators assessed in a patient by both nurses. Agreement was deemed to exist if the information collected by BOTH nurses led us to deem that the indicator criteria had been met OR if the information collected by BOTH nurses led us to deem the indicator criteria had not been met. If information collected by both nurses did not lead to the same judgment, there was no agreement. The kappa value for this type of agreement (overall for the 65 indicators) was 0.57 or moderate (Table 16.2).

Table 16.2

Interobserver reliability for the 65 quality indicators assessed

	Agreement on QI Met for a Subject out of the 65 QIs	Agreement on QI Applicability for a Subject out of the 65 QIs
Kappa for Interobserver Reliability	0.57	0.53
Proportion of Occurrences with Agreement between the Two Observers	79.3 %	77.5 %

Discussion and Conclusion

The data sources (clinical and medical records) as well as telephone interviews with the elderly, caregivers, or legal representatives were appropriate for the pilot project. Taken in isolation, clinical and medical records cannot report all the information relating to care or services, because they less frequently contain entries about prevention and counseling activities, and could therefore influence the quality of care[29, 30, 36]. Confidence in records alone could lead to mistaken conclusions about the care process and its quality[37]. Despite this caveat, records are nonetheless considered as the gold standard for many quality measures. Indeed, it is preferable to use them rather than only administrative data, particularly when attempting to measure geriatric conditions (dementia, end of life, malnutrition, pressure sores, urinary incontinence)[38].

The telephone interview about satisfaction carried out with the elderly, their caregivers, or their legal representatives—in conjunction with the review of clinical and medical records—yield a more overall assessment of quality. The telephone questionnaire was successful and proved to be an effective tool for rounding out the information in the records. It was all the more important to use this method because what the respondents report about the quality of inter-actions with caregivers can be different from the technical quality of care measured by reviewing records. Indeed, the satisfaction reported is not auto-matically associated with the technical quality of care, but can be related to the degree of communication during interpersonal relations[39].

Except for the hitches relating to anonymizing at the beginning of the project, getting copies of the records was easy. Physician practicing in their offices were quite quick in responding. In contrast to the concerns we had about fast access to medical records, the physicians were more than helpful and very prompt in responding to our requests for copies of patient records. As men-tioned above, anonymizing records generated significant delays and costs. If a similar project were carried out on a larger scale, much more care would have to go into the wording of the consent form: the text must be adequately clear and leave no room for interpreting that the files must be anonymized. Moreover, the involvement of several ethics committees, as was the case in this pilot project, can bog down the process and jeopardize the completion of a larger project.

The interobserver agreement, expressed as a moderate kappa value, applies to the 61 quality indicators assessed by the two nurses. Given that 22 quality indicators occurred in 10 or more subjects and that other indicators were never detected (3 were never assessed because they didn't occur in the records), there is reason to either increase the number of records reviewed using the same num-ber of quality indicators or reduce the number of indicators to be assessed.

These outcomes, coupled with comments from the nurses, also point to the need to improve working tools and nurse training. For example, the technical sheets need to be made more user-friendly and their contents reviewed. The training offered to the nurses should be longer. Moreover, participants in the training must develop a common understanding of the sheet contents and the information to be collected. Nurse performance and knowledge should also be checked frequently and regularly, particularly at the start of the review process. Periodic assessments could also be put on the schedule.

Costs stand out as a major obstacle in this type of study because the work is highly intensive. As stated above, the average cost for reviewing a subject's records and administering the satisfaction survey amounts to $184. This means that a project intending to review 1000 records would require a large budget for data collection alone. Furthermore, a large project would face some serious hur-dles in getting funding. Nevertheless, the suggestion improvements could help cut costs somewhat. The development of electronic clinical records and their widespread use would be quite beneficial in reducing the costs involved in assessing quality indicators. The pilot project proved critical in determining the scope of the task in a process to assess quality. It opens the door for a more ambitious research project, with the express condition that certain changes be made to the data-collection instruments.

Acknowledgments

The pilot project was funded by the Canadian Institutes of Health Research (CIHR – Project # 29188). The research team would like to thank Marie-Andrée Leblanc, coordinator of home-care services with the Centre de santé et de services sociaux de la Vieille-Capitale and the ten social workers involved. We are also grateful to the people responsible for the CSSS/VC archives as well as to the consulting archivist who reviewed the information sheets and assisted the nurses in preparing the review work. We deeply appreciate the contributions of Édith Picard-Marcoux and Sophear Sar, the two nurses who reviewed the records. Our thanks also go out to the general physicians who cooperated with the pilot project.

References

1. World Health Organization. *The World Health Report 2000: health systems, improving performance*. Geneva: WHO, 2000.

2. Hurtado MP, Swift EK, Corrigan JM. (eds). *Envisioning the National Health Care Quality Report*. Washington, D.C., 2001; Institute of Medicine, Board on Health Care Services: 234 p.

3. National Health Services (NHS). *Quality and performance in the NHS: High level of performance indicators*. London, 1999; 76 p.

4. Gouvernement du Québec. *Projet de loi no 38: Loi sur le Commissaire à la santé et au bien-être*. Québec, 2003.

5. Wenger NS, Solomon DH, MacLean C, Saliba D, Roth C, Kamberg C, Rubenstein L, Schnelle J, Young RT, Skekelle PG. Vulnerable elders receive worse quality care for geriatric conditions than for medical conditions. *Journal of General Internal Medicine*. 2001; 16: 222.

6. Wenger NS, Solomon DH, Roth CP. The Quality of medical care provided to vulnerable community older patients. *Annals of Internal Medicine*. 2003; 139: 740-747.

7. Jencks SF, Cuerdon T, Burwen DR, Fleming B, Horick PM, Kussmaul AF, Nilasena DS, Ordin DL, Arday DR. Quality of medical care delivered to Medicare beneficiaries. *Journal of the American Medical Association*. 2000; 284 (13): 1670-1676.

8. Jencks SF, Cuerdon T. Change in the quality of care delivered to Medicare beneficiaries 1998-1999 to 2000-2001. *Journal of the American Medical Association*. 2003; 289: 305-312.

9.   Brook RH, McGlynn EA, Shekelle PG. Defining and measuring quality of care: a perspective from US researchers. *International Journal for Quality in Health Care*. 2000; 12: 281-295.

10. Marshall CL, Bluestein M, Chapin C, Davis T, Gersten J, Harris C, Hodgin A, Larsen W, Rigberg H, Krishnaswami V, Darling B. Outpatient management of diabetes mellitus in five Arizona Medicare managed care plans. *American Journal of Medical Quality*. 1996; 11: 87-93.

11. Sloss EM, Solomon DH, Shekelle PG, Young RT, Saliba D, MacLean CH, Rubenstein LZ, Schnelle JF, Kamberg CJ, Wenger NS. Selecting target conditions for quality of care improvement in vulnerable older adults. *Journal of the American Geriatrics Society*. 2000; 48: 363-369.

12. Fahey T, Montgomery AA, Barnes J, Protheroe J. Quality of care for elderly resident in nursing homes and elderly people living at home: controlled observational study. *British Medical Journal*. 2003; 326: 580-585.

13. Marciniak TA, Ellerbeck EF, Radford MJ, Kresowik TF, Gold JA, Krumholz HM, Kiefe CI, Allman RM, Vogel RA, Jenck SF. Improving the Quality care for Medicare patients with acute myocardial infarction. *Journal of the American Medical Association*. 1998; 279 (17): 1351-1357.

14. Kane RL. Improving the quality of long-term care. *Journal of the American Medical Association*. 1995; 273: 1376-1380.

15, Dickinson E, Brocklehurst J. Improving the quality of long term care for older people: lessons from the CARE scheme. *Quality in Health Care*. 1997; 6: 160-164.

16. Brook RH, McGlynn EA, Cleary PD. Quality of health care. Part 2: measuring quality of care. *New England Journal of Medicine*. 1996; 335: 966-970.

17. Donabedian A. *Exploration in quality assessment and monitoring*. Volume 1: The definition of quality and approaches to its assessment. Michigan: Health Administration Press, Ann Arbor, 1980.

18. Irvine D. *Managing for quality in general practice*. London: King's Fund Centre, 1990.

19. Higashi T, Shekelle PG, Adams JL, Kamberg CJ, Roth CP, Solomon DH, Reuben DB, Chiang L, MacLean CH, Chang JT, Young RT, Saliba DM, Wenger NS. Quality of Care Is Associated with Survival in Vulnerable Older Patients. *Annals of Internal Medicine*. 2005; 143 (4): 274-281

20. Donabedian A. Methods for deriving criteria for assessing the quality of medical care. *Medical Care Review*. 1980; 37: 653-698.

21. Lohr KN. Medicare: A Strategy for Quality Assurance. In: Lohr KN. *Committee to design a strategy for quality review and assurance in Medicare*. Institute of Medicine, ed. Vol. II: Sources and Methods: National Academy Press, 1990: 476.

22. MSSS. *Priorités nationales de santé publique 1997-2001. Vers l'atteinte des résultats attendus: 3ᵉ bilan.* Québec, MSSS, 2001.

23. Durand PJ, Tourigny A, Bonin L, Paradis M, Lemay A, Bergeron P. *Mécanisme de coordination des services géronto-gériatriques des Bois-Francs – QC 403. Rapport final sur les résultats présentés au Fonds d'adaptation des services de santé.* Québec, avril 2001.

24. Tourigny A, Durand PJ, Bonin L, Hébert R, Rochette L. Quasi-experimental Study of the Effectiveness of an Integrated Service Delivery Network for Frail Older People. *Canadian Journal of Aging.* 2004, 23 (3): 231-246.

25. Capital Health Authority. *Program description for the comprehensive home option of integrated care for the elderly.* (Working document). Edmonton: Capital Health Authority. 1995.

26. Eng C, Pedulla J, Eleazer GP, McCann R, Fox N. Program of All-inclusive Care for the Elderly (PACE): an innovative model of integrated geriatric care and financing. *Journal of the American Geriatrics Society.* 1997; 45 (2): 223-232.

27. National Advisory Committee on Health and Disability. Summary of the National Health Committee Quality Workshop. National Advisory Committee on Health and Disability, Wellington, New Zealand, 2001: 53.

28. Tourigny A, Côté L, Kröger E, Lebel P, Kergoat MJ, Morin D, Tousignant M. Framework for the Evaluation of the Quality of Care and Services Provided to Vulnerable Elder Persons. In Hébert R, Tourigny A, Gagnon M. éd. *Integrated service delivery to ensure person' functional autonomy.* Québec: Édisem, 2004: 291-309.

29. Min LC, Reuben DB, MacLean CH, Shekelle PG, Solomon DH, Higashi T, Chang JT, Roth CP, Kamberg CJ, Adams J, Young RT, Wenger NS. Predictors of Overall Quality of Care Provided to Vulnerable Older People. *Journal of the American Geriatrics Society.* 2005; 53 (10): 1705-1711.

30. McGlynn EA, Asch SM, Adams J, Keesey J, Hicks J, DeCristofaro A, Kerr EA. The Quality of Health Care Delivered to Adults in the United States. *The New England Journal of Medicine.* 2003; 348 (26): 2635-2645.

31. Higashi T, Shekelle PG, Solomon DH, Knight EL, Roth C, Chang JT, Kamberg CJ, MacLean CH, Young RT, Adams J, Reuben DB, Avorn J, Wenger NS. The Quality of Pharmacologic Care for Vulnerable Older Patients. *Annals of Internal Medicine.* 2004; 140 (9): 714-720.

32. Haan MN, Wallace R. Can Dementia Be Prevented? Brain Aging in a Population-Based Context. *Annual Review of Public Health.* 2004: 25: 1-24.

33. Wenger NS, Shekelle PG. Assessing care of vulnerable elders: ACOVE project overview. *Annals of Internal Medicine.* 2001; 135 (8Pt2): 642-646.

34. Website CSSS de la Vieille-Capitale http://www.csssvc.qc.ca

35. Gagnon M. *Satisfaction et autonomisation des personnes âgées face aux soins et services de santé: instruments de mesure et variables associées.* Thèse de doctorat présentée à l'Université du Québec à Trois-Rivières, février 2004.

36. Luck J, Peabody JW, Dresselhaus TR, Lee M, Glassman P. How Well Does Chart Abstraction Measure Quality? A Prospective Comparison of Standardized Patients with the Medical Record. *The American Journal of Medicine*. 2000, 108: 642-649.

37. Schnelle JF, Osterweil D, Simmons SF. Improving the Quality of Nursing Home Care and Medical-Record Accuracy With Direct Observational Technologies. *The Gerontologist*. 2005, 45 (5): 576-582.

38. MacLean CH, Louie R, Shekelle PG, Roth CP, Saliba D, Higashi T, Adams J, Chang JT, Kamberg CJ, Solomon DH, Young RT, Wenger NS. Comparison of Administrative Data and Medical Records to Measure the Quality of Medical Care Provided to Vulnerable Older Patients. *Medical Care*. 2006, 44(2): 141-148.

39. Chang JT, Hays RD, Shekelle PG, MacLean CH, Solomon DH, Reuben DB, Roth CP, Kamberg CJ, Adams J, Young RT, Wenver NS. Patients' Global Ratings of Their Health Care Are Not Associated with the Technical Quality of Their Care. *Annals of Internal Medicine*. 2006, 144 (9): 665-672.

Indicator :

T6 IF a vulnerable elderly person has mild to moderate Alzheimer's disease, THEN the attending physician must discuss with the patient and his/her caregiver (if available) the possibility of treatment with cholinesterase inhibitors.

Elements to Consider: :	Element Present	
	Yes	No
Vulnerable elderly person: See E1	☐	☐
Alzheimer's disease		
Diagnostic of Alzheimer's disease noted in the record	☐	☐
Note in the record indicating that the disease is mild to moderate AND	☐	☐
Score of the MMSE (between 15 and 27)	☐	☐
Attending physician Physician from: ☐ CLSC ☐ Physician's office ☐ Hospital		
Inhibitor therapy Node in record about prescription of a cholinesterase inhibitor: Rivastigmine – Exelon (registered trademark); Galantamine – Remynil (registered trademark); Donazepil – Aricept (registered trademark); Memantine hydrochloride – Ebixa, new medication – marketing authorized station subject to conditions OR	☐	☐
Discussion Nodes in the record indicating discussion with the elderly person or caregiver about medication	☐	☐

Indicator assessment:
Indicator met: Yes ☐
                           No   ☐

Comments :
_____
_____
_____
_____
_____

Research nurse's name _____ Date____ d____ m____

Chapter 17
Validation of Process Quality Indicators for the Integrated Care of Frail Older Adults[*]

Edeltraut Kröger, André Tourigny, Diane Morin,
Lise Côté, Marie-Jeanne Kergoat, Paule Lebel,
Line Robichaud, Shirley Imbeault, and Solange Proulx

Highlights

1. A rigorous quality-assessment method needs to be developed before the quality of care and services to frail older adults can be improved.
2. Process quality indicators were assembled to assess the quality of care and services to older adults affected by cognitive impairment or dementia.
3. These indicators came from abroad and had not been developed for an integrated services network; thus, selected indicators had to be validated by a multidisciplinary research team.
4. A Delphi panel of 33 clinicians from nine health-care disciplines or specialties judged the majority (88 %) of the indicators submitted for validation as acceptable for quality assessment within an integrated service system.
5. These indicators will be used experimentally in a pilot project in order to evaluate their feasibility and reliability for assessment of the quality of ambulatory services delivered to older adults affected by cognitive impairment or dementia in Quebec.

KEYWORDS: Validation, process indicators, quality improvement

OBJECTIVES: To validate process quality indicators developed elsewhere for care and services offered to frail older adults, as part of a research program on the improvement of care quality in an integrated service system.

---

[*] Parts of the content of this chapter can be found in the publication: Kröger E, Tourigny A, Morin D, Côté L, Kergoat MJ, Lebel P, Robichaud L, Imbeault S, Proulx S, Benounissa Z. Selecting process quality indicators for the integrated care of vulnerable older adults affected by cognitive impairment or dementia. BMC Health Serv Res 2007;7:195. weblink: http://www.biomedcentral.com/1472-6963/7/195

DESIGN: Modified RAND®/University of California at Los Angeles appropriateness method, a two-round Delphi panel.

SETTING: Three major urban centers in Quebec, Canada.

PARTICIPANTS: A total of 33 expert panellists representing two medical specialties (family medicine, geriatrics) and seven health or social services specialties (nursing, occupational therapy, psychology, neuropsychology, pharmacy, nutrition, and social work), from the primary and secondary levels of care, including long-term care.

MAIN OUTCOME MEASURES: Face and content validity of process quality indicators, as assessed by the interpercentile range (IPR) statistical measure adjusted for symmetry, measuring agreement with three criteria (median rating of 7–9, on a nine-point scale) and among panellists.

RESULTS: Of the initial 82 indicators for care of frail older adults with cognitive impairment/dementia, which were submitted to the panellists, 72 (88 %) were accepted after two rounds. The discarded indicators involved the treatment (1), follow-up (4), consent (1 PQI), satisfaction (3), and access domains (1). The accepted indicators covered all of the dimensions of the conceptual framework for quality: safety (13), effectiveness (27), patient-centeredness (16), access (3), and continuity (13).

CONCLUSION: A multidisciplinary panel of experts judged a large majority of the initial indicators valid for use in integrated care systems for frail older adults in Quebec, Canada. These indicators are to be measured using patient files, patient or caregiver interviews, and administrative data.

Although large variations in the quality of health care and services may affect all parts of the population,[1] such variations are particularly worrisome for frail older adults[2-4]. Increased quality of care for this population is associated with longer survival.[5] Furthermore, the demand for care and services for older adults, a rapidly increasing segment of the population, is overburdening the capacity of the health-care system[6]. Under funded healthcare services, common to many industrialized countries, including Canada,[7] may accentuate quality problems for this group. Therefore, initiatives were aimed at improving the quality and efficiency of health care for older and disabled populations[8].

Integration of care and service delivery is one promising approach designed to improve access, quality, user satisfaction, and efficiency[9-11]. Derived from a variety of demonstration projects,[6, 12, 13] the main features of an effective integrated service system for frail older adults are a single point of entry into the system, case management, geriatric assessment, and a multidisciplinary care team[14]. Based on these principles, an innovative model, the Program of Research to Integrate Services for the Maintenance of Autonomy (PRISMA), has been underway in the province of Quebec since 1999, aimed at ensuring the independence of community-dwelling older adults[13, 15].

Specific research projects, as part of the PRISMA program, investigated patient satisfaction and patient perception regarding integrated service systems[16, 17]. Since quality improvement is one of the main objectives of service integration, one specific project is aimed at assessing and improving the quality of health care and services provided to frail older adults within integrated service systems[15]. Quality assessment, with the help of process quality indicators (PQIs), is an essential first step of quality improvement and the reduction of its variability[4, 18].

In the United States, a large-scale research program called the Assessing Care of Vulnerable Elders (ACOVE) project evaluated the quality of care for older adults with the help of PQIs[19, 20]. The ACOVE research team developed and validated 236 PQIs for 22 clinical conditions for vulnerable community-dwelling people, 65 years of age and older[21]. However, PQIs cannot be transferred between countries without prior validation, and often translation, to take into account variations in language, culture, and practice[22]. Thus, PQIs developed by ACOVE and elsewhere had to be validated before implementation in integrated service systems in Quebec. To our knowledge, previous reports on validation of indicators for transfer between countries[4, 22, 23] do not consider these systems. We report how this study developed and validated PQIs for frail older adults in an integrated service system.

Methods

Quality framework

The research project on quality assessment and improvement for frail older adults in integrated service systems, of which the present study is part, relies on the US Institute of Medicine's (IOM) definition of quality[24]. It is also guided by a conceptual framework to ensure a meaningful and rigorous quality evaluation and improvement[25]. We modified a published version of the IOM's conceptual framework, which is a four-by-four matrix of quality dimensions (safety, effectiveness, patient-centeredness, and access) and patients' perspectives of health care during different life stages (staying healthy, getting better, living better with illness or disability, and coping with the end of life)[25]. Within the IOM framework, equity is a cross-cutting dimension of quality, integral to all of its aspects. Continuity is a quality dimension essential to integrated service systems, especially for frail older adults[10, 26]. We therefore added this dimension as a second cross-cutting element to the framework. We also considered the perspectives of the caregivers of frail older patients, along with the patients' perspectives, and enlarged the concept of patient-centeredness to include the patient's community, an important element within an integrated service system (see Figure 17.1)[15]. We translated the resulting framework into French to guide the whole quality improvement project.

Figure 17.1
Conceptual framework, adapted from the Institute of Medicine[25]

Patients' and caregivers' perspectives on health-care needs	Safety	Effectiveness	Patient and community centered care	Access
Staying healthy	Cross-cutting dimension: Continuity			
Getting better				
Living with illness or disability				
Coping with the end of life	Cross-cutting dimension: Equity			

Selecting PQIs

Quality can be measured by process or outcome indicators[27]. Process indicators were chosen because they assess the actual care given and its quality[28] and help to detect care and service processes needing improvement. Compared with outcome indicators, they are also less influenced by case-mix and other confounding factors[29]. To limit the scope of the present study, we developed a set of PQIs for one clinical condition. We based our choice of this condition on two criteria: highly prevalent among frail older adults and requiring integrated services, namely, interventions across the whole care continuum (i.e. ambulatory, short- and long-term care)[30] and from different health-care disciplines. We chose to develop PQIs for cognitive impairment/dementia because this condition affects about 16.8 % and 8.0 % of adults 65 years of age and older, respectively,[31] and requires interventions from several types of healthcare providers. Some PQIs for other medical problems that frequently affect patients with cognitive impairment/dementia, such as incontinence, pressure ulcers, multiple medications and malnutrition, were also included, so that the final indicator set captures most of the care required by these patients.

We selected appropriate PQIs from published and grey literature, including PQIs for social work and occupational therapy. Choices were discussed within the multidisciplinary research team, composed of investigators from public health, medicine, geriatrics, nursing, occupational therapy, psychology, and pharmacy. We compiled a list of 82 PQIs: 62 ACOVE PQIs applicable to patients with the chosen condition[32] and 20 additional indicators to make sure all dimensions of the conceptual framework, the whole care continuum and the full range of services were covered (see Table 17.1).

Table 17.1

**Process Quality Indicators from the ACOVE Project OR
Adapted from Other Sources and Submitted for Validation**

Process quality indicator	Modified*	Result of validation
Indicators from the ACOVE project		
E1) † ALL vulnerable elders newly admitted to a hospital or to a physician's practice should receive, within 6 months, the elements of a comprehensive geriatric assessment, including assessment of cognitive ability and functional status[32].	No	Accepted
E 2) IF a vulnerable elder is admitted to the hospital for any acute or chronic illness or any surgical procedure, THEN the evaluation should include, within 24 hours, 1) diagnoses, 2) prehospital and current medications, and 3) cognitive status[32].	No	Accepted
E 6) ALL vulnerable elders should be screened at least once to detect problem drinking and hazardous drinking by taking a history of alcohol use or by using standardized screening questionnaires[32].	No	Accepted
E 7) IF a vulnerable elder uses tobacco regularly, THEN he or she should be offered counseling and/or pharmacologic therapy at least once to stop tobacco use.	No	Accepted
E 8) ALL vulnerable elders should receive an assessment of their level of physical activity *at least once a year and, if necessary, be provided with counseling about appropriate resources*[32].	After 1st round‡	Accepted
E 9) ALL vulnerable elders should have documentation that they were asked at least annually about the occurrence of recent falls[32].	No	Accepted
E 13) IF a vulnerable elder is admitted to an intensive care unit or a medical or surgical unit of a hospital and cannot reposition himself or herself or has limited ability to do so, THEN risk assessment for pressure ulcers should be done on admission[32].	No	Accepted
E 14) ALL vulnerable elders should have documentation of the presence or absence of urinary incontinence during the initial evaluation and annually[32].	No	Accepted

Table 17.1 (*suite*)
**Process Quality Indicators from the ACOVE Project OR
Adapted from Other Sources and Submitted for Validation**

Process quality indicator	Modified*	Result of validation
E 15) IF a vulnerable elder has a new urinary incontinence that persists for more than 1 month or urinary incontinence at the time of a new evaluation, THEN a clinical conduct based on evidence and including targeted history, physical exam, diagnostic tests, and discussion of treatment options should be offered[32].	Adapted	Accepted
E 16) IF a vulnerable elder has dementia, THEN he or she should be screened for depression during the initial evaluation.[32]	No	Accepted
E 17) IF a vulnerable elder presents with new onset of one of the following symptoms: *anxiety, somatic problems*, sad mood, feeling down, insomnia or difficulties with sleep, apathy or loss of interest in pleasurable activities, complaints of memory loss, unexplained weight loss greater than 5 % in the past month or 10 % over 1 year, or unexplained fatigue or low energy, THEN the patient should be asked about or treated for depression, or referred to a mental-health professional within 2 weeks of presentation[32].	After 1st round‡	Accepted
E 18) IF a vulnerable elder presents with onset or discovery of one of the following conditions: stroke, myocardial infarction, dementia, malignancy (excluding skin cancer), chronic pain, alcohol or substance abuse or dependence, anxiety disorder or personality disorder, THEN the patient should be asked about or treated for depression, or referred to a mental health professional within 2 months of diagnosis of the condition[32].	No	Accepted
E 19) IF a vulnerable elder receives a diagnosis of a new depression episode, THEN the medical record should document on the day of diagnosis the presence or absence of suicidal ideation and psychosis (consisting of, at minimum, auditory hallucinations or delusions)[32].	No	Accepted
E 20) IF a vulnerable elder has thoughts of suicide, THEN the medical record should document, on the same date, that the patient either has no immediate plan for suicide or that the patient was referred for evaluation for psychiatric hospitalization[32].	No	Accepted
E 21) IF a vulnerable elder is being treated for depression, THEN, at each treatment visit, suicide risk should be documented if he or she had suicidal ideation during a previous visit[32].	No	Accepted

Table 17.1 (*suite*)
Process Quality Indicators from the ACOVE Project OR
Adapted from Other Sources and Submitted for Validation

Process quality indicator	Modified*	Result of validation
E 22) IF a hospitalized vulnerable elder has a definite or suspected diagnosis of delirium, THEN an evaluation for potentially precipitating factors must be undertaken and identified causes treated[32].	No	Accepted
E 23) ALL community-dwelling vulnerable elders should be weighed *at least every 6 months* and these weights should be documented in the medical record (*doctor's office, outpatient clinic or CLSC §*)[32].	After 1st round‡	Accepted
E 24) IF a community-dwelling vulnerable elder has documented involuntary weight loss (greater than or equal to 10 % of body weight) or hypoalbuminemia (< 3.5 g/dL), THEN he or she should receive an evaluation for potentially relevant comorbid conditions, including medications that might be associated with decreased appetite (for example, digoxin, fluoxetine, anticholinergics), depressive symptoms, and cognitive impairment and for potentially reversible causes of poor nutritional intake[32].	Adapted	Accepted
E 25) IF a vulnerable elder is hospitalized, THEN his or her nutritional status should be documented during the hospitalization by evaluation of oral intake or serum biochemical testing (for example, albumin, prealbumin, or cholesterol)[32].	No	Accepted
E 26) IF a vulnerable elder presents with symptoms of dementia, THEN the physician should review the patient's medication list (*prescriptions, over the counter, or supplements*) for initiation of medications that might correspond chronologically to the onset of dementia symptoms[32].	After 1st round‡	Accepted
E 27) IF a vulnerable elder presents with symptoms of dementia that correspond in time with the initiation of new medications (prescriptions, over the counter, or supplements) then the physician should discontinue or justify the necessity of continuing these medications[32].	After 1st round‡	Accepted
E 28) ALL vulnerable elders should be screened for chronic pain during the initial evaluation period and regularly thereafter[32].	No	Accepted

Table 17.1 (*suite*)
**Process Quality Indicators from the ACOVE Project OR
Adapted from Other Sources and Submitted for Validation**

Process quality indicator	Modified*	Result of validation
E 29) IF a vulnerable elder has a newly reported chronic painful condition, THEN a targeted history and physical examination should be initiated within 1 month and treatment should be offered[32].	No	Accepted
E 30) IF a vulnerable elder has newly diagnosed dementia, THEN serum levels of vitamin B12 and thyroid-stimulating hormone should be measured[32].	No	Accepted
E 31) IF a vulnerable elder has signs of dementia and focal neurologic findings that suggest an intracranial process, THEN he or she should be offered neuroimaging (brain computed tomography or magnetic resonance imaging)[32].	No	Accepted
T1) † IF a vulnerable elder has newly diagnosed dementia, THEN the diagnosing physician should ask the patient *whether he drives a motor vehicle and, if yes, should inquire at follow-up visits about the patient's capacity to safely continue this activity*[32].	After 1st round‡	Accepted
T 2) IF a hospitalized vulnerable elder is unable to take foods orally for more than 72 hours, THEN alternative enteral alimentation should be offered[32].	No	Rejected
T 5) IF a vulnerable elder is identified as at risk for pressure ulcer development or a pressure ulcer risk score indicates that the person is at risk, THEN a preventive intervention addressing repositioning needs and pressure reduction (or management of tissue loads) must be instituted within 12 hours[32].	No	Accepted
T 6) IF a vulnerable elder has mild to moderate Alzheimer disease, THEN the treating physician should discuss treatment with a cholinesterase inhibitor with the patient and the primary caregiver (if available)[32].	No	Accepted
T 7) IF a vulnerable elder with dementia has cerebrovascular disease, THEN he or she should be offered appropriate prophylaxis against stroke[32].	No	Accepted
T 8) ALL vulnerable elders should not be prescribed a medication with strong anticholinergic effects if alternatives are available[32].	No	Accepted
T 10) IF a vulnerable elder is prescribed a new drug, THEN the prescribed drug should have a clearly defined indication documented in the record[32].	No	Accepted

Table 17.1 (*suite*)
**Process Quality Indicators from the ACOVE Project OR
Adapted from Other Sources and Submitted for Validation**

Process quality indicator	Modified*	Result of validation
T 11) IF a vulnerable elder is prescribed a new drug, THEN the patient (or, if incapable, a caregiver) should receive education about the purpose of the drug, how to take it, and the expected side effects or important adverse reactions[32].	No	Accepted
T 12) IF a vulnerable elder with chronic pain is treated with opioids, THEN he or she should be offered a bowel regimen or the medical record should document the potential for constipation or explain why bowel treatment is not needed[32].	No	Accepted
T 14) IF a vulnerable elder with dementia has depression, THEN he or she should be treated for the depression[32].	No	Accepted
I 15) IF a vulnerable elder with dementia has a caregiver (and, if capable, the patient assents), THEN the physician should discuss or refer the patient and caregiver for discussion about patient safety, provide education on how to deal with conflicts at home, and inform them about community resources for dementia[32].	No	Accepted
T 16) IF a vulnerable elder with dementia is to be physically restrained in the hospital, THEN the target behavioral disturbance or safety issue justifying use of the restraints must be identified to the consenting person (patient or legal guardian) and documented in the chart[32].	No	Accepted
T 17) IF a vulnerable elder is physically restrained and the target behavioral disturbance requiring restraint is identified, THEN the health-care team should include methods other than physical restraints in the care plan[32].	No	Accepted

Table 17.1 (*suite*)
Process Quality Indicators from the ACOVE Project OR
Adapted from Other Sources and Submitted for Validation

Process quality indicator	Modified*	Result of validation
T 18) IF a vulnerable elder is placed in physical restraints, THEN each of the following measures should be enacted: 1. Consistent release from the restraints at least every 2 hours; 2. Face-to-face reassessment by a physician or nurse at least every 4 hours and before renewal of the restraint order; 3. Observation at least every 15 minutes, and more frequently if indicated by the patient's condition, while the patient is in restraints; 4. Interventions every 2 hours (or as indicated by patient's condition or needs) related to nutrition, hydration, personal hygiene, toileting, and range of motion exercises[32].	No	Accepted
T 19) IF a vulnerable elder presents with a pressure ulcer, THEN the pressure ulcer should be assessed for location, depth and stage, size, and presence of necrotic tissue, and managed using evidence-based measures (ulcer care guidelines), such as debridement, cleansing, and topical dressings[32].	Adapted	Accepted
FU1) † IF the elements of a comprehensive geriatric assessment are performed, THEN follow-up should assure the implementation of recommendations[32].	No	Accepted
FU 3) IF a vulnerable elder has an advance directive in the outpatient, inpatient, or nursing home medical record or the patient reports the existence of an advance directive in an interview, and the patient receives care at a second venue, THEN 1) the advance directive should be present in the medical record at the second venue or 2) documentation should acknowledge its existence, its contents, and the reason that it is not in the medical record[32].	No	Accepted
FU 4) IF a vulnerable elder has specific treatment preferences (for example, a do-not-resuscitate order, no tube feeding, or no hospital transfer) documented in a medical record, THEN these treatment preferences should be followed[32].	No	Accepted
FU 5) IF a vulnerable elder enters the hospital, THEN discharge planning should begin *in the days following admission, as soon as the patient's condition stabilizes.*[32]	After 1st round‡	Accepted

Table 17.1 (*suite*)
Process Quality Indicators from the ACOVE Project OR
Adapted from Other Sources and Submitted for Validation

Process quality indicator	Modified*	Result of validation
FU 6) For ALL vulnerable elders, the patient's medical record (*doctor's office, CLSC§, hospital and community pharmacy*) should contain an up-to-date medication list[32].	After 1st round‡	Accepted
FU 8) EVERY new drug that is prescribed to a vulnerable elder on an ongoing basis for a chronic medical condition should have a documentation of the response to therapy, *including side effects*[32].	After 1st round ‡	Accepted
FU 9) ALL vulnerable elders should have a drug regimen review at least annually[32].	No	Accepted
FU 10) IF a vulnerable eldor has boen prescribed a cyclo-oxygenase nonselective nonsteroidal anti-inflammatory drug (NSAID) for the treatment of chronic pain, THEN the medical record should indicate whether he or she has a history of peptic ulcer disease and, if a history is present, justification of NSAID use should be documented[32].	No	Accepted
FU 11) ALL vulnerable elders (or their caregivers) should be able to identify a provider or a clinic that they could call when in need of medical care or should know the phone number or other mechanism by which they can reach a source of care[32].	After 1st round	Rejected
FU 12) IF an outpatient vulnerable elder is started on a new prescription medication and he or she has a follow-up visit with the prescribing physician, THEN the medical record at the follow-up visit should document one of the following: 1) the medication is being taken *and* the physician asked about the medication (for example, side effects, adherence, or availability), or 2) the medication was not started because it was not needed or was changed[32].	After 1st round	Accepted
FU 13) IF a vulnerable elder is under the outpatient care of two or more physicians, and one physician has prescribed a new prescription medication or a change in medication (medication termination or change in dosage), THEN subsequent medical record entries by the nonprescribing physician should acknowledge the medication change[32].	No	Rejected

Table 17.1 (*suite*)
Process Quality Indicators from the ACOVE Project OR
Adapted from Other Sources and Submitted for Validation

Process quality indicator	Modified*	Result of validation
FU 14) IF an outpatient vulnerable elder is referred to a consultant physician, THEN the reason for consultation should be documented in the consultant's note[32].	No	Accepted
FU 15) IF an outpatient vulnerable elder is referred to a consultant and subsequently visits the referring physician after the visit with the consultant, THEN the referring physician's follow-up note should document the consultant's recommendations, or the medical record should include the consultant's note, within 6 weeks or at the time of the follow-up visit, whichever is later[32].	No	Accepted
FU 16) IF the outpatient medical record documents that a diagnostic test was ordered for a vulnerable elder, THEN the medical record at the follow-up visit should document one of the following: 1) the result of the test, 2) the test was not needed or reason why it will not be performed, or 3) the test is still pending[32].	No	Accepted
FU 17) IF a vulnerable elder is discharged from a hospital to home and he or she received a new prescription medication or change in medication (medication termination or change in dosage) before discharge, THEN his or her medical record (*doctor's office, CLSC §, or long term care facility*) should acknowledge the medication change within 6 weeks of discharge[32].	After 1st round	Accepted
FU 18) IF a vulnerable elder is discharged from a hospital to the home or to a nursing home and the transfer form or discharge summary indicates that a test result is pending, THEN his or her medical record (*doctor's office, CLSC §, or long-term care facility*) should include the test result within 6 weeks of hospital discharge[32].	After 1st round	Rejected
FU 19) IF a vulnerable elder is discharged from a hospital to home or to a nursing home and the hospital medical record specifies a follow-up appointment for a physician visit or a treatment (for example, physical therapy or radiation oncology), THEN the medical record (*doctor's office, CLSC §, or long-term care facility*) should document that the visit or treatment took place or that it was postponed or not needed[32].	After 1st round	Accepted

Table 17.1 (*suite*)
Process Quality Indicators from the ACOVE Project OR
Adapted from Other Sources and Submitted for Validation

Process quality indicator	Modified*	Result of validation
FU 20) IF a vulnerable elder is discharged from a hospital to the home and survives at least 4 weeks after discharge, THEN he or she should have a follow-up visit or documented telephone contact within 6 weeks of discharge AND the physician's medical record documentation should acknowledge the recent hospitalization[32].	No	Rejected
FU 21) IF a vulnerable elder is transferred between emergency departments or between acute-care facilities, THEN the medical record at the receiving facility should include medical records from the transferring facility or should acknowledge transfer of such medical records[32].	No	Accepted
FU 22) IF a vulnerable elder is discharged from a hospital to the home or to a nursing home, THEN there should be a discharge summary in the medical record (*doctor's office, CLSC §, or long-term care facility*) within 6 weeks[32].	After 1st round	Accepted
FU 23) IF a vulnerable elder is deaf or does not speak English, THEN an interpreter or translated materials should be employed to facilitate communication between the vulnerable elder and the health-care provider[32].	No	Accepted
C1)† IF a vulnerable elder is to have inpatient or outpatient elective surgery, THEN the medical record should document the patient's ability to understand risks, benefits, and consequences of the proposed surgical operation before the operative consent form is presented for signature[32].	No	Accepted

Indicators from sources other than the ACOVE project

E 3) If a patient has early stage dementia, then his or her performance in productive activities, leisure and everyday activities as well as his or her ability to drive a car should be evaluated[33].	No	Accepted
E 4) If a patient has intermediate stage dementia, then his or her performance in communicating and personal care should be evaluated[33].	No	Accepted
E 5) If a patient has advanced stage dementia, then his or her performance in swallowing and his or her positioning should be evaluated[33].	No	Accepted

Table 17.1 (*suite*)
**Process Quality Indicators from the ACOVE Project OR
Adapted from Other Sources and Submitted for Validation**

Process quality indicator	Modified*	Result of validation
E 10) All vulnerable elders living in psychosocial circumstances presenting a high-risk for their health should be identified as soon as possible[34].	Adapted	Accepted
E 11) If a vulnerable elder is assessed, then language barriers, needs of persons with disabilities (including sensory impairment) or ethnic, cultural, and religious preferences should be taken into account[35].	Adapted	Accepted
E 12) All caregivers of patients with dementia must be asked about their needs for support services[36].	No	Accepted
T 3) *If a service plan is necessary, then this plan should be elaborated with the vulnerable elder or his or her respondent or caregiver*[37].	After 1st round	Accepted
T 4) If a confidential discussion has to take place with a vulnerable elder, then it should take place in private[35].	Adapted	Accepted
T 9) No person with dementia should be taking long-acting sedatives (hypnotics, anxiolytics), unless there is an explicit justification for this medication in the medical record[36].	No	Accepted
T 13) In order to manage behavioral and psychological aspects of dementia, *no drug management strategies should be considered before drug treatment is started*[89].	After 1st round	Accepted
FU 2) If a vulnerable elder has symptoms of cognitive impairment but has not received a diagnosis of dementia, then it should be documented that the provider inquired again about those symptoms within 12 months of the first presentation[36].	Adapted	Accepted
FU 7) All vulnerable elders with complex medication regimens who are returning to community living *should be evaluated whether they are able to maintain a self-medication program*[33].	After 1st round	Accepted
C 2) All vulnerable elders should be informed about the legal and organizational implications of their situation, they should receive the necessary explanations and be informed about measures to take[37].	Adapted	Rejected
SA1)† When appropriate, the opinion of the older adults or their caregivers should be obtained at the end of all interventions[37].	After 1st round	Rejected

Table 17.1 (*suite*)
**Process Quality Indicators from the ACOVE Project OR
Adapted from Other Sources and Submitted for Validation**

Process quality indicator	Modified*	Result of validation
SA 2) If the opinion of the older adult or his or her caregiver has been obtained, then it has to be considered and practices have to be revised and changed, if applicable[37].	Adapted	Rejected
SA 3) If a vulnerable elder requests access to his or her records, then this request should be treated promptly and appropriately[38].	No	Rejected
A1)† All vulnerable elders should receive primary care when needed[39].	No	Accepted
A 2) If a vulnerable elder has an appointment in a clinician's office, then the waiting time in this office should be less than one hour[40].	Adapted	Rejected
A 3) If a vulnerable elder has to consult a specialist, *then the delay between making the appointment and the time of the visit should be a maximum of 8 weeks*[40].	Adapted and modified	Accepted
A 4) If a vulnerable elder needs services or health care at home (nursing care, rehabilitation care, domestic services) then he or she should receive them, according to a previously established order of priority[40].	Adapted	Accepted

* Some indicators were modified upon panellists' comments after the 1st round of the validation process and some were adapted for use in Quebec from the original version found in the literature before the validation process.

† Indicators were grouped according to their respective care domain: E 1 to E 31 for evaluation, T1 to T 19 for treatment, FU 1 to FU 23 for follow-up, C1 and C2 for consent, Sa 1 to SA 3 for satisfaction and A1 to A 4 for access.

‡ Text in italic letters indicates modified part of the indicator.

§ The *Centre local de services communautaires* (CLSC) is the local Quebec community center for health and social services.

Validating the Indicators

The authors (SP, EK) translated the 82 indicators into French, with revision by the research team. No back-translation method was used since some modifications of the indicators were to be expected during the validation process. The validation process followed a slightly modified version of the RAND® University of California, Los Angeles (UCLA) appropriateness method, a modified Delphi panel[41, 42]. This method was privileged since it has successfully been used to develop indicators[21, 42] and to validate PQIs transferred from another country[4]. To facilitate the validation process for the clinical experts on the panel, we arranged the PQIs according to domains of care, namely, clinical evaluation (31 PQIs); treatment (19 PQIs); follow up (23 PQIs); satisfaction with, and consent and access to care (9 PQIs).

Given our interdisciplinary approach, we formed a panel with 33 clinical experts who were identified and recruited by the investigators. These expert practitioners came from three major urban centers in Quebec, i.e. Montreal, Sherbrooke, and Quebec City and worked in ambulatory, hospital and long-term care settings. Recruitment criteria were a minimum of five years of clinical experience with a geriatric clientele and ongoing involvement in integrated care for older adults (75 years and older). Panel members received an honorarium of CAN$50 per hour, corresponding to the estimated number of hours needed to validate the assigned indicators. They represented nine clinical fields, namely medicine or geriatric medicine (n=9), nursing (n=6), occupational therapy (n=3), psychology (n=3), neuropsychology (n=2), pharmacy (n=4), nutrition (n=3), and social work (n=3). The PQIs were validated during two rounds of consultation with the panellists.

Validation Process

The panellists were asked to validate the PQIs that corresponded to their field of expertise, using a form for each PQI assessed. Physicians were asked to validate all 82 PQIs. The forms contained the original English version and the French version of the PQI, its source, the criteria, the judging scale, and a summary of the scientific evidence supporting its use. Panellists were asked to indicate their agreement with five statements on a scale from one to nine (see Figure 17.2): four about the validity of the indicator and one about the necessity to document information relating to the indicator in the patient's file. They were also invited to comment on, or suggest additional PQIs, and 29 out of 33 panellists commented on some PQIs (78 of 82) after the first round, which helped to modify 23 of them. A discussion among the research team took place between the two rounds to decide on these modifications. The complete validation process took place from April to November 2004 and is presented in Figure 17.3.

Statistical Analyses

Scores and comments were analyzed after each of the two rounds. The methods for determining consensus and judging indicators were based on the RAND®/ UCLA method and required (a) the panellists' agreement with the statement (median score, 7–9, upper tertile of the scale) and (b) agreement among the panellists. This type of agreement was assessed with a statistical measure of dispersion, the interpercentile range adjusted for symmetry[42]. This measure was developed by RAND®, is based on the interpercentile range, a commonly used continuous statistical measure of dispersion, and was modified to apply to any size of panel.

Figure 17.2
Criteria submitted to the panellists for scoring

In the context of your clinical practice, please indicate for the above indicator, how much you agree, on a scale from 1 to 9, with each of the following five statements:	
	I completely Disagree .... Agree 1 .... 5 9
C1 Adequate scientific evidence or professional consensus supports a link between the care process specified by the indicator and a health benefit to the patient.	
C2 This indicator is relevant for the assessment of the quality of health care and services to vulnerable elderly patients.	
C3 A health professional with high rates of adherence to this indicator can be considered as a higher quality provider.	
C4 The care and service provider can influence a majority of factors that determine adherence to this indicator.	
C5 It is essential that information on this indicator is present in the patient's file.	

Judgment on Indicators

Judgment on an indicator was based on the panellists' scoring of this PQI for the first three criteria, namely, (1) scientific evidence for a link between process and outcome, (2) clinical relevance to the care of frail older adults, and (3) ability to discriminate between a high- and a low-quality provider. The fourth criterion, concerning the provider's influence on factors affecting adherence to the indicator, was not included in the final analyses, since a number of panellists reported problems in scoring this criterion due to the interdisciplinary nature of their work. The fifth criterion was mainly used to guide the next steps of the research program. Three judgment results were possible: *appropriate*, *uncertain*, and *inappropriate*. If an indicator was judged appropriate and modifications were only minor corrections to wording, it was accepted without resubmission. If the modification was major or if the indicator was judged *uncertain* (median score 4–6 or disagreement among panellists), it was automatically resubmitted for a second round of validation. Indicators judged *inappropriate* (median score 1–3 and agreement among panellists) were rejected.

Figure 17.3
Validation process and results

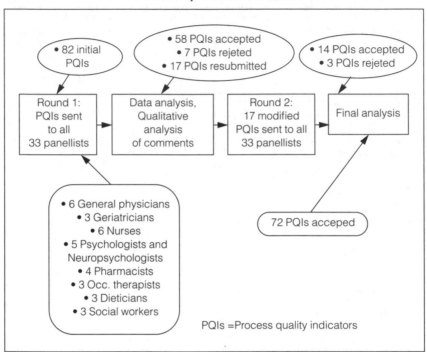

Final acceptance of an indicator after the second round was limited to those judged *appropriate*. However, if, after the second round, an indicator was judged *uncertain* only by physicians and *appropriate* by the other health-care professionals, or vice versa, an additional statistical measure was calculated. This measure was the rate of acceptance, i.e., the number of panellists in agreement with the indicator (score 7 to 9 on the agreement scale) divided by the number of panellists that rated this indicator). If this rate of acceptance was above 80 % in the group having judged the indicator as *uncertain* and the other group had rated it *appropriate*, the indicator was accepted.

Results

All 33 panellists completed the two rounds of validation. Of the initial 82 indicators submitted to the panel, 72 (88 %) were accepted after two rounds of submissions (see Table 17.2). The rejected indicators concerned all care stages, except evaluation. Regarding the PQIs' sources, 92 % from ACOVE, 67 % from the National Health Service, UK, and 20 % from the American Association of Social Workers were accepted. All PQIs from the other sources were accepted. The resulting indicator set covered all the dimensions of the conceptual

Table 17.2
**Results of Process Quality Indicator Validation according to Source,
Quality Dimension, and Care Domain**

Indicator characteristic	Number submitted	Number accepted	(%)
Source of indicator			
ACOVE[32]	62	57	92
AASW[37, 38]	5	1	20
NASW[34]	1	1	100
AOTA[33]	4	4	100
RAND®[36]	3	3	100
Shield and colleagues[35]	2	2	100
Scottish collegiate[39]	1	1	100
NHS[40]	3	2	67
IOM[25]	1	1	100
Quality dimension covered by indicator			
Safety	13	13	100
Effectiveness	33	32	97
Patient-centeredness	17	13	76
Access	4	3	75
Continuity	15	11	73
Care domain to which indicator applies			
Evaluation	31	31	100
Treatment	19	18	95
Follow-up	23	19	83
Consent	2	1	50
Patient satisfaction	3	0	0
Access to care	4	3	75
All indicators	82	72	88

framework. Specifically, 13 indicators related to safety, 33 to effectiveness, 13 to patient-centeredness, 3 to access, and 11 to continuity.

Discussion

In this study, panellists judged the face and content validity of a large majority (88 %) of the translated PQIs appropriate for use in the clinical context of integrated service systems in Quebec, Canada. These validated indicators can be measured using patient files, patient or caregiver interviews, and administrative data from the Quebec Health Insurance Board.

Other studies[4, 22, 23] have validated the transfer of PQIs from one country to another. Notably, Marshall reported on the transfer of RAND®/UCLA quality indicators for primary care from the US to the UK and 56.3 % of the US indicators could be validated for use in the UK[22]. In a study by Morris on the transfer of indicators of preventable drug-related morbidity from the US to the UK, after two Delphi panel rounds, 19 of 57 US indicators could be transferred and 10 out of 16 new indicators were accepted, illustrating differences in clinical perspectives and professional attitudes between the two countries[23]. Steel *et al*[4] studied the transfer of ACOVE indicators from the US to the UK and found that 86 % of PQIs were valid, a result comparable to that of the present study. This may be explained by the careful and thorough development of the ACOVE indicators and a reasonable similarity in the clinical practices of geriatric medicine among the US, the UK, and Canada, as reflected by the high level of agreement for PQIs related to safety and effectiveness.

However, to our knowledge, no other study has validated PQIs for use within an integrated service system. The indicator set reported here covered all dimensions of the comprehensive conceptual framework for quality guiding this research, although coverage for access was somewhat limited, since few PQIs for this dimension could be identified in the literature. Furthermore, to fully explore the dimension of patient- and caregiver-centeredness, satisfaction of patients and caregivers should be assessed as well. To this purpose, the ongoing quality assessment and improvement project intends to use a validated questionnaire from the PRISMA project[43]. Thus, combining PQIs with the assessment of satisfaction will permit a broad, comprehensive evaluation of the quality of integrated service systems for frail older adults in the province of Quebec.

The next step of this project concerns the evaluation of measurement feasibility and reliability of the PQIs, as well as the elaboration of strategies to support indicator implementation and continuous quality improvement. A pilot study involving 60 patients with cognitive impairment or dementia is underway. Furthermore, PQIs are currently being validated for problems of mobility/falls, using the same validation process.

Acknowledgements

This research was supported by the *Réseau Québécois de recherche sur le vieillissement*, a Quebec Health Research Fund (FRSQ) supported research network; the Canadian Institutes of Health Research; the Canadian Health Services Research Foundation; and the PRISMA Research Group. The authors gratefully acknowledge the collaboration of all the panellists. They thank Mr Louis Rochette and Ms Zohra Benounissa for statistical analyses and Dr. Sharon Nancekivell, Guelph, Ontario, Canada, for editorial assistance.

References:

1. Brook RH, McGlynn EA, Shekelle PG. Defining and measuring quality of care: a perspective from US researchers. *Int J Qual Health Care 2000*; 12(4): 281-95.

2. Wennberg JE. Understanding geographic variations in health care delivery. *N Engl J Med* 1999; 340(1): 52-3.

3. Reuben DB, Shekelle PG, Wenger NS. Quality of care for older persons at the dawn of the third millennium. *J Am Geriatr Soc* 2003; 51(7 Suppl): S346-50.

4. Steel N, Melzer D, Shekelle PG, Wenger NS, Forsyth D, McWilliams BC. Developing quality indicators for older adults: transfer from the USA to the UK is feasible. *Qual Saf Health Care* 2004; 13(4): 260-4.

5. Higashi T, Shekelle PG, Adams JL, et al. Quality of care is associated with survival in vulnerable older patients. *Ann Intern Med* 2005; 143(4): 274-81.

6. Johri M, Beland F, Bergman H. International experiments in integrated care for the elderly: a synthesis of the evidence. *Int J Geriatr Psychiatry* 2003; 18(3): 222-35.

7. Tousignant M, Hébert R, Dubuc N, Coulombe C. Public funding of home care services for frail older adults: are the needs being met? In: Hébert R, Tourigny A, Gagnon M, eds. Integrated service delivery to ensure persons' functional autonomy: Edisem; 2005:225-40.

8. Kodner D, Kyriacou K. Fully integrated care for frail elderly: Two American models. *Int J of Integrated Care* 2000;1(November):1-26.

9. Gröne O, Garcia-Barbero M. Integrated care: A position paper of the WHO European office for integrated health care services. *Int J of Integrated Care* 2001; 1(April-June): 1-14.

10. Ouwens M, Wollersheim H, Hermens R, Hulscher M, Grol R. Integrated care programmes for chronically ill patients: a review of systematic reviews. *Int J Qual Health Care* 2005; 17(2): 141-6. Epub 2005 January 21.

11. Tourigny A, Durand P, Bonin L, Hebert R, Rochette L. Quasi-experimental Study of the Effectiveness of an Integrated Service Delivery Network for the Frail Elderly. *Can J Aging* 2004; 23(3): 231-46.

12. Budetti PP, Shortell SM, Waters TM, et al. Physician and health system integration. *Health Aff* (Millwood) 2002; 21(1): 203-10.

13. Hébert R, Durand PJ, Dubuc N, Tourigny A. Frail elderly patients. New model for integrated service delivery. *Can Fam Physician* 2003; 49:992-7.

14. Kodner D, Spreeuwenberg C. Integrated care: meaning, logic, applications and implications - a discussion paper. *Int J of Integrated Care* 2002; 2 (November): 1-9.

15. Tourigny A, Côté L, Kröger E, et al. Framework for the evaluation of the quality of care and services provided to vulnerable elder persons. In: Hébert R, Tourigny A, Gagnon M, eds. Integrated service delivery to ensure persons' functional autonomy. Quebec: Edisem; 2005: 291-309.

16. Morin D, Tourigny A, Pelletier D, et al. Seniors' views on the use of electronic health records. *Inform Prim Care* 2005; 13(2): 125-33.

17. Gagnon M. Satisfaction et autonomisation des personnes âgées face aux soins et services de santé: instruments de mesure et variables associées. Trois-Rivières: Université du Québec à Trois-Rivières; 2004.

18. Mainz J. Developing evidence-based clinical indicators: a state of the art methods primer. *Int J Qual Health Care* 2003; 15 (Suppl 1): i5-11.

19. Wenger NS, Shekelle PG. Assessing care of vulnerable elders: ACOVE project overview. *Ann Intern Med* 2001; 135 (8 Pt 2): 642-6.

20. Wenger NS, Solomon DH, Roth CP, et al. The quality of medical care provided to vulnerable community-dwelling older patients. *Ann Intern Med* 2003; 139(9): 740-7.

21. Shekelle PG, MacLean CH, Morton SC, Wenger NS. Assessing Care of Vulnerable Elders: Methods for Developing Quality Indicators. *Ann Intern Med* 2001; 135 (8 Pt 2): 647-52.

22. Marshall MN, Shekelle PG, McGlynn EA, Campbell S, Brook RH, Roland MO. Can health care quality indicators be transferred between countries? *Qual Saf Health Care* 2003; 12(1): 8-12.

23. Morris CJ, Cantrill JA, Hepler CD, Noyce PR. Preventing drug-related morbidity--determining valid indicators. *Int J Qual Health Care* 2002; 14(3): 183-98.

24. Lohr KN, Donaldson MS, Harris-Wehling J. Medicare: a strategy for quality assurance, V: Quality of care in a changing health care environment. *Qual Rev Bull* 1992; 18(4): 120-6.

25. Hurtado MP, Swift EK, Corrigan JM. Envisioning the National Health Care Quality Report. Washington, D.C.: Institute of Medicine, Board on Health Care Services; 2001.

26. Haggerty JL, Reid RJ, Freeman GK, Starfield BH, Adair CE, McKendry R. Continuity of care: a multidisciplinary review. *BMJ* 2003; 327 (7425): 1219-21.

27. Brook RH, McGlynn EA, Cleary PD. Quality of health care. Part 2: measuring quality of care. *N Engl J Med* 1996; 335 (13): 966-70.

28. Mainz J. Defining and classifying clinical indicators for quality improvement. *Int J Qual Health Care* 2003; 15 (6): 523-30.

29. McGlynn EA, Asch SM, Adams J, et al. The quality of health care delivered to adults in the United States. *N Engl J Med* 2003; 348 (26): 2635-45.

30. Sloss EM, Solomon DH, Shekelle PG, et al. Selecting target conditions for quality of care improvement in vulnerable older adults. *J Am Geriatr Soc* 2000; 48 (4): 363-9.

31. Lindsay J, Sykes E, McDowell I, Verreault R, Laurin D. More than the epidemiology of Alzheimer's disease: contributions of the Canadian Study of Health and Aging. *Can J Psychiatry* 2004; 49 (2): 83-91.

32. Shekelle PG, MacLean CH, Morton SC, Wenger NS. Acove quality indicators. *Ann Intern Med* 2001; 135 (8 Pt 2): 653-67.

33. AOTA. Standards for continuing competence. The American Occupational Therapy Association, Inc. *Am J Occup Ther* 1999; 53 (6): 599-600.

34. NASW Commission on Health and Mental Health. NASW Clinical Indicators for Social Work and Psychosocial Services in the Acute Psychiatric Hospital: NASW; 1990.

35. Shield T, Campbell S, Rogers A, Worrall A, Chew-Graham C, Gask L. Quality indicators for primary care mental health services. *Qual Saf Health Care* 2003; 12 (2): 100-6.

36. RAND. Measuring General Practice - A demonstration project to develop and test a set of primary care clinical quality indicators. Santa Monica: National Primary Care Research and Development Centre; 2003.

37. AASW. Practice Standards for Social Workers: Achieving Outcomes: Australian Association of Social Workers; 2003.

38. AASW. Draft - Outcome Practice Standards for Social Workers – Direct Practice & Service Management. Kingston: Australian Association of Social Workers; 2001 November 12, 2001.

39. Draft National Care Standards Consultation Document – First Tranche. Scottish Executive, 2000. (Accessed 02-27, 2003, at www.researchweb.org.uk/ncsc/ncscontents.html.)

40. NHS Performance Indicators: July 2000. NHS Executive, 2000. (Accessed 04-08, 2002, at http://www.doh.gov.uk/nhsperformanceindicators/hlpi2000/foreword.html.)

41. Hasson F, Keeney S, McKenna H. Research guidelines for the Delphi survey technique. *J Adv Nurs* 2000;32(4):1008-15.

42. Fitch K, Bernstein SJ, Aguilar MD, et al. The RAND/UCLA Appropriateness Method User's Manual: RAND; 2001.

43. Gagnon M, Hébert R, Dubé M, Dubois M. Development of an instrument to measure satisfaction with health care and services and validation in an elderly population: The Health Care Satisfaction Questionnaire (HCSQ). *J of nursing measurement,* 2006; 14 (3): 190-204.

Chapitre 18
The Selection of Essential Variables to Establish the Psychological and Social Needs of Residents and the Social Service Workload in Long-Term Care Hospital Centers

Nathalie Delli-Colli, Nicole Dubuc, Réjean Hébert, Catherine Lestage

Abstract

This study reports the results of a Delphi-type consultation of experts conducted in Quebec in 2006. Sixty experts—including social –work practitioners, managers, and researchers interested in the psychological and social needs of the frail elderly and the workload of social workers in long-term care hospital centers—completed two postal questionnaires. The study resulted in the selection of 105 variables considered to be essential for creating a portrait of the needs of residents and for establishing the social service workload in the hospitals that care for them over an extended period.

The context

As a group, the frail elderly are very heterogeneous with different levels and types of disabilities resulting from various chronic illnesses and comorbidities. While institutions and the community offer a range of care and services to respond to their varied needs, seniors generally prefer to receive services in their homes. But despite their desire to remain at home, home care is no longer an option for some and the need to move to a facility for the elderly arises. Usually this alternative is considered because the elderly person has experienced a significant loss of independence, their safety is threatened, their family and social network are limited, or their home is inadequate for the care and services they require.

In Quebec, institutional facilities such as long-term care hospital centers (CHSLD) are important resources: 71 % of funding for long-term care are devoted to them. Yet, in recent decades, the profile of their residents has changed considerably. Some 25 years ago, the CHSLDs provided hotel-type services for seniors. Now they accommodate residents with major physical disabilities, complex health problems, and significant cognitive deficits. In addition to these changes, the implementation of new policy measures has greatly modified the nature of the work they do. These include the creation of an accreditation organization, visits to assess the quality of life in long-term care environments and the establishment of a "living environment" approach.

The Ministère de la Santé et des Services Sociaux's 2005-2010 action plan for seniors who have lost autonomy advocates living environments conforming to high quality standards[2]. These standards must take into account the multiple and complex needs of seniors, be founded on evidenced-based practices, and be fulfilled with effective and efficient interventions.[2] To achieve all this, several professionals must be consulted and well-known evaluation tools must be used. Among these professionals, CHSLD social workers are important actors in assessing and implementing interventions aimed at best meeting psychosocial needs.

The Multiclientele Assessment Tool (outil d'évaluation multiclientèle or OEMC) has been used in Quebec since November 2001 to assess the needs of the frail elderly.[5] Its core component is the Système de mesure de l'autonomie fonctionnelle (functional autonomy measurement system or SMAF), the only standardized tool used in the OEMC[5]. A classification system called Iso-SMAF profiles was developed from the 29 items of the SMAF. The system represents the needs of the frail elderly and is a good predictor of nursing resources (80 %)[6]. Nevertheless, functional autonomy and medical diagnoses are inadequate as indicators for determining resource requirements in social services, which requires taking into account other variables such as psychosocial considerations[7, 8]. It is well-known that the Multiclientele Assessment Tool does gather some information about psychosocial needs, but this information is not standardized by precise indicators. Such indicators are needed to support clinical processes as well as to improve human resources and financial management in social services. Currently, the number of social workers required in CHSLDs is determined by an arbitrary formula based solely on the number of beds. Resident characteristics and CHSLD physical and organizational aspects are not taken into account, despite their considerable impact on the delivery of social services[9].

Objectives

The main objective of this study is to identify the variables related to resident and environment characteristics that are essential to assessing psychological and social needs and that could influence the social service workload in long-term care hospital centers.

The results will be used in a later study aimed at developing a model for predicting social service resource requirements according to resident needs and to the physical and organizational environments in long-term care centers.

Theoretical framework

The features of a model for predicting social services resource requirements in long-term care hospital centers have been studied using the Quality Health Outcomes Model (QHOM)[10, 11]. This general model for measuring the use and quality of services is based on Donabedian's traditional linear "structure-process-outcome" framework. While developed by researchers in nursing, the QHOM has also been studied in other disciplines. The premise is that specific interventions result from relations among interventions, patient characteristics, health care system characteristics, and patient outcomes. The QHOM takes into account professional practices and the full set of elements needed to develop a complete system. Moreover, it takes into account factors that resist measurement, such as psychosocial ones.

The review of the literature focuses on management systems and predictive models used in social services past and present, in Quebec and elsewhere. The following summarizes the systems according to the QHOM framework's four dimensions: resident characteristics, the environment, social-service activities, and the outcomes of those activities.

Literature review

A review of the scientific literature about social services shows that there has not always been a consensus about the use of management systems. On one hand, authors in favor of such systems argue that the practice gives added value because it provides for standardized data, quality assessment, and adequate financing[7, 8]. On the other hand, updating management systems has met with skepticism from some authors because of the complexity of factors to measure (e.g. multiple psychosocial problems) and because of resistance by workers to these systems. Nonetheless, five social service management systems have been developed in the last twenty-five years: 1) The Berkman-Rehr classification of psychosocial problems and outcomes,[12, 13] 2) the classification by types in long-term care and service environments (CTMSP 87), assessment of services and social service resources required by beneficiaries,[14] 3) the Person-in-Environment Classification System,[15, 16, 17] 4) the Australian National Classification System for Social Work Practice in Health Care (ANCS),[7, 18, 19] and 5) the Workload Analysis Scale (WAS)[20].

Resident Characteristics

An important component of a management system is its ability to determine user needs, which means being able to identify and measure resident character-istics—such as psychosocial needs—that require social-service interventions. The management systems listed above deal with a wide variety of populations, but currently none has addressed specifically the psychosocial needs of people with impaired independence living in placement settings. The WAS system is used to study the particular needs of people in rehabilitation or undergoing assessment, while the others—the Berkman-Rehr, and the ANCS—have attempted to grasp the psychosocial needs of hospitalized patients in intensive care. Overall then, a broad variety of variables could be measured. In the case of the Person-in-Environment system, only social roles are considered as charac-teristics, while the ANCS attempts to measure several dimensions of the indi-vidual, including physical, nutritional and social needs. Only the WAS considers functional independence, since it is an essential element in geriatric assessment.

Environment Characteristics

The above systems give very little consideration to environmental factors even though, according to Chernesky and Grube (1999), these have a significant impact on workload[21]. Only the WAS is interested in an environmental aspect, specifically staff characteristics, such as the number of years of experience and perceived occupational stress.

Social-Service Activities

A social-service department needs a list of activities carried out by social work-ers to estimate resource requirements. The CTMSP alone estimates the services required upon CHSLD admission of frail individuals; it does not, however, include all the professional activities actually performed. Moreover, the time required is estimated by the worker and reports vary greatly. The WAS and ANCS use a list of 10 to 16 activities. Only the WAS has demonstrated a rela-tionship between patient psychosocial needs and the resources required for social services. Nevertheless, the system's time estimates are based on statistics compiled by the workers in their normal activities. Among the methods for esti-mating time related to professional activities, it would appear that continuous time and motion studies would provide the most reliable and valid data[22, 23, 24].

Outcome Indicators

Once the characteristics of the resident and environment have been examined and the resources required estimated, can the outcomes of the services provided be established? As things now stand, only the ANCS has broached the measure-ment of certain performance indicators such as accessibility, relevance, and effectiveness. ANCS authors have stated, however, that the measurement method should be reviewed. Moreover, the authors did not publish their results.

System Reliability and Validity

Reliability and validity are major considerations in the development and use of management systems, yet few researchers have considered the importance of validating each stage of a system's development. Only the Berkman-Rehr and WAS researchers have verified their systems' interjudge reliability, which they report as good and high, respectively. They have also ensured that their systems actually measured the concept under study. In fact, the Berkman-Rehr researchers actually studied the system's construct validity, while WAS researchers measured its predictive validity.

In conclusion, even though there is little information about how these systems are used, it appears that the Berkman-Rehr, ANCS, and WAS systems were developed in response to the underfunding of professional services in the health-care system, mainly in order to demonstrate the importance of social services. Nevertheless, the systems offer little support to daily practice. In some Quebec acute-care hospitals affiliated with McGill University, the Person-in-Environment Classification System is used for clinical purposes to standardize assessment of patient functioning. Currently, none of the systems deals with all the psychological and social needs of residents in long-term care or the impact of these needs on social-work practice. Moreover, none attempts to reconcile clinical needs with those of management.

Methodology

We used a Delphi-type expert consultation, modified to include the RAND/UCLA method to select essential variables. The method combines evidence from the literature with expert opinion. Initially, a review of the literature allowed us to identify two lists of variables. The first included variables useful for the assessment of psychosocial needs of seniors living in long-term care. The second contained physical and organizational environmental factors that could potentially influence the social services workload. We then proceeded with two rounds of Delphi-type consultations using a postal questionnaire sent to social workers, managers, and researchers known for their expertise on the subject of the frail elderly and CHSLDs.

The Delphi Method

The Delphi method uses postal questionnaires to structure a communication process and gather expert opinion. Our experts were practitioners, managers, professors, and researchers with an interest in social work. They are knowledgeable about the research topic (practice of social work), but this opinion is not necessarily informed by their area of specialization (the development of management systems). Moreover, our informants are relatively impartial regarding expected results[25]. The main characteristics of the Delphi method are anonymity among the participants, statistical synthesis of the responses, regular feedback and reduced group pressure towards uniformity[26]. Basing its consultations on mail questionnaires, the method also has an economic advantage, because it avoids the expense and challenges of bringing together experts from various regions to a discussion group[26]. The Delphi method is used in several areas of health care to develop items and standards related to training, skills assessment, and research priorities as well as to design, plan, and evaluate programs[26, 27].

In order to identify the key variables in geriatric assessment, a 1998 study by Saltz and collaborators used the Delphi method to document social, environmental, and economic factors to consider in assessing the needs of elderly patients[28]. The Delphi method was also used in nursing to study workload management[29, 30]. The traditional Delphi method usually includes nine steps, although the procedure and content of the steps can vary from one study to the next[29].There is therefore no single way to carry out a study using the Delphi method[29, 30]. With the Rand method, since a literature review is done beforehand, two to three rounds of consultations are usually enough, depending on the subject under study.[31]

Procedure

Phase 1: Preparation of the postal survey

For the questionnaire, we drew up a list of variables related to psychosocial needs and workload following a review of the literature. Several sources of information were consulted to compile this list of variables: databases (CINAHL, social service, social work abstracts), existing management systems, and documentation from professional associations (e.g. the *Ordre professionnel des travailleurs sociaux du Québec*, the Canadian Association of Social Workers, the National Association of Social Workers (US), and the Australian Association of Social Workers). Variables known to be useful in the assessment of psychosocial needs or for their potential to influence the social service workload were selected. As for patient characteristics, in particular, their psychosocial needs, 111 variables were identified and included in the first part of the questionnaire. The second list in the first questionnaire included 66 environmental variables associated with the social service workload. For clarity, the terms used for the variables were accompanied by a short definition from the scientific and professional literature or a dictionary, or were created by the research team[26]. Open questions were included in both lists so that experts could add variables not on our list. As recommended by the RAND/UCLA method,[32] a Lickert scale from 1 to 9 was used to group responses into categories. This method facilitates analysis and the grasp of the sometimes subtle differences between experts' opinions. It also allowed us to observe changes of opinion during the course of the consultation[29, 30]. The questionnaire was previously tested using eight experts with characteristics similar to those of the participants we recruited[27, 29, 30].

Example 1 (question on psychosocial needs)

To what degree is this factor essential to drawing a portrait of a patient's psychosocial needs?

VULNERABILITY

Not essential   Absolutely essential

| 1 | 2 | 3 | 4 | 5 | 6 | 7 | 8 | 9 |

Vulnerability: Someone who is vulnerable is someone who is easily hurt or who has weak defenses. Examples of elements of vulnerability include advanced age, exploitation, bereavement or loss, poverty, abuse, and isolation. (OEMC and *Rapport sur l'exploitation des personnes âgées,* October 2001)

NOT ESSENTIAL: the factor is useful. It contributes quality, but it isn't necessary or indispensable in creating a portrait of the patient's psychosocial needs.

ABSOLUTELY ESSENTIAL: the factor is of the utmost importance and is indispensable in creating a portrait of the patient's psychosocial needs.

Example 2 (question on workload)

To what degree do you believe this factor influences your workload, either positively or negatively?

BALANCE BETWEEN CLINICAL ACTIVITIES AND OTHER TASKS

Does not   Greatly
influence   influences

| 1 | 2 | 3 | 4 | 5 | 6 | 7 | 8 | 9 |

BALANCE: Time devoted to tasks directly related to casework as opposed to administrative, teaching, research, or other tasks. (Research team)

Phase 2: Recruitment of experts

There is no consensus regarding the type of experts that should be invited to participate in a Delphi study. In this one, which targeted identifying clinical variables, the experts recruited were social-work practitioners, managers, and researchers. All were given the same questions. They were chosen for their expertise with the target population and their credibility in the subject area[25].

The experts were recruited from different regions of Quebec. In order to ensure wide representation of different fields, particular attention was paid to finding experts from rural, urban and suburban areas working in small, medium and large establishments[25]. The target was 60 experts (n = 60).

There is no single way to recruit using the Delphi method[29, 30]. Since we don't know the whole expert population, the sample was chosen out of convenience and the experts were recruited according to the above criteria[29, 30]. The principal investigator used several recruitment strategies: advertising at provincial conferences on care for the very frail elderly and e-mails sent by the *Ordre professionnel des travailleurs sociaux* to 70 % of its 6000 members. We also contacted key informants working in health and social services agencies, health and social services centers and social-work schools and departments in Quebec universities. These key informants identified experts who met our criteria in their organizations and in other establishments in their areas. By recruiting in a variety of ways, we were able to create a list of experts interested in participating in the project. We sent an explanatory document by fax or by email with information on the research objectives, the expected task, the estimated time needed to complete the consultation and our intended use of the results. If the experts were still interested after reading this document, they were sent the first questionnaire.

Phase 3: Sending the first questionnaire

The 60 experts received the questionnaire along with the following documents: 1) a letter reminding them of the project's goal and instructions for completing the questionnaire; 2) two consent forms (one to return and one to keep); 3) a short questionnaire to gather socio-demographic information; and 4) a pre-addressed, pre-paid return envelope. The experts were given three weeks to respond and return the documents. A reminder was sent at the end of the second and the third weeks. For the experts who had not returned their questionnaire within the prescribed time, we followed up with a request that they either estimate how much additional time they needed to complete the questionnaire or explain their reasons for withdrawing from the study.

Phase 4: Analysis of the results of the first questionnaire

As illustrated in Table 18.1, we used two methods to decide whether a variable would be retained and whether there was agreement: the median and the spread of responses.

FIRST PROCEDURE: A median of 7 is generally used to decide on the relevance or the degree to which a given variable is essential[32]. Nonetheless, this criterion is less appropriate for single-discipline panels of experts, since they tend to assign high value to certain variables[33]. A stricter criterion, such as a median of 8, is therefore recommended. The results analysis for each element was interpreted as follows: if the median score was higher than or equal to 8, the variable was retained. If the median ranged from 4 to 7, the variable was subject to discussion. Lastly, if the median was less than or equal to 3, it was rejected.

<u>SECOND PROCEDURE:</u> The formula proposed in the RAND/UCLA appropriateness method document was used to measure the level of agreement among the experts[32]. The scattering of expert responses must be taken into consideration in order to conclude that the experts agreed that a variable was essential. Initially, the Rand method was used with small panels (maximum of 15 people), which makes it easy to verify the data polarity visually. For example, we would conclude there was significant disagreement (using a strict definition of agreement) if one expert in a 9-member panel ranked an item 1 and another member ranked it 9.

Table 18.1
Data analysis using the RAND/UCLA method

Median	IPR[1] < IPRAS[2]	IPR > IPRAS
≤ 3	Agree	Disagree
	NOT ESSENTIAL	NOT ESSENTIAL
>3 and 7	Agree	Disagree
	UNCERTAIN	UNCERTAIN
≥8	Agree	Disagree
	ESSENTIAL	ESSENTIAL

[1] IPR: Interpercentile Range
[2] IPRAS Interpercentile Range Adjusted for Symmetry

In cases with a large group of experts, the interpercentile range (IPR) cannot incontrovertibly prove agreement among the participants. Another measure has therefore been developed to detect agreement on panels with subgroups located opposite ends of the scale. The asymmetry index (the distance between the IPR central point and the scale's central point, which is 5 in this case) is calculated and included in the IPRAS formula. Agreement is evidenced by the IPR being smaller than the IPRAS, as illustrated in Table 18.1. Figure 18.1 shows that, when expert opinions aggregate at the extremities of the scale, the boundaries of the observation area must be shifted to take into account the asymmetry in order to bring agreement, if present. Table 18.2 shows the elements to consider relative to the data in Figure 18.1 when calculating the IPR and the IPRAS.

Finally, the research team analyzed the content of the experts' written comments.

Figure 18.1
Example of data asymmetry when determining agreement

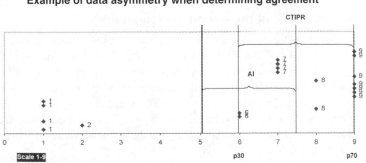

Table 18.2
Elements to consider in calculating the IPR and IPRAS

Element	Value
p30 (30th percentile)	6
p50 (50th percentile)	7
p70 (70th percentile)	9
IPR: p70-p30	3
CTIPR: Central point of IPR: p70+p30 / 2	7.5
AI: Asymmetry index: distance between 5 and the central point of IPR	2.5
IPRAS: 2,35 + (AI x 1.5 fixed correlation factor)	6.1
IPR < IPRAS = agreement	Yes

Phase 5: Sending the second questionnaire

The second questionnaire includes the items that were categorized as "uncertain" (median between >3 and ≤ 7) and those that were selected by the experts. It was decided to modify the questions because of the large number of elements selected in the first round of consultation, the significant number of elements deemed uncertain, and the high level of consensus. We therefore a firmer stand with the experts to foster specificity of the data[25]. Instead of asking the experts to rank the uncertain elements in order of importance, we asked them to answer whether a given element should be added to the list of variables already selected. In this second mailing, the experts received the results of the first round of consultation and their feedback about the group's opinion was requested[26]. A letter explaining the objectives of the second round of the consultation was also sent out. Consequently, the experts had to think about how to make the measurement of these variables operational, or in other words, how they might be measured in a clinical environment. The 8 new variables formulated by the experts in Phase One were submitted with a definition and a Lickert-type scale from 1 to 9 as in the first questionnaire. The participants had 2 weeks to complete the questionnaire. They received reminders; arrangements were made (e.g. extensions given due to illness) to accommodate the largest possible number of experts.

Phase 6: Analysis of the second questionnaire

Our analysis of the responses to the yes/no questions used a threshold of 80 %,[25] retaining only those variables for which 80 % of the experts had judged their addition to be absolutely essential. The proposed variables that obtained a median superior or equal to 8 and that demonstrated a satisfactory level of agreement among the experts were kept. The variables that did not meet these two criteria were rejected. By the end of this phase, we had established a list of variables essential for the assessment of psychosocial needs and identified a list of variables influencing workload.

Phase 7: Sending the final list of selected variables to all the experts

We mailed the list of selected variables to the experts who participated in the various steps of the Delphi process[26].

Results

Selection of experts

After the study was announced, more than 100 people showed interest in participating. After we distributed the explanatory document, 60 experts indicated their interest in taking part in the study and met the criteria for inclusion. The experts had the following characteristics: 71 % were clinical specialists working in social services, 10 % were managers, and 4 % were researchers. The rest (15 %) were clinicians or managers who had recently retired. The average participant was 44 years old (with a spread of 11.8 years) and the average time spent working with seniors was 11.6 years (with a spread of 8.4 years). The experts came from 14 of Quebec's 18 administrative regions.

Round 1

Of the 60 questionnaires distributed in round 1, 53 were returned and analyzed, for a response rate of 88 %. With the median serving to determine the essential character of an element and the scattering of responses to determine the level of agreement between experts, we considered the median number and the spread of responses, 100 out of the 177 variables were retained (56 %). Sixty-seven of the 111 psychological and social variables were retained (about 60 %). The greatest number of elements retained came from the category dealing with perceptions of users, principal caregivers, and family members. Forty-nine percent of variables linked to the physical and organizational environment were retained (32 out of 65). The largest number of variables retained related to organizational environment in the health and social service centers and social-service departments. A single element was deemed non-essential. The experts disagreed on only once on the 177 elements, which related to the human environment category. A content analysis of experts' comments enabled us to formulate 8 new variables for the second round (see Table 18.3).

Round 2 (Table 18.4)

Fifty out of the 53 questionnaires distributed were received and included in the analysis, for a participation rate of 94 %. By making experts aware of the feasibility of measuring these variables in the context of current social-service practice, and by establishing a threshold of 80 % of experts in agreement to retain variables, only 4 variables were added to the existing list generated during the first round. Out of the 8 new variables proposed by the panel of experts after round 1, only 1 met the requirement of a median equal to or greater than 8, and sufficient agreement among experts according to IPR and IPRAS results.

Table 18.3
Results of Round 1

	Initially submitted	Retained	Not retained	Uncertain	New	
Is essential to establish a portrait of psychological and social needs	111	67 (60%)	0 (0%)	44 (40%)	3	Round 1
Influences the workload	66	33 (50%)	1 (2%)	32 (48%)	5	
	177	100 (56%)	1 (1%)	76 (43%)	8	

Table 18.4
Results of Round 2

	Submitted (n = 84)	Retained	Rejected	
Is essential to establish a portrait of psychological and social needs	47	5	42	Round 2
Influences the workload	37	0	37	
	84	5 (6%)	79 (94%)	

After two rounds, 105 variables (57 %) constituted the final list, as illustrated in Table 18.5. Eighty variables (43 %) were rejected because they were considered "uncertain" in round 1 and "not essential" in round 2. The detailed lists of variables for the 2 categories (psychological and social needs, and physical and organizational environment) are presented in Appendices 18.1 and 18.2.

Table 18.5
Final results after Rounds 1 and 2

	Submitted + new	Retained	Rejected	
Is essential to establish a portrait of psychological and social needs	114	72 (63%)	42 (37%)	Final Results
Influences the workload	71	33 (46%)	38 (54%)	
	185	105 (57%)	80 (43%)	

Discussion

Using the Rand-type modification of the Delphi method made it possible to select variables linked to the characteristics of residents and the environment that are essential for assessing psychological and social needs and that can influence the social services workload in long-term care hospital centers. The high number of experts, their origins, and the various strategies used to recruit them for our study assures sound representation of social-work stakeholders in placement centers and long-term care facilities[29]. Other professionals in psychological and social services, the elderly, and the people around them could have been consulted in the part of the study dealing with the psychological and social needs of the aged. Since one of our aims was to develop a tool that could predict the resources required in social services and management, we thought it better to rely on experts with knowledge in the field.

Use of the Quality Health Outcome Model as a conceptual framework in this case allowed optimal coverage of the variables linked to characteristics of patients and the environment[10, 11]. We must also emphasize that the experts suggested only eight variables be added to those already presented. Finally, the results of this study are similar to those of other studies with regard to the behavior of the experts. It is generally recognized that panels composed of experts form the same profession tend to consider many more variables as essential and to reach a high level of consensus[33]. In this regard, it must be noted that only one element was considered "not essential," that a disagreement among the experts was observed, and that only two rounds of consultation were needed.

In all, the experts retained 105 variables, constituting 57 % of those submitted. These variables have been measured or discussed as pertinent in other environments, with other patient populations or in different areas of care. The purpose of this exercise was to select the most essential psychological and social needs of residents, and the physical and organizational environment in Quebec's placement centers and long-term care facilities.

Regarding psychosocial needs, the experts selected essential variables relating to different aspects of the person, reflecting that it is a multidimensional concept. Experts assigned weight to the resident motivation and adaptability, resident state of health, psychological and social situations, and the situation faced by those who help them. They expressed that these dimensions are essential to developing a portrait of the resident's needs and can influence the way that treatment plans are designed. Certain variables linked to a patient's state of health that were selected by the experts in our study are similar to those found in the ANCS and the WAS, such as the diagnosis on admission and the number of former hospitalizations[7, 8, 19, 20]. As in the WAS, functional independence was important to our experts, particularly in the areas of communication and cognitive functions, because these two dimensions impact directly on how social workers intervene.

Other dimensions of functional independence—such as activities of daily living, activities of domestic life, and mobility—obtained a median of seven, so they were not retained. This choice by our experts perhaps reflects that either they dealt rarely with these issues or that the great majority of residents of long-term care hospital centers suffer from a serious lack of independence in daily and domestic life, so that precise information in these areas is less pertinent.

Finally, the experts concluded, as did the WAS study, that family support is essential as far as psychological and social variables are concerned. This also holds true for the capacity for motivation, self-criticism, adaptation, and the resolution of residents' problems[20].

No other system has taken into account variables linked to the physical and organizational environment. Only WAS measured the influence of variables such as age and years of experience on the workload of professionals[20]. In our study, the experts believed that an establishment's work environment and the organization of work in the social-services department should be examined for their influence on the workload of social workers in placement facilities.

Future impacts

As stated above, this study fits into a much wider research proposal to develop a model for predicting social-service resources requirements according to resident needs and the particular physical and organizational environments in placement centers and long-term treatment facilities.

Further work is required to determine which variables can be used effectively within this model. Some studies are underway to identify the tools that would allow us to measure the variables in a clinical context. Accordingly, one or several questions have been compiled emerging from a measuring instrument validated in French for each variable or group of variables associated with a common concept. We have paid particular attention both to those tools already used within the health-care network and those developed and validated in Quebec. So far, we have established that 83 % of the variables selected could be measured with existing tools. The definitive choice of tools that are appropriate within the Quebec context will be made by a focus group. Afterwards, preliminary testing will be undertaken to estimate the time required, access, possible data sources, and the feasibility of acquiring data from this set of tools. This will allow us to prepare a broader study in different long-term care hospital centers across the province that will simultaneously combine measurement of patient characteristics and their physical and organizational environment, and time and motion studies among the social workers in these institutions.Moreover, the prediction model that emerges will be the core of a clinical and administrative management system that will support decision-making that will more effectively organize psychological and social resources so as to better meet the needs of residents. Lastly , it will enhance professional practice and communication through the use of standardized tools.

Acknowledgements

We would like to thank all the panelists who participated in the Delphi process. Nathalie Delli-Colli holds a master training award from the Fonds de la Recherche en Santé du Québec (FRSQ) and the programme-

réseau de Formation interdisciplinaire en recherche Santé et Vieillissement (FORMSAV)

References

1. Dubuc, N., Hébert, R., Desrosiers, J., Buteau, M., and Trottier, L. (2006). Disability-based classification system for older people in integrated long-term care services: the Iso-SMAF profiles. Archives of Gerontology & Geriatrics. 42(2); 191-206.

2. Ministère de la santé et des services sociaux. "Les services aux aînés en perte d'autonomie: Un défi de solidarité." Plan d'action 2005-2010, Gouvernement du Québec, Québec, 2005.

3. Ministère de la santé et des services sociaux. "Un milieu de vie de qualité pour les personnes hébergées en CHSLD." Orientations ministérielles, gouvernement du Québec, 2003.

4. Association des CLSC et des CHSLD du Québec. "Une vision pour les ressources publiques d'hébergement et de soins de longue durée." Association des CLSC et des CHSLD du Québec, Montréal, 2004.

5. Kaufman, T., Asselin, F., Boyer, M.L., Corriveau, A., Couture, J., Flynn, L., Girard, S., Mercier,L., Normandeau, L. and Quintal, J. "Comité aviseur sur l'adoption d'un outil d'évaluation Intégré des besoins des personnes en perte d'autonomie et de détermination des services requis notamment en institution ou à domicile," Ministère de la santé et des services sociaux du Québec, Québec, 2000.

6. Dubuc, N., Hébert, R., Desrosiers, J., Buteau, M., and Trottier, L. *Système de classification basé sur le profil d'autonomie fonctionnelle*. In Hébert R and Kouri K. *Autonomie et vieillissement*, Institut universitaire de gériatrie de Sherbrooke, Edisem, St-Hyacinthe, 1999.

7. Cleak H. (2002). A model of social work classification in health care. Australian Social Work, 55 (1); 38-49.

8. Pockett R., Lord B., & Dennis J. (2001). The Development of an Australian National Classification System for Social Work Practice in Health Care. Social Work Health and Mental Health, 34 (1-2); 177-193.

9. McGuire, J., Bikson, K., and Blue-Howells, J. (2005). How many social workers are needed in primary care? A patient-based needs assessment example. Health and Social Work, 30(4); 305-313.

10. Mitchell P., Ferketich S., and Jennings B. (1998). Quality Health Outcomes Model. Journal of Nursing Scholarship, 30 (1); 43-46.

11. Mitchell P. and Lang N. (2004). Framing the Problem of Measuring and Improving Healthcare Quality: Has the Quality Health Outcomes Model been Useful? Medical Care, 42 (2); 4-11.

12. Berkman B. (1980). Psychosocial Problems and Outcome: An External Validity Study. Health and Social Work, 5 (3); 5-21.

13. Berkman B. and Rehr H. (1972). Social needs of the hospitalized elderly: a classification. Social Work, 17; 80-88.

14. Tilquin, C. and Coupal, M. (1987). *C.T.M.S.P. 87.* "La détermination des services requis et la mesure des ressources requises par le bénéficiaire, extrait des services sociaux." Ministère de la santé et des services sociaux, Québec, 127-207.

15. Karls J., Lowery C., Mattaini M., and Wandrei K. E. (1997). The use of the PIE (Person-In-Environment) System in Social Work Education. Journal of Social Work Education, 33 (1); 49-58.

16. Karls, J.M. and Wandrei, K.E. (1992). PIE: a new language for social work. Social Work, 37(1); 80-85.

17. Ordre professionnel des travailleurs sociaux. (1996). Système de classification du fonctionnement de la personne dans son environnement. Manuel du système CFPE.

18. Pockett R., Lord B., and Dennis J. (2001). The Development of an Australian National Classification System for Social Work Practice in Health Care. Social Work Health and Mental Health, 34 (1-2);177-193.

19 . National Allied Health Casemix Committee. (2001). An Australian standard describing the range of activities provided by health professionals. Health Activity Hierarchy, version 1.1, 1-11. www.dlsweb.rmit.edu.au/bus/nahcc/.

20. Gathercole, M.F. and De Mello. L.R. (2001) Development of the workload analysis scale (WAS) for the assessment and rehabilitation services of Ballarat health services. Social Work Health and Mental Health. 34(1/2); 143-160.

21. Chernesky, R.H.&Grube B. (1999) HIV/AIDS case management: views from the frontline. The Care Management Journals. 1(1); 19-28.

22. Fein, E. and Saff.E. (1991). Measuring the use of time. Administration in Social Work. 15(4); 81-93.

23. McHugh, M.L. and Dwyer, V.L. (1992). Measurement issues in patient acuity classification for prediction of hours in nursing care. Nursing Administration Quarterly, 16 (4); 20-31.

24. Niebal, B.W. and Frievalds, A. (2003). *Methods, Standards, and Work Design.* Eleventh Edition. Mc Graw Hill. New-York.

25. Powell, C. (2003). The Delphi technique: myths and realities. Journal of advanced nursing, 41(4); 376-382.

26. Mayer, R. and Ouellet, F. (1991). *Méthodologie de recherche pour les intervenants sociaux*. Gaétan Morin ed., ltée. Boucherville, Québec, Canada.

27. Burnette, D., Morrow-Howell, N., and Chen, L-M. (2003). Setting priorities for gerontological social work research: a national delphi study. The Gerontologist. 43(6); 828-838.

28. Saltz, C., Shaefer, T., and Weinreich,D. (1998). Streamlining outpatient geriatric assessment: essential social, environmental and economic variables. Social Work in Health Care, 27(1);1-14.

29. Mead, D. and Moseley, L. (2001). Considerations in using the Delphi approach: design, questions and answers. Nurse Research, 8(4); 24-37.

30. Mead, D. and Moseley, L. (2001). The use of the Delphi as a research approach. Nurse Research, 8(4); 4-23.

31. Washington, D.L, Bernstein, S.T., Kahan, J.P., Leape, L.L., Kamberg, C.J., and Shekelle, P.G. (2003). Reliability of clinical guideline development using mail-only versus in-person expert panels. Medical Care, 41(12); 1374-1381.

32. Brook, R.H. (1994). *The RAND/UCLA Appropriateness Method*. In Mc Cormick, K.A. Moore, S.R., and Siegal, R.A., eds. *Methodology perspectives*. Rockville, MD. Public Health Service, US. Department of Health and Human Services, AHCPR Pub. No. (95-009); 59-70.

33. Coulter, I., Adams, A., and Shekelle, P.(1995) Impact of varying panel membership on ratings of appropriateness in consensus panels: a comparison of a multi- and single disciplinary panel.; Health services research, 30;577-591.

Appendix

Appendix 18.1
List of Variables – Psychosocial Needs

	First Round: Median[1]	First Round: IPR < IPRAS = agreement	Second Round: Retained variable = agreement ≥ 80%[3]
Category 1: Health status			
Current diagnosis and upon admission	9	1< 7.60	
Emotion state	9	1< 7.60	
Level of psychological distress	9	0< 8.35	
Personal and family health history	9	1< 6.85	
Stage of illness	8	1< 7.60	
Prognosis for recovery	8	1< 6.10	
Personal and family mental-health history	8	1< 7.60	
Personality traits	8	1< 7.60	
Modification of state	8	1< 7.60	
Patient's mental capacity	7	1< 6.10	80.4
Stability of state	7	1< 6.10	56.5
Management of symptoms	7	1< 6.10	54.3
Recent and past hospitalizations	7	1< 4.60	56.5
Comorbidity	7	1< 6.10	43.5
Presence of specific care	7	2< 5.35	52.2
Professional health-care services required	7	1< 6.10	73.9
Medication	6	2.81<2.96	43.5
Category 2: Lifestyle			
Personal and leisure activities	8	1< 6.10	
Sleep	7	1< 4.60	52.2
Alcohol use	7	2< 5.35	78.3
Drug use	7	2< 5.35	67.4
Tobacco use	6	1.81< 2.49	60.9
Nutrition	6	2.81< 3.24	45.7
Category 3: Functional autonomy			
Mental functions	9	1< 7.60	
Communication	8	1< 7.60	
Activities of daily living (ADL)	7	1< 6.10	
Mobility	7	1< 6.10	
Instrumental activities of daily living (IADL)	7	2< 3.85	
Category 4: Psychosocial situation			
History of social problems	9	1< 7.60	
History of legal problems (victim)	9	1< 7.60	
Vulnerability	9	0.8< 7.74	
Protection of property	9	0< 8.35	
Protection of the individual	9	0< 8.35	
Age	8	1< 5.35	
Need for an interpreter	8	1< 7.60	
Past life situation	8	2< 6.85	
Change in living environment required	8	1< 7.60	

	First Round: Median[1]	First Round: IPR < IPRAS = agreement	Second Round: Retained variable = agreement ≥ 80%[3]
Category 4: Psychosocial situation			
Social hardship	8	1.81< 6.71	
istory of legal problems (offender)	8	1< 7.60	
Relationship between the social problem and the past	8	1< 7.60	
Civil status	7.5	1.81< 5.49	89.1
Occupation	7	2< 5.35	84.8
Ethnic group	7	1< 6.10	80.4
Level of integration, if immigrant	7	1< 6.10	50.0
Type of residence before admission	7	1< 6.10	67.4
Level of education	6	1<4.60	60.0
Category 5: Patient's family situation			
Family dynamics	9	1< 7.60	
Marital dynamics	9	1< 7.60	
Social resources	8.5	1< 7.60	
Satisfaction with family network	8	1< 7.60	
Composition of family network	8	1< 7.60	
Problems experienced by the family with respect to patient orientation	8	1< 7.60	
Significant events in family's collective history	8	1< 7.60	
Frequency of visits by family members	7.5	1< 6.10	67.4
Perception of having a family network (scope)	7.5	1< 6.10	58.7
Frequency of family interactions, from a distance	7	1< 6.10	43.5
Category 6: Main caregiver			
Presence of significant other	9	0< 8.35	
Number of caregivers	8	1< 6.10	
Availability of caregivers	8	1< 7.60	
Caregiver's personal coping strategies	8	1< 6.10	
Caregiver's state of health	8	1< 6.10	
Caregiver-helpee-family relationship	8	1< 7.60	
Caregiver's stress level	8	2< 6.85	
Description of assistance provided	8	1< 6.10	
Caregiver's perception of role	8	1< 6.10	
Caregiver's satisfaction with living environment	8	1< 6.10	
Relationship between caregiver and staff	8	1.81< 6.71	
Caregiver's satisfaction with relationship with patient	8	1< 6.10	
Relationship between caregiver and promoters of formal services	8	1.81< 6.71	
Portrait of main caregiver	7.5	1< 6.10	41.3
Need for support and services from the formal network to fulfill caregiver role	7	1< 6.10	65.2
onciliation of roles	7	1< 6.10	50.0
Financial costs	6	1< 4.60	30.4

	First Round: Median[1]	First Round: IPR < IPRAS = agreement	Second Round: Retained variable = agreement ≥ 80%[3]
Category 7: Patient's social network			
Proximity of relationships	8	1< 6.10	
Patient's ability to maintain a relationship	8	0< 6.85	
Patient's satisfaction with social network during interactions	7	1< 6.10	63.0
Perception of having a social network (scope)	7	1< 5.35	30.4
Composition of social network	7.5	1< 6.10	65.2
Number of visits from members of social network	7	1< 4.60	39.1
Frequency of social interactions, from a distance	6	1< 4.60	23.9
Category 8:Community and private resources			
Patient's use of services	7	1< 4.60	41.3
Past experience with services	7	1< 4.60	34.8
Category 9: Patient perceptions and capacities			
Decision-making capacity	9	1< 7.60	
Patient's expectations of system	9	1< 7.60	
Patient's satisfaction with living environment	9	1< 7.60	
Adjustment strategies	8	1< 7.60	
Problem-solving capacity	8	0.81< 7.46	
Capacity for self-criticism	8	1< 7.60	
Level of motivation	8	1< 7.60	
Perceived level of well-being	8	1.81< 6.99	
Degree of change anticipated by patient	8	1< 6.10	
Empowerment	8	1< 6.10	
Cooperation of client system with staff	8	0< 6.85	
Client-system level of participation	8	0< 6.85	
Patient satisfaction with the care and services delivered	8	1.81< 6.99	
Category 10: Psychosexual functioning			
Inappropriate sexual behaviors	8	1.81< 6.99	
Sexual activity or loving behavior	6	2.62< 3.10	23.9
Sexual satisfaction	6	2< 3.85	43.5
Frequency of sexual activity	5	2< 2.35	2.2
Category 11: Personal values and beliefs			
Religion	8	1< 6.10	
Culture	8	1< 6.10	
Religious beliefs	7	3< 4.60	28.3
Category 12: Other psychosocial variables			
Capacity to participate in end-of-life decisions	9	1< 7.60	
Feelings about his/her end of life	9	1< 7.60	
End-of-life arrangements	8	1< 6.10	
Accomplishment of primary social roles	8	1< 6.10	
Social skills	7	1< 6.10	43.5
Patient's and family's level of knowledge	7	1< 6.10	28.3
Educational needs	7	1.81< 5.21	28.3

	First Round: Median[1]	First Round: IPR < IPRAS = agreement	Second Round: Retained variable = agreement ≥ 80%[3]
Category 13: Economic conditions			
Patient's capacity to meet financial obligations	8	1< 7.60	
Responsible financial management	8	1 < 7.60	
Sources of income	7	1< 6.10	65.2

Appendix 18.2
List of Variables – Physical and Organizational Environment

	First Round: Median	First Round: IPR < IPRAS = agreement	Second Round: Retained variable = agreement ≥ 80%
Category 14: Physical environment			
Size of living environment	8	2< 6.85	
Living environment is safe.	8	1.81< 5.49	
Living environment provides opportunities for social interactions.	8	1< 6.10	
Living environment is more residential than institutional.	8	1< 6.10	
Living environment is flexible and adaptable.	8	1< 7.60	
Living environment is stimulating.	8	1< 7.60	
Living environment provides for grouping of patients.	8	1< 6.10	
Living environment can be personalized.	7.5	1< 6.10	65.2
Living environment fosters orientation.	7	2< 5.35	
Living environment offers comfort.	7	2< 5.35	39.1
Living environment is open to the community.	7	1.81< 5.49	47.8
Living environment provides for privacy.	7	1< 6.10	67.4
Living environment fosters access to outdoors.	7	1< 4.60	56.5
Living environment has a garden.	6	2.81< 3.24	26.1
Geographic location	6	2< 3.85	39.1
Proximity of services	6	2< 3.85	45.7
Category 15: Human Environment			
Practitioner's professional skills	9	1< 7.60	
Practitioner's personal skills	9	1< 7.60	
Practitioner's level of comfort with the issue	8	0.81< 7.46	
Practitioner's job satisfaction	8	0< 6.85	
Practitioner's identification with the Living environment	8	1< 6.10	
Practitioner's framework	8	1< 6.10	
Practitioner's perception of the health-care network's efficacy	7	1< 6.10	37.0
Number of years of experience with patients	7	0< 5.35	52.2
Number of years of experience in the network	7	1< 4.60	30.4
Practitioner's level of education	6	2< 3.85	34.8
Number of years of experience as practitioner	6	2< 4.60	30.4
Practitioner's age	5	2.81 < 2.96	4.3
OPTSQ member	3	4.81> 4.46	

	First Round: Median	First Round: IPR < IPRAS = agreement	Second Round: Retained variable = agreement ≥ 80%
Category 16: Organizational Environment (social-work team)			
No. of social workers ÷ No. of beds	9	1< 7.60	
Relative weight of workload	9	1< 7.60	
Number of site served by the social worker	8	1< 7.60	
Balance between clinical activities and other tasks	8	0.81< 7.46	
Presence of other psychosocial professions in the institution	8	1< 6.10	
Mandate and definition of social work in the CSSS	8	1< 7.60	
Practitioner has a private office	8	1< 7.60	
Number of practitioners in the file	7.5	1< 6.10	60.9
Territory served by the CSSS	7	2< 5.35	37.0
Number of sites constituting the CSSS	6	1.81< 3.99	30.4
Category 17: Organizational Environment (CSSS)			
Program of care and services	8	1< 6.10	
Presence of intervention plan	8	1< 7.60	
Access to and availability of specialized services	8	1< 6.10	
Institutional context	7	1< 4.60	30.4
Level of technologies present	7	1< 6.10	52.2
Organization of basic services	7	1< 4.60	37.0
Justice and fairness of health care in the CSSS	7	1< 6.10	45.7
Organization of food services	5	2<2.35	21.7
Category 18: Work Organization in the CSSS			
Presence, composition, and effectiveness of the work of the multidisciplinary team	9	1< 7.60	
Lack of time	8.5	1< 7.60	
Staff turnover	8	1< 6.10	
Lack of health-care and other staff	8	1< 7.60	
Lack of training	8	1.81< 6.71	
Access to supervision	8	1< 6.10	
Access to consultation	8	1.62< 6.85	
Access to managerial staff	8	1< 6.10	
Work-group dynamics	8	1< 7.60	
Human resources	7	1< 6.10	23.9
Use of private agency	7	2< 3.85	34.8
Access to and availability of support staff	7	1< 6.10	65.2
Recruitment problems	7	1.81< 5.49	43.5
Category 19: Organizational Environment in the Health-Care Network			
Accessibility and availability of specialized services	8	1< 6.10	
Accessibility and availability of primary-care services	7	2< 5.35	39.1
Ministerial policy directions	7	1< 6.10	56.5
Justice and fairness in health care	7	2< 5.35	37.0
Organization complexity	7	1.81< 5.49	39.1
Accessibility and availability of community resources	6	1< 4.60	58.7

[1,2] Retained variable = in first round if median ≥ 8 and IPR < IPRAS

[3] Retained variable = in second round if = agreement ≥ 80%

Chapter 19
Assessment of the Adequacy of the Home Support Program's Services Offered Versus User Needs: Bridging the Gap between a Research Project and the Harnessing of Administratively Valuable Data

Danielle Benoit, Michel Tousignant, Guylaine Allard, Myriam Bergeron, Nicole Dubuc, and Réjean Hébert

Introduction

In 2003, it became possible for the first time in Quebec to draw a picture of the long-term clientele receiving home-support services (French acronym: SAD) for the entire region of one Agence de santé et de services sociaux (ASSS; formerly Régie régionale). This description has been operationalized by a classification, stemming from information integrated into the Multi-clientele Assessment Tool (French acronym: OEMC). Through the use of a classification based on standard profiles (Iso-SMAF), needs and services can be objectified, the required services can be standardized to a certain extent, and budgets can be adjusted based on the distribution of users in each profile. It was therefore possible to obtain clinical information also valuable for administrative purposes. Based on the results of the 2003 study, we were able to document that the public-health system meets 8.3 % of the nursing, support, and assistance care and that the intensity of these services varies from one Centre local de services communautaires (CLSC) region to another.

Two impacts arise from this study. First, the Iso-SMAF profiles can be used to compare clienteles of SAD services within a single region, in different regions of a given province, and in different provinces. Second, the data are now available as decision-making tools intended for the distribution of financial resources for the program *Perte d'autonomie liée au vieillissement* (PALV).

This study represents a big step in the right direction. In general, CLSCs are relatively familiar with their users individually. At the same time, they know their clientele poorly as a whole and are even less aware of the extent of client needs for services. This hampered CLSC efforts to provide decision-makers and administrators with valuable information about the provision of home-support services.

Research findings are seldom used in day-to-day administration. It is thus reasonable to examine the appeal of such an approach and the use of data by clinicians and Centre de santé et de services sociaux (CSSS) administrators. This chapter outlines the follow-up activities undertaken by those involved in the initial study.

The Strengths and Limitations of the 2003 Study

One of the strengths of the 2003 study was the consolidation of the activities undertaken in November 2000 intended to harmonize practices across service delivery sites. This endeavor was a valuable asset in the adjustment of services offered according to the needs of the clientele. This project was also pivotal in the implementation of a vision shared by all stakeholders of the 19 CLSCs offering home-support services in the Montérégie region. The result is a similar range of services that better targets specific clienteles. Various tools were developed and implemented over this period such as an evaluation quality management guide, prioritization guidelines, and waiting list generating guidelines.

Another strength was that we were able to ascertain the quality of the administrative database of the Client Information System (French acronym: SIC). Through sustained effort, timely and reliable data were produced. The information provided a solid foundation for the findings generated. In this respect, the Montérégie is recognized province-wide for the quality of its SIC data related to home support.

Yet the most significant limitation recognized by the agencies involved in research and administration was the use of a three-month period to produce the adequacy ratios. These quarterly data were subsequently extrapolated for an annual figure. Nevertheless, seasonal effects may impact both service supply and demand.

This limitation as recognized served to establish the agenda: To carry out a study on adequacy between services provided versus those required on an annual basis. The challenge was considerable. To calculate the Iso-SMAF profiles, the 2003 study required that the SMAF items be entered for all the users by rather rudimentary electronic methods. Over 8,000 files were input by CLSC personnel. It was clear that a better system would be needed to ensure project sustainability.

Rate of Adequacy of the Offer of Services to Needs of Users of the Home-Support Program for 2004: from the Three-Month Period to Continuous Data

Computerizing SMAF Data

To facilitate obtaining the Iso-SMAF profiles, the research team developed and implemented software known as eSMAF.[2] This software's architecture is based on four overlapping levels: 1) user group (three subgroups: active, inactive, and institution); 2) client; 3) client clinical information; 4) report production. Each level provides a different view of the database, with each view providing access to specific retrievable information such as the number of users per group, the user's file, and reports in figure or table form.

Interrelation of the Databases

Five databases are used to obtain all the information required to calculate the rate of adequacy of response versus needs (Figure 19.1). The key (identifier) used to create a link between the various databases is the user file number as it appears in the SIC. The first database is derived through retrieving information from the SIC at the local level. This database contains various data (e.g., reason for intervention, actions, durations), each describing the interventions carried out among users receiving services under the PALV Program (intervention profile 710) in a given period. This database is merged with a second database compiled by each CLSC (using *Access* software) containing data on each of the services provided according to two criteria: direct allocation and family support. The results of this step enable us to establish the complete list of active, long-term users to be considered. For each user, we search for an Iso-SMAF profile in the eSMAF database. If the user is absent, we then search a third database, also compiled (*Access*) by each CLSC, for justification of the absence of the SMAF. Based on the final database derived through retrieving information from the SIC, we search for various service episodes of home-support programs for users under consideration for whom we have an Iso-SMAF profile. These episodes enable us to determine the number of days when the user was under home-support care by a CLSC and therefore likely to receive services.

Methodology

Study Population

This study focuses on the frail elderly who receive home-support services from CSSS in the Montérégie (the CLSCs are subsumed by the various CSSSs). To be eligible for the study, subjects must fit the intervention profile, i.e., *aging-related functional decline* and meet the following two criteria:

Figure 19.1
The databases

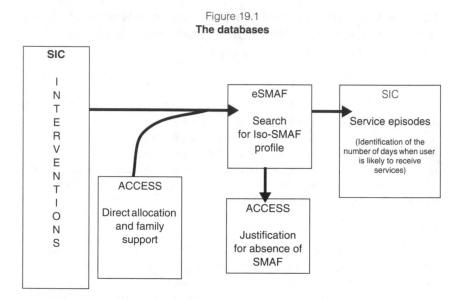

- Be an "active user," i.e., someone who has received at least one instance of care or a service from the CLSC and/or received one direct allocation or family-support service during the study's observation window.
- Have been evaluated during the preceding year with the Functional Autonomy Measurement System (French acronym: SMAF).

Clinical Measurement

The OEMC's focal point—the SMAF[3-5]—is a clinical scale of functional autonomy. It consists of 29 items that rate functional skills in five areas: activities of daily living (7 items), mobility (6 items), communication (3 items), mental functions (5 items), and instrumental activities of daily living (8 items). Each item is scored on a 4- or 5-point scale, ranging from -3 (dependent) to 0 (autonomous). The total score ranges from 0 to -87, where -87 indicates a high level of dependence.

Based on the scores on the SMAF components, a classification was developed under a previous study in order to categorize individuals according to mutually exclusive characteristics. Through statistical validation procedures and consultation of a group of experts, we were able to establish 14 Iso-SMAF profiles,[6] arranged in order from low incapacity (profile 1) to very high incapacity (profile 14). Based on the main impairment, five profile categories are observed: 1) individuals with a significant disability related to instrumental activities of daily living (profiles 1, 2, and 3); 2) individuals whose impairment is primarily mobility-related, with mental functions relatively unaffected (profiles 4, 6, and 9); 3) those whose impairment is primarily mental (profiles 5, 7,

8, and 10); 4) individuals with serious mobility impairments and incontinence problems (profiles 11 and 12); and 5) individuals exhibiting severe incapacity (generally bed-ridden; profiles 13 and 14).

The Rate of Adequacy of Response to Needs: Measuring the Disparity between User Needs and Services Available

The measurement of the disparity between the services provided by the SAD programs in the public-health system and the needs of frail individuals is expressed by an adequacy ratio of response to needs, which is defined as:

Adequacy ratio of response to needs= $\dfrac{\text{Number of hours of services provided by the SAD}}{\text{Number of hours of service required based on the Iso-SMAF profiles}}$

Duration of Care Provided (numerator)

The duration of care provided is represented by the duration of home interventions dispensed by SAD personnel (nurses, homemakers, social-services assistants). Information can be extracted from the SIC database on the duration of each of the interventions dispensed for a given user during the observation window. This direct time obtained is subsequently added together for all users to determine the total number of care/service hours provided per year for the CLSC's entire clientele for two care components: nursing, support, and assistance care. This study also covers care provided through direct allocation and family support. The direct allocation mechanism attributes the service hours (hourly rate, minimum wage, privately contracted employee paid by vouchers). Through this mechanism the individual can obtain assistance required in performing the activities of daily living (ADL) and instrumental activities of daily living (IADL) necessary for them to remain at home. The family support program allocates money to the individual. This program enables families to assume their specific responsibilities towards the individual while pursuing their personal, social, and professional activities as well as enjoying the same conditions as other families. For the purposes of this study, the monetary allocations were converted into hours based on an hourly rate of $7.30 (the equivalent of the minimum wage at the time).

Duration of Care Needed (denominator)

The estimate of the direct period of care needed in nursing / assistance and support services is based on the Iso-SMAF profiles. More specifically, the determination of the median number of hours required per day for the 14 Iso-SMAF profiles was determined under a previous study[7]. For the purposes of this study, these hours required are attributed to each of the users based on their Iso-SMAF profiles. This individual time is subsequently added together for the entire client group to calculate the total number of care/service hours required per year to serve the CSSS's clientele for the two care/service components: nursing, support, and assistance care.

Data Collection Procedures

Each CSSS (through the CLSCs) is responsible for providing all data required by the study. Tools have been made available to each for data input and retrieval. Two requests were created in *Impromptu* (software used to extract data in various formats) to facilitate extraction from the two SIC-derived databases. An *Access*-based program, designed to record justifications for the absence of SMAFs, also limits justifications to a predefined list. A second *Access*-based program was designed for the input of direct allocation and family-support data. Once completed and validated, these five databases are sent to the Research Centre on Aging (French acronym: CRV), where a second validation procedure is performed. The second validation is primarily concerned with data coherence across the five databases. This step generates 13 validation files, which are returned to the institution concerned for correction of the original databases. Once completed, the CSSS returns the five corrected databases. They are subsequently merged to calculate the adequacy ratio.

Findings

Description of the Study Population

Table 19.1 presents the descriptive statistics of the study population. They show that the majority of active PALV users are women with an average age of 82 years. Moreover, the average age of the direct allocations subgroup is 25 years, which suggests that this clientele is largely made up of individuals with intellectual impairments.

Table 19.1
Descriptive statistics of the population studied (N = 14,265)

	Sex % Male	Average age (standard deviation)	Average SMAF score (standard deviation)
Age-related functional decline (N=12,816)	32 %	82.0 (7.5)	-23.6 (14.5)
Direct allocation or family support (N = 1,449)	54 %	25.0 (23.3)	-34.5 (14.0)

Figure 19.2 provides the findings on the distribution of Iso-SMAF profiles. A look at it leads us to conclude that the Iso-SMAF profiles of the SAD program's long-term clients are distributed heterogeneously. In general, the overall

client portrait is consistent with the CLSC's mission of serving a very high proportion of the individuals with impairments related to instrumental activities of daily living (45 %), individuals affected by largely movement-related impairments with relative preservation of mental function (36 %), and individuals with predominantly mental impairments (15 %). On the other hand, 4 % of the individuals have the profile of patients regularly placed in institutions in Quebec.

Figure 19.2
Relative proportions of Iso-SMAF profiles (long-term SAD, Montérégie 2004-2005)

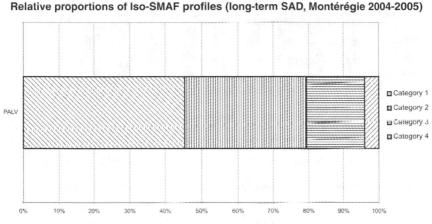

n= 12 816
Category 1: profiles 1, 2, and 3; Category 2: profiles 4, 6 and 9; Category 3: profiles 5, 7, 8, and 10; Category 4: profiles 11, 12, 13, and 14.

Figure 19.3 presents the average rate of adequacy of response to needs for nursing, support, and assistance care in Montérégie as well as the rate of adequacy of response to needs for the 11 CSSSs. Two institutions show a result more than 2 % higher than the regional average (D and K), while two institutions show a result of more than 2 % lower (H and C).

Harnessing Administratively Valuable Data

The data stemming from this research project are used at both the local and regional levels. Since 2000, we observe a marked change in the availability of information relative to the needs of PALV clientele served in all districts of the Montérégie. Figure 19.4 clearly illustrates this progression.

The Iso-SMAF profiles allow for multidimensional administration. From a clinical point of view, the SMAF can be used to identify largely similar characteristics requiring the same general types of services and resources for a given group. The Iso-SMAF profiles provide the clinician with a portrait of the individual (brief representation) that can be used as a *benchmark to guide decision-making* on an individual basis. Moreover, they allow for an ongoing assessment of needs and required services.

Figure 19.3
Rate of adequacy of response to needs by CSSS

Nursing, Assistance, and Support Care

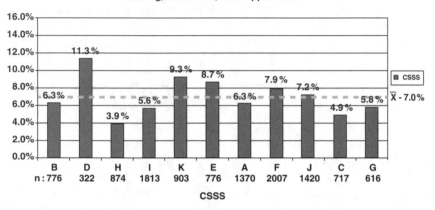

Figure 19.4
Progression in administratively valuable data

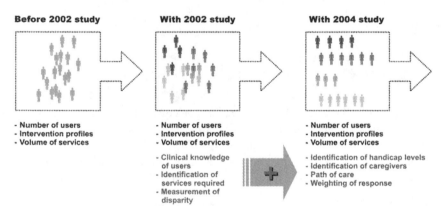

The availability of this information helps to improve planning of services (type, quantity, quality, timeliness), regardless of the delivery location. Since the profiles are independent of current structures, they are easily adaptable to new practices and technologies.

From an operational standpoint, the administrators have already launched a more exhaustive analysis of the findings in order to better pinpoint the resources needing development in their regions. Since their creation, the CSSSs have had a responsibility to the population. Consequently, they must, within the scope of their clinical approach, ensure the integration of services in their jurisdictions. By combining information provided by the profiles with other data (e.g., index of patient load, personal status, location of intervention, hours worked), analyses can be performed for the purposes of human resources and financial planning.

With respect to financial management, the project in the Montérégie has served as a trailblazer in the province in terms of using data in developing a budgetary allocation method. Since fiscal 2004–2005, the Agence de la santé et des services sociaux de la Montérégie has been using these data to allocate financial resources. Fiscal 2006–2007 has retained two components: the relative weighting of the PALV program (30 %) and the relative weighting of the SAD program (70 %). The weighting of the SAD program was calculated using a composite index: 40 % for the rate of adequacy of response to needs, 40 % for the patient load index, and 20 % for the inclusion rate.

The analysis of the data in its entirety should continue. Yet Montérégie policymakers and administrators are already in a position to reexamine practices and to make adjustments in services offered by CSSSs since the information is now available. This information enables them to reexamine actions to be taken at all levels, as illustrated below:

- Applicability: Should complete bathing assistance be given to an individual when only partial assistance is required?
- Effectiveness: Ensure that each intervention is effective.
- Equality: Meet the critical needs of one individual before meeting another person's less pressing needs.
- Efficiency: When faced with two efficient services, choose the one requiring fewer resources.
- Preferences: Try to respect the wishes of the individual.
- Saturation: Maintain a balance between the service offered and the ability of the person to receive it.

It is now possible to establish a link between measuring results, the quality of care and services, and client satisfaction.

Conclusion

Armed with these six years of collaborative work between the Agence de la santé et des services sociaux de la Montérégie, PALV program administrators and the professionals involved in the care and services of the Centre de recherche sur le vieillissement, we have clearly demonstrated the feasibility of using these research findings for administrative purposes. The success of this project was tied to the Agence's commitment, clearly demonstrated not only by its financial support, but also by its clear and firm stance favorable to this clinical undertaking and through the participation of the CSSSs.

Acknowledgements

Members of the research committee: Chantal Arsenault, Céline Charest, Marie-Christine Letellier, Murielle Savignac and Jean-Pierre Beaudry (the authors

Guylaine Allard, Danielle Benoit, Myriam Bergeron and Michel Tousignant were also members). From the ASSS: Claire Pagé and Robert Johnson. From the CSSSs, all administrators, workers, and managers responsible for the application of the SIC normative framework.

References

1. Tousignant M., Hébert R., Dubuc N., and Coulombe C. Home care programmes for disabled older adults: How can we assess the adequacy of services provided compared to the needs of users? Health and Social Care in the Community 2007; 15:1-7.

2. Boissy P., Brière S., Tousignant M., and Rousseau E. The eSMAF: a software for the assessment and follow-up of functional autonomy in geriatrics. BMC Geriatrics (www.biomedcentral.com/1471-2318/7/2) 2007; 7:2, 1-14.

3. Hébert R., Carrier R., and Bilodeau A. The Functional Autonomy Measurement System (SMAF): description and validation of an instrument for the measurement of handicaps. Age and Ageing 1988; 17:293-302.

4. Desrosiers J., Bravo G., Hébert R., and Dubuc N. Reliability of the revised Functional autonomy measurement system (SMAF) for epidemiological research. Age and Ageing 1995; 24: 402-6.

5. Hébert R., Guilbault J., Desrosiers J., and Dubuc N. The functional autonomy measurement system (SMAF): A clinical-based instrument for measuring disabilities and handicaps in older people. Geriatrics Today: Journal of the Canadian Geriatrics Society 2001; 4:141-147.

6. Dubuc N., Hébert R., Desrosiers J., Buteau M., and Trottier L. Disability-based classification system for older people in integrated long-term care services: the Iso-SMAF profiles. Archives of Gerontology and Geriatrics 2006; 42: 191-206.

7. Hébert R., Dubuc N., Buteau M., Desrosiers J., Bravo G., Trottier L., St-Hilaire C., and Roy C. Ressources and costs associated with disabilities of elderly people living at home and institutions. Canadian Journal on Aging 2001; 20:1-21.

Chapter 20
Profiles of the Functional Independence of the Clientele in Private Residences for the Elderly in Estrie

Pauline Gervais, Réjean Hébert, and Michel Tousignant

Highlights

In Quebec, private residences for the elderly (RPHs, for "résidences privées d'hébergement") house twice as many elderly as do facilities in the public system. Little is known about the needs of these residents. The purpose of the present study is to sketch a portrait of the RPH clientele. Four hundred seventy-nine residents inventoried in the territories of Coaticook and Granit in Estrie were assessed using the Functional Independence Measurement System (SMAF, for "Système de mesure de l'autonomie fonctionelle"). Iso-SMAF profiles confirmed the presence in this group of significantly frail individuals, as well as the mixed nature of the clientele. A comparison with residents in public facilities revealed that private and public facilities complement each other. In RPHs, we found limited service delivery by local community service centres (CLSCs, for "centres locaux de services communautaires") and varying ranges of service offered to residents by the RPHs themselves.

Introduction

Quebec's population in residential facilities numbers about 120,000,[1, 2] of which 80,000 are housed in private residences for the elderly (RPH).[2] Under Quebec legislation, this type of facility is defined as "a congregate residential facility where rooms or apartments intended for elderly persons are offered for rent along with a varied range of services relating, in particular, to security, housekeeping assistance and assistance with social activities, except a facility operated by an institution [as defined by the Act Respecting Health Services and Social Services, RSQ c. S-4.2] and a building or residential facility where the services of an intermediate resource or a family-type resource [as defined by the same statute] are offered" (RSQ c. S-4.2, Section 346.0.1; RSQ c. A-19.1).

RPHs represent a way point commonly passed through (8.2 %) by the elderly on the trajectory of assisted living. For many, these are the final dwelling place; for others, they constitute a transition to public facilities such as family-type residences (RAs, for "résidences d'accueil") (0.32 %), intermediate-type residences (RIs, for "résidences de type intermédiaire") (0.26 %), and, at the end of the continuum, residential and extended care centres (CHSLDs, for "centres d'hébergement et de soins de longue durée") (5.37 %)[3, 4]. The private network of residences for the elderly, numbering 2,400, has become the main player in residential services in Quebec,[5] a result of the aging of the population and the reduction over the past fifteen years in the number of beds available in CHSLDs[6]. The situation is the same in other provinces of Canada[7]. Given the general aging of the population and current policies that promote home care, this trend towards growth in the private sector is likely to persist and indeed gain momentum.

Little is known about RPH clientele. Unlike the situation in public facilities, these residences are not required to follow an assessment protocol with the individuals they house[8]. Although the majority of RPHs do not hold a permit from the Quebec Department of Health and Social Services allowing them to house frail individuals, studies show that close to half of their residents have obvious disabilities[9-13]. In raising questions about the quality of services provided in these facilities,[7, 14] we considered it essential to begin by investigating client profile. This is the framework for the study. Our objectives were 1) to inventory the residents of RPHs over an entire territory; 2) to determine their degree of functional independence; 3) to compare this clientele's independence profiles with those for clienteles in other settings; and 4) to evaluate the level of services provided.

Methodology

Population

The study was carried out in two regional municipal counties (MRCs, for "municipalité régionale de comté") of the Estrie region, Coaticook and Granit. There are twelve rural municipalities in Coaticook's territory and its population of 18,463 accounts for 6.3 % of the population of Estrie as a whole. Of these inhabitants, 41.1 % are aged 65 and over (n = 2,610). The MRC is served by one CHSLD, which has 93 beds and also oversees two RI beds.

In geographic territory, the Granit MRC is the largest in Estrie and rural in character. With 22 municipalities on its territory, it has 22,278 inhabitants, representing 7.5 % of the population of Estrie. Of these, 15 % are aged 65 and over (n = 3,336). Service is available from one CHSLD, which has 109 beds on its premises and oversees another 48 places in RIs and RAs[13, 14].

In both these MRCs, French is the main language of use.

Recruitment

The first stage of recruitment consisted of drawing up a list of RPHs that qualified for the study. To this end, we consulted the *Registre des résidences pour personnes âgées en Estrie – 2002-2003*[15] (the Estrie register of residences for the elderly for 2002-2003) and the individuals in charge of home care services in the two territories' local community services centres (CLSCs, for "centre local de services communautaires"). Low-cost housing facilities and housing cooperatives were excluded from the study because they provide no personal assistance or care services. The RPHs included in the study were grouped under three headings: 1) RPHs with nine housing units or fewer, which are not required to comply with regulations enforced by the Quebec Department of Agriculture, Fisheries, and Food or the Quebec Construction Board; 2) midsized RPHs, with 10 to 29 places; and 3) large RPHs with 30 places or more.

All residents aged 65 and over who had lived in an RPH for at least three months were eligible for this study. Residents whose placement was funded by the public sector as they awaited a CHSLD or palliative care bed were excluded.

Instruments

Two of the four data-collection instruments were borrowed from similar studies and adapted to the needs of this one:[9, 10, 18] the form for number of RPH places available and filled, and the form on residents' socio-demographic characteristics. A questionnaire was developed on services available to residents.

Residents' functional independence was measured using the Functional independence Measurement System (SMAF, for "système de mesure de l'autonomie fonctionnelle")[19]. This assessment scale is included in the Multiclientele Assessment Tool adopted by the Department of Health and Social Services for assessing adults who receive home-care services or are referred to public facilities[8]. Next, each resident's functional independence profile (Iso-SMAF profile)[20] was determined. Each profile corresponds to a given "Iso-ressources" group, i.e., a group of similar subjects requiring similar services and incurring similar costs, and is linked to a level of disability ranging from very low (Profile 1) to significant (Profile 14). Profiles are grouped under four disability levels. Subjects with profiles 1, 2, and 3 have disabilities related exclusively to domestic tasks; subjects with profiles 4, 6, and 9 present with motor impairment but have comparatively well-preserved mental function; in subjects with profiles 5, 7, 8, and 10, mental disability predominates; and subjects with profiles 11, 12, 13, and 14 have impaired mobility, are dependent as regards activities of daily living (ADL), or present with cognitive deficits and almost total communicative disability. Each profile is associated with a daily budget, in dollars, and an average number of care and service hours[21].

Data Collection

The study was conducted from November 2, 2003 to December 5, 2003 by two health/social-service professionals assigned to the task by the MRCs' CLSCs. They received specific training on the use of the assessment instruments and the data-gathering procedures. Continuous monitoring was provided during the study. In each RPH, the information was obtained from service providers. This methodological choice made it possible to assess all residents without requiring them to attend individual meetings. Prior to the meetings, the providers were informed of the questions they would be asked, especially regarding their residents' functional abilities. They were also alerted to the impact that over- or under-assessment of their residents' independence could have on the study's findings.

Analyses

Descriptive statistics were obtained for the characteristics of the RPHs and their residents. An index of level of required care (ILRC) was calculated for each RPH. This index made it possible to draw up a quantitative portrait of subjects' needs and compare the units studied with each other[22]. This was calculated using coefficients determined as follows. For each Iso-SMAF profile, the median of the number of hours needed daily to meet nursing, assistance, and support needs was divided by the median of total hours needed for the profile associated with the highest required-care level, Profile 14. The coefficient thus obtained was multiplied by the number (n) of subjects for the profile in question. This calculation was performed for each of the 14 profiles, and the sum of these coefficients was then divided by the total number (N) of subjects.

$$\left[\frac{\bar{x} \text{ profile hours } 1}{\bar{x} \text{ profile hours } 14} \right] \times n + \dots \frac{\bar{x} \text{ profile hours } 14}{\bar{x} \text{ profile hours } 14} \times n = \frac{\Sigma}{N}$$

T-tests were done comparing different groupings. All the analyses were performed with SPSS software version 12.0.

In order to place RPH residents on the continuum of services for frail individuals, we had recourse to data from other studies carried out with the same instrument. These had been in 2003 during annual assessments of the clienteles attending a day centre (run by Les CHSLD Estriade); living in CHSLDs, RIs, and RAs (under the Estrie Health and Social Services Agency); and receiving home care[23].

Findings

As can be seen in Table 20.1, we identified 41 residences for the elderly in the 2 MRCs studied. Of these, twelve low-cost housing facilities and one residence that offered its clients no supervision at all were excluded. Of the other RPHs, three had no clients at the time of data gathering. Thus, 25 RPHs were visited. All owners or managers agreed to provide the information needed for the studies we carried out. Altogether, the RPHs surveyed offer 528 residential places; 33 of these were funded by a CHSLD. The 595 remaining private places are distributed as follows: 61 % in large RPHs, 27 % in medium-sized ones, and 12 % in small ones. The occupancy rate was 86 %; the residents represent 9.7 % of inhabitants aged 65 and over in Coaticook and 6.8 % in Granit.

Table 20.1
RPH Recruitment

	Coaticook	Granit	2 MRC
Number of residences for the elderly	16	25	41
– Listed in the *Registre des résidences*	14	23	37
– Added by the CLSC	2	2	4
Excluded residences	6	7	13
– Low cost housing	6	6	12
– Those offering no supervision		1	1
Number of RPHs eligible for the study	10	18	28
– Small (9 or fewer places)	4	7	11
– Medium (10 to 20 places)	1	9	10
– Large (30 or more places)	5	2	7
No of RPHS visited	9	16	25
– Small (9 or fewer places)	3	6	9
– Medium (10 to 20 places)	1	8	9
– Large (30 or more places)	5	2	7

A total of 541 individuals were inventoried. Of these, 62 were ultimately excluded: 25 had come to live in the RPH less than three months previously, 33 occupied a place funded by a CHSLD, 4 were waiting for a place in the public sector. Four hundred seventy-nine (479) subjects participated in the study: 253 from Coaticook and 226 from Granit.

The average age of residents was 83.3 years. Nine out of ten were aged 75 or older; 70 % of participants were women. The mother tongue of almost all participants was French. Nearly half the participants had been living in an RPH for over two years; 80 % of participants had been living in the same MRC before coming to the RPH. Table 20.2 presents subjects' characteristics.

Table 20.3 shows how Iso-SMAF profiles were distributed among the different groupings. The profiles reveal the heterogeneousness of the RPH clientele. Over half of the residents assessed present with an impairment related to instrumental activities of daily living, or IADL (Category 1: profiles 1, 2, and 3). One quarter (26.3 %) present with a predominant motor impairment (Category 2: profiles 4, 6, and 9) and 15.9 % with a predominant mental impairment (Cate-

Table 20.2
Subject Sociodemographic Characteristics

	Coaticook n = 253	Granit n = 226	2 MRC n = 479
Number of women	184(73%)	153 (68%)	337 (70%)
Average age	83.9 (6.8)*	82.5 (7.1)*	83.3 (7.0)*
Women	84.4 (6.5)*	83 (7.1)*	83.8 (6.6)*
Men	82.6 (7.4)*	81.6 (7.0)*	82 (7.2)*
Aged less than 65	2 (1%)	2 (1%0	4 (0.8%)
65 to 74 years	18 (7%)	27 (12%)	45 (10%)
75 to 84 years	116 (46%)	103 (45%)	219 (46%)
85 or older	117 (46%)	94 (42%)	211 (44%)
Average length of stay in years	1.9 (1)*	1.9 (0.8)*	1.9 (0.8)*
3 to 23 months	88 (34%)	79 (35%)	167 (35%)
2 to 5 years	115 (45%)	103 (46%)	218 (46%)
6 to 10 years	38 (15%)	35 (15%0	73 (15%)
11 years or older	12 (%)	9 (4%)	21 (4%)
Provenance Same MRC as that of RPH	175 (69%)	207 (92%)	382 (80%)
Another Estrie MRC	20 (8%)	3 (1%)	23 (5%)
Not from Estrie	19 (8%)	12 (5%)	31 (6%)
Unknown	39 (15%)	4 (2%)	43 (9%)

* Average (standard deviation)

gory 3: profiles 5, 7, 8, and 10). A very small proportion (2.1%) of subjects have significant disabilities of both kinds (Category 4: profiles 11, 12, 13, and 14). These data show that close to half (44.3%) of these RPH residents need assistance performing ADL, with moving, with communicating, or in relation to their mental disabilities. The gap of 0.06 between ILRCs makes clear there is a difference between the two MRCs' clienteles as regards degree of reduced functional independence: The Granit's clientele would appear to be less frail, and a chi-square test confirmed that Granit had fewer RPH residents classed as having motor impairments (Category 2; $p < 0.001$).

Small and large RPHs house a larger proportion of residents with motor impairment than medium-sized ones ($p < 0.01$). Indeed, the small RPHs house the cases requiring the most care, as indicated by the ILRC of 0.47 (Table 20.4). Age would appear to affect residents' Iso-SMAF profiles. Analysis by age group, as shown in Table 20.5, reveals a significant difference with respect to mental disabilities ($p < 0.01$) between the 75-to-84 age group and other age groups.

Comparison of the RPH residents' Iso-SMAF profiles with those for clients of other care and housing facilities on the continuum of services for frail individuals shows how the level of service needs rises as this clientele moves along the trajectory from home to CHSLD. As well, the complementary nature of private and public residential facilities is observable. It is noteworthy that the

Table 20.3
Distribution of Iso-SMAF Profiles across MRCs

Profile	Coaticook	Granit	2 MRC
1	26 (10.3 %)	44 (19.5 %)	70 (14.6 %)
2	46 (18.2 %)	51 (22.6 %)	97 (2.03 %)
3	37 (14.6 %)	63 (27.9 %)	100 (20.9 %)
4	27 (10.7 %)	7 (3.1 %)	34 (7.1 %)
6	71 (28 %)	15 (6.6 %)	86 (18.0 %)
9	5 (2.0 %)	1 (0.4 %)	6 (1.3 %)
5	6 (2.4 %)	22 (9.7 %)	28 (5.8 %)
7	4 (1.6 %)	10 (4.4 %)	14 (2.9 %)
8	25 (9.9 %)	6 (2.7 %)	31 (6.5 %)
10	2 (0.8 %)	1 (0.4 %)	3 (0.6 %)
11	0 (0 %)	3 (1.3 %)	3 (0.6 %)
12	3 (1.2 %)	3 (1.3 %)	6 (1.3 %)
13	0 (0 %)	0 (0 %)	0 (0 %)
14	1 (0.4 %)	0 (0 %)	1 (0.2 %)
ILRC	0.45	0.39	0.42

Table 20.4
Distribution of Iso-SMAF Profiles by RPH Size

Profile	Small 9 places and more	Medium 10 to 29 places	Large 30 places and more
1	1 (2.4 %)	15 (9.6 %)	54 (19.1 %)
2	10 (24.4 %)	37 (23.7 %)	50 (17.7 %)
3	10 (24.4 %)	46 (29.5 %)	44 (15.6 %)
4	1 (2.4 %)	7 (4.5 %)	26 (9.2 %)
6	8 (19.5 %)	11 (7.1 %)	67 (23.8 %)
9	0 (0 %)	2 (1.3 %)	4 (1.4 %)
5	2 (4.9 %)	18 (11.5 %)	8 (2.8 %)
7	6 (14.6 %)	5 (3.2 %)	3 (1.1 %)
8	0 (0 %)	8 (5.1 %)	23 (8.2 %)
10	0 (0 %)	3 (1.9 %)	0 (0 %)
11	0 (0 %)	2 (1.3 %)	1 (0.4 %)
12	3 (7.3 %)	1 (0.6 %)	2 (0.7 %)
13	0 (0 %)	0 (0 %)	0 (0 %)
14	0 (0 %)	1 (0.6 %)	0 (0 %)
ILRC	0.47	0.44	0.40

Table 20.5
Distribution of Iso-SMAF Profiles According to Residents' Ages

Profile	65 to 74 years	75 to 84 years	85 years or older
1	5 (11.1%)	39 (17.8%)	26 (12.3%)
2	13 (28.9%)	62 (28.3%)	21 (10.0%)
3	5 (11.1%)	44 (20.1%)	51 (24.2%)
4	2 (4.4%)	12 (5.5%)	20 (9.5%)
6	2 (4.4%)	33 (15.1%)	51 (24.2%)
9	1 (2.2%)	4 (1.8%)	1 (0.5%)
5	9 (20.0%)	9 (4.1%)	9 (4.3%)
7	1 (2.2%)	3 (1.4%)	10 (4.7%)
8	5 (11.1%)	8 (3.7%)	16 (7.6%)
10	0 (0%)	2 (0.9%)	1 (0.5%)
11	1 (2.2%)	0 (0%)	2 (0.9%)
12	0 (0%)	3 (1.4%)	3 (1.4%)
13	0 (0%)	0 (0%)	0 (0%)
14	1 (2,2%)	0 (0%)	0 (0%)
ILRC	0.44	0.39	0.44

clientele for RPHs and that for in-home services present similar independence profiles.

The responses received from RPH managers made it possible to identify the range of services provided by RPH staff and their cost. We considered only services associated with ADL, IADL, and nursing care, because they are personalized and often subject to extra charges for housing. We observed that the supply of services varied from one RPH to another but that, generally speaking, 58.2 % of residents relied on assistance with ADL, which corresponds to the percentage of individuals with an Iso-SMAF profile of four and over (54.3 %). In this category, hygiene and personal care services predominate; they are followed by assistance with elimination and then help with dressing and feeding. Almost all residents require assistance with IADL, in particular for meals, housekeeping, and laundry. Nursing services consist mainly of monitoring and supervision. The cost of these services is generally included in the monthly rent. CLSC services are not much in evidence in RPHs. According to the data provided by the residences, only ten percent of their residents received CLSC in-home services during the study's window of observation, and these consisted mainly of nursing care.

Discussion

This study consisted in conducting an inventory of elderly individuals living in RPHs in two Estrie MRCs, with a view to sketching a portrait of this target group's degree of functional independence and comparing it with that of clients of other (public) care and residential facilities. Our findings show that the RPH clientele is largely female (70 %), which reflects the distribution of the sexes in

Figure 20.1
**Distribution of Iso-SMAF Profiles in Various Types of Settings
(Different Territories)**

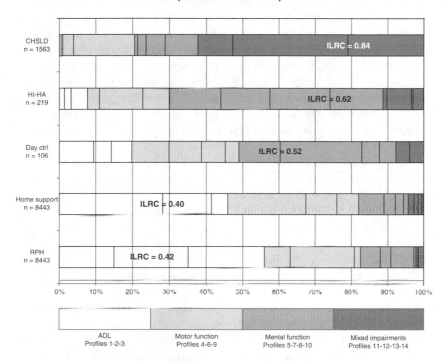

the elderly population as a whole. As is found in the public sector's CHSLDs, the functional independence profiles of residents varied significantly.[23]

These findings are in line with those of an earlier study[19] conducted in the various care settings served by a CLSC. Close to half (44.3 %) of RPH residents need assistance performing ADL, compensating for motor and communicative disabilities, and compensating for impaired mental function (corresponding to Iso-SMAF profiles 4 and higher). The percentage of residents with motor (26.3 %) and mental (15.9 %) impairment is lower than that found in the Bravo studies[10, 11]. The divergences in findings may be accounted for by the fact that our study covered the whole of the clientele and all the residences in the territory rather than using samples based on criteria associated with frailty or CLSC-service use. Comparison of Iso-SMAF profiles and ILRCs based on RPH size revealed the presence of a clientele with a higher level of care needs in the small and large residences. This feature also emerged from the Bravo studies.[9, 10]

Although the whole range of Iso-SMAF profiles is found among RPH residents, it is nevertheless possible to discern a kind of complementarity among the various life settings, with the clientele requiring ever increasing care as the continuum is followed from CLSC-service delivery at home to residence in a CHSLD. The degree of functional independence of those living in RPHs is similar to that of individuals in the public sector's RIs and RAs. A comparison of the ILRCs for different settings with those for RPHs confirms the impression that the level of required care is higher in the public sector, except as regards CLSC in-home services, whose ILRC is slightly lower than that of the RPHs.

According to the responses to the questionnaire on services, RPH residents are receiving most of the services they need. We observed however that the range of services available varied from one RPH to another. As well, the degree of CLSC penetration in this setting is comparatively low. In a future study, it would be worth investigating the adequacy of the response to this target group's service needs.

Questions may be raised about this study's internal validity, but numerous measures were taken to ensure our findings would be accurate. One of the strengths of the study is that it avoided selection bias altogether by inventorying all RPHs and their residents in two CLSC territories. Particular attention was paid to controlling for information bias. To this end, data gathering was entrusted to experienced health/social-service professionals from the territories' CLSCs, who were familiar with the SMAF assessment instrument. We also ensured all the data-gathering instruments were used consistently. Assessments were checked upon reception; any missing or imprecise data resulted in systematic follow-up with the person who performed the assessment. Measures were also taken to reduce possible bias associated with social desirability. In order to ensure the accuracy of the information supplied and that assessments reflected reality, RPH owners and managers were alerted to the potential for unintended consequences for the study's findings if their clientele's disabilities were under- or over-assessed. Nevertheless, we are aware our data is subject to potential weakness, since we obtained our information from secondary sources and our methodology did not include a mechanism for validating the information provided. To back up the validity of the SMAF assessments, we used the tried method of Euclidean distance[19, 21] Only 4 of the 479 assessments, i.e., 1 %, had a Euclidean distance greater than 5. This threshold reflects one profile's deviation from its group[20]. Given the efforts we made to reduce the risk of bias, we are confident of the study's sound internal validity.

Conclusion

The primary goal of this study was to draw up a portrait of the clientele for privately managed residential facilities in two Estrie MRCs. To our knowledge, this is the first study that has relied on Iso-SMAF profiles to describe the functional independence of the elderly living in RPHs. The study allowed us not just to establish functional independence profiles for RPH residents, but also to compare this target group with that of other (public) care and residential settings, namely day centers, CLSCs, RIs and RAs, and CHSLDs.

The study throws fresh light on a segment of the elderly population about which the public health and social services system has known comparatively little until now. Our findings confirm that frail individuals are living in RPHs, and they reveal the heterogeneous nature of the functional independence profiles for the residents of such facilities. They also reveal that the range of services provided by RPHs is broad, while CLSC service delivery to these facilities is minimal. In light of the attraction of RPHs for the elderly public, we consider it necessary to continue studying the sector and draw up a more extensive portrait of its clientele, one that would reflect Quebec reality, measure the adequacy of the response to needs, and estimate public and private funding of the costs associated with this type of residential care.

References

1. Ministère de la Santé et des Services sociaux du Québec. (2003). Nombre de places internes dressées pour de l'hébergement et des soins de longue durée au sein du réseau d'établissements publics et privés conventionnés du Québec, selon la région socio sanitaire, situation observée au 31 mars, de 1991 à 2002.

2. Ministère de la Santé et des Services sociaux du Québec. (2005). Bulletin d'information présentant certaines statistiques extraites du Registre des résidences avec services pour personnes âgées. INFO-RRASPA.

3. Ministère de la Santé et des Services sociaux du Québec. (2004). Bulletin d'information présentant certaines statistiques extraites du système d'information des ressources intermédiaires et de type familial – INFO-SIRTF.

4. Ministère de la Santé et des Services sociaux du Québec. (2003). Bulletin d'information présentant certaines statistiques sur les lits dressés, les places internes, les usagers admis et les jours-présence, dans le réseau socio sanitaire québécois. Info-Stats.

5. Charpentier, M. (2004). De l'institution au marché: transformation de l'hébergement des personnes âgées et enjeux actuels. Vie Et Vieillissement, 3(2):2-8.

6. Boucher, G. (1998). Hébergement privé: un développement exponentiel. Le Magazine De L'Association Des CLSC Et CHSLD Du Québec, (10):17.

7. Canada Housing and Mortgage Corporation. (2000). Le logement-services pour les aînés.

8. Ministère de la Santé et des Services sociaux du Québec. (1997). Les mécanismes régionaux d'orientation et d'admission – Une mise à jour. Government of Quebec.

9. Bravo, G., Charpentier, M., Dubois, M.-F., De Wals, P., & Émond, A. (1997). La qualité des soins dispensés aux personnes âgées en perte d'autonomie par les ressources d'hébergement avec et sans permis ministériel. Research Centre on Aging, Sherbrooke Geriatric University Institute.

10. Bravo, G., Dubois, M.-F., Tardieu, F., De Wals, P., & Tessier, S. (2001). La qualité des soins dispensés dans les ressources d'hébergement de la Montérégie. Research Centre on Aging, Sherbrooke Geriatric University Institute.

11. Dugal, L. (1996). Portrait des résidences privées et de leur clientèle en milieu rural - MRC l'Islet. Faculté des lettres et sciences humaines, Université de Sherbrooke.

12. Désilets, I., & Gervais, P. (2001). Profils d'autonomie des personnes âgées de 65 ans et plus vivant en résidence privée d'hébergement. Rapport remis au CLSC-CHSLD du Haut-St-François.

13. Charpentier, M. (2001). La position des acteurs du secteur public et du secteur privé sur la pertinence d'une régulation des résidences pour personnes âgées au Québec. Research Centre on Aging, Sherbrooke Geriatric University Institute.

14. Ministère de la famille et de l'enfance du Québec. (2001). Le Québec et ses aînés: engagés dans l'action – Engagements et perspectives 2001-2004. Direction des communications, Government of Quebec.

15. Agence de la santé et des services sociaux de l'Estrie. (2004). La population de la MRC de Coaticook. Direction de la santé publique et de l'évaluation.

16. Agence de la santé et des services sociaux de l'Estrie. (2004). La population de la MRC du Granit. Direction de la santé publique et de l'évaluation.

17. Régie régionale de la santé et des services sociaux de l'Estrie. (2003). Registre des résidences pour personnes âgées avec services – Liste régionale des résidences 2002-2003.

18. Dubuc, N., Tousignant, M., Buteau, Hébert, R., & Coulombe, C. (2002). Services requis parles personnes âgées en perte d'autonomie – Évaluation clinique et estimation des coûts sur le territoire de la Régionale de la santé et des services sociaux de Laval. Research Centre on Aging, Sherbrooke Geriatric University Institute.

19. Hébert, R., Guilbeault, J., Desrosiers, J., & Dubuc, N. (2001). The functional autonomy measurement system (SMAF): A clinical-based instrument for measuring disabilities and handicaps in older people. Geriatrics Today: Journal of the Canadian Geriatrics Society, (September): 141-7.

20. Dubuc, N., & Hébert, R. (2002). Les profils Iso-SMAF: Un système de gestion clinico-administratif pour la planification des services de longue

durée dans un système de soins intégrés. SMAF: Quoi de neuf? Expertise Centre of the Sherbrooke Geriatric University Institute.

21. Hébert, R., Dubuc, N., Buteau, M., Desrosiers, J., Bravo, G., Trottier, L., St-Hilaire, C., & Roy, C. (2001). Resource and costs associated with disabilities of elderly people living at home and in institutions. Canadian Journal on Aging, 20(1):1-22.

22. Tousignant, M., Hébert, R., Dubuc, N., & Coulombe, C. (2003). Détermination du profil d'autonomie fonctionnelle et du taux de réponse aux besoins de la clientèle long-terme du programme soutien à domicile des CLSC de la Montérégie. Research Centre on Aging, Sherbrooke Geriatric University Institute.

23. Tousignant, M., Hébert, R., Dubuc, N., & Coulombe, C. (2004). Détermination du profil d'autonomie fonctionnelle et de la mesure de l'écart entre les services requis et fournis de la clientèle desservie par le programme de soutien à domicile des CLSC de la Montérégie. Research Centre on Aging, Sherbrooke Geriatric University Institute.

24. Tousignant, M., Hébert, R., Dubuc, N., Simoneau, F., & Dieleman, L. (2003). Application de la classification des profils Iso-SMAF à la détermination des profils d'accueil et à la répartition d'allocation budgétaire à l'intérieur de la méthode d'équité – volet hébergement de la région de l'Estrie. In: Hébert R, Tourigny A, Gagnon M, eds. Intégrer les services pour le maintien de l'autonomie des personnes. Québec: Edisem; 207-19.

Chapter 21
The PRISMA-Estrie Study: Determining the Cost of Health Services

Danièle Blanchette, Suzanne Durand, and Réjean Hébert

Highlights

In this chapter, we present the method by which we determined the costs of social and health services whose use is likely to be influenced by the integrated services network for frail elders (RISPA; *réseau intégré de services pour personnes âgées*). Services were evaluated in a societal perspective, in accordance with the principles of opportunity cost and replacement cost. The services whose cost was assessed included residential placement/housing, administrative support, user-support activities, nursing and assistance care, surveillance, respite services, professional consultations, medications, hospital stays, day hospital visits, day center visits, and travel for medical purposes. Translating social and health services into cost terms makes it possible to create a shared measurement system for the overall impact of the integrated services network. In addition, knowing the value of these services may prove useful to managers, who will be able to gauge their relative significance when making management decisions. The study makes an original contribution to knowledge about health costs, taking a societal perspective.

Introduction

The integrated services network for frail elders (RISPA; *réseau intégré de services pour personnes âgées*) is intended to enhance the accessibility, continuity, and coordination of services delivered to the elderly. Among other things, it aims to reduce service duplication and delay institutionalization. It is expected that it will have an impact on the types and the quantity of services used by the elderly, as well as on the costs of residential placement.

To measure the economic impact of RISPA, we gathered information about the services used by 1501 participants in the PRISMA-Estrie study. These data are available expressed as quantities and types of service used. Conversion of the quantities into costs made it possible to arrive at a shared measurement system in order to identify the overall impact of RISPA on use of these many social and health services. Cost measurement was arrived at by multiplying the quantity of services used by a unit cost[1]. Given the variety of services examined, determining unit costs was a major challenge, especially because few of the costs had been calculated prior to the study and services whose cost had not previously been calculated entailed a complex process of assessment. To perform this exercise we relied on existing studies but we also had to carry out several ourselves. The objective of this text is to explain how we determined unit costs for the purposes of measuring RISPA's economic impact.

The costs came under two broad categories. The first, which we designated as "RISPA costs," relates to the resources deployed to create the integrated network and the consequent restructuring of the way services to the elderly were managed, as well as resources invested in the network's operation. The second category, "service costs," covered the cost of health and social services delivered to the elderly. The methodology devised to identify the implementation and operational costs of RISPA is presented separately in Chapter 10 of this volume (Durand, Blanchette, and Hébert). This chapter focuses on service costs.

The first part of this chapter presents the context in which data were collected and the principles of economic assessment in the health field that guided our methodology. We then briefly describe our main data sources for services use and costs. Last, we present the methodology used to determine unit costs for services delivered to the elderly. We describe different types of costs, presenting some of our findings for each. The order in which these types of costs are presented respects the classification used in the two tables (21.10 and 21.11) at the end of this chapter, which provide an overview of our methodology. The types of costs consist of: (A), (B) residential placement / housing, including infrastructure and operations; (C) administrative support; (D) user-support activities; (E) nursing and assistance care; (F) surveillance; (G) respite services; (H), (I) consultations with physicians and other health and social services professionals; (J), (K) medications and pharmaceutical services; (L), (M), (N) hospital stays, including emergency room visits and surgeries; (O), (P) day hospital and day center visits; and (Q) travel for medical purposes. We classified life settings in 10 categories: 1) private dwelling, user-owned; 2) private dwelling, user-rented; 3) private dwelling, user as sole lodger; 4A) foster home, nine residents or fewer; 4B) private residential facility housing nine residents or fewer; 5A) facility attached to a larger institution and housing ten residents or more; 5B) private residential facility housing ten residents or more; 6- residential and long-term care center (CHSLD; *centre d'hébergement et de soins de longue durée*), private and under agreement; 7) CHSLD, private and not subject to an agreement; 8- public CHSLD, including long-term care units in hospitals (USLD; *unité de soins de longue durée*). We classified service-providing organizations into 7 headings: 1) public organization or institution; 2) volunteer organization; 3) private agency; 4) cooperative agency; 5) direct benefits; 6) residential facility with services optional; 7) residential facility or foster family with services included.

Context of the Study

The elderly people who were followed for this study lived in very diverse settings. Some occupied their own homes, whether as owners or tenants, while others lived in intermediate-type facilities or public or private CHSLDs, some of which are licensed by Quebec's department of health and social services (MSSS; *Ministère de la Santé et des Services sociaux*) and some of which are not. The elderly person's degree of frailty and place of residence both influence the cost of services[2]. Place of residence also had an impact on our methods of collecting data useful for cost determination, as well as the amount of data we could obtain. This was taken into account when we developed and applied our methodology.

Economic Assessment

To measure costs, we adopted the principle of opportunity cost advocated in the scientific literature on health economy[1,3,4]. Opportunity cost consists of the value that a given resource could have yielded if it had been put to the "best available alternative use"[3,4].

It is sometimes difficult to identify and measure opportunity cost[3]. For example, what would the opportunity cost be of work carried out by an employee transferred from a different service sector to that of services to elders under RISPA? How could we identify the value of this work before the transfer? In practice, market price was used[1,5]. According to economic theory, prices as found in the competitive marketplace reflect the opportunity cost of resources. Market price is thus a suitable method for conducting an economic assessment of reassigned resources. If the market price proves not to reflect opportunity cost sufficiently well because of market distortion, it must be adjusted[3]. In the example above, the value of the employee's work was determined on the basis of salary, which we considered to be representative of the work's opportunity cost.

When the amount spent on delivering a service can no longer be known or is no longer representative of the service's value, value is determined by replacement cost. Replacement cost corresponds to what it would cost to receive the same service from similar existing services that are easily accessible. Replacement cost can be assessed according to market value or gross replacement cost, depending on the type of resource and how available the information is. For example, it is not informative to estimate the value of a building several years old based on its cost at construction. We chose to use the municipal appraisal (market value), which more closely reflects its current value. We took the same approach with equipment, which was assessed at its current replacement cost rather than cost at the time of purchase.

In assessing costs, we adopted a societal perspective[1]. This means we took into account costs borne by all service providers: public, private, and volunteer.

The assignment of value to volunteer services, however, is not presented here, because the relevant analyses had not yet been completed when this book went to press.

RISPA's economic impact was measured based on differential costs[1, 3, 5]. We only considered services whose use might have been impacted by the presence or absence of an integrated services network and whose use could thus be subject to variation in costs from region to region.

We opted to value care and services using normalized costs applied to both the project experimental and control zones. This approach favored a more accurate measurement of RISPA's impact on service costs by highlighting differences in use while avoiding the need to take regional disparities and institutional performance differentials in various regions into account[5, 6].

Finally, it should be noted that we assessed costs in constant 2002 dollars in order to offset the possible effects of inflation.[1]

Services Use

A telephone survey conducted with participating elders allowed us to determine the frequency of use of the various services other than residential placement and related expenditures. For some types of services, such as meals-on-wheels, cost is directly related to frequency of use. On the other hand, for most of the services examined in this study, cost is also a function of the time invested in delivering the service or the nature of the service itself. Cases in point are nursing care, services delivered by health professionals, and assistance care. To estimate costs it is therefore necessary to first determine the duration and nature of each service (for example, for a visit to the dentist: annual check-up, cleaning, fillings, etc.). The information was difficult to get directly from the elders we surveyed because it was so specific. We therefore decided to estimate the average time or settle on a paradigm case for each of the services involved. We used numerous approaches to this end. In some cases, we conducted telephone surveys with health and social services workers. The number of contacts varied, depending on the type of service and the availability of service-provider respondents. Based on these surveys, we constructed a paradigm profile of services delivered to the elderly. For example, three dentists in the Estrie region were questioned about services usually delivered to this target group. In other instances, discussions with local professionals or a review of previous studies provided us with the information we needed.

Studies

The sources of the data that underlay our findings are numerous; but some stood out for their usefulness, and we therefore deemed it appropriate to offer a summary presentation of their contents so that readers are better able to grasp their role in our cost determination process.

HÉBERT ET AL. (1997):[2] Services requis par les personnes âgées en perte d'autonomie – Évaluation clinique et estimation des coûts selon le milieu de vie [Services needed by frail elders – A clinical assessment and an estimate of costs according to life setting]

This study conducted across various sectors used the Function Autonomy Measurement System (SMAF; *Système de mesure d'autonomie fonctionnelle*)[7] to assess the degree of disability of 1 977 frail elders living in nine different settings (at home; in family– and intermediate-type facilities; in CHSLDs). It then determined the resources needed to offset frailty and estimated the costs engendered by the care and services provided. The services assessed included residential placement: nursing, assistance, and support care; surveillance; transport; and administration. An estimate of costs and a determination of how cost financing was distributed across the public, private, and volunteer sectors was conducted based on financial data obtained from the institutions involved in the study and information gathered during interviews with the subjects.

For family- and intermediate-type facilities, the person who managed the residence was invited to fill in a questionnaire which gathered information on the residence's characteristics (number of rooms, inventory of furnishings and equipment, municipal assessment of lot and building values, operating expenses); the paid staff; expenses related to administering the residence; number of beds; occupancy rate; and, when appropriate, those living in the residence besides frail elders in placement. In the case of public institutions, most of the necessary information was obtained from AS-471 audited financial statements and AS-478 statistical reports or, in cases where more detailed information was needed, internal reports and specific questionnaires.

DUBUC ET AL. (2002):[8] Services requis par les personnes âgées en perte d'auto-nomie – Évaluation clinique et estimation des coûts sur le territoire de la Régie régionale de la santé et des services sociaux de Laval [Services needed by frail elders – A clinical assessment and an estimate of costs in the region covered by the Laval regional health and social services board]

In the region governed by the Laval regional health and social services board, Dubuc et al. conducted a study along essentially the same lines as that of Hébert et al. However, they enhanced their population sample by including private residential facilities among the life settings studied.

Survey on private residential facilities conducted by PRISMA – Estrie

Dubuc et al. (2002) did not provide sufficiently detailed data on the costs of services in private residential facilities to meet the needs of our study. We therefore conducted a study similar to theirs in 17 private residential facilities in the experimental zone. To determine the costs of different services, we used the same instruments as were used in the two previous studies.

DURAND ET AL. (2001):[9] Développement et implantation d'un système de prix de revient des soins et services à domicile dans le cadre du projet de démonstration d'un réseau intégré des services dans les Bois-Francs avec une coordination de services par gestion de cas (case-management) [Developing and implementing a system of cost assessment of in-home care and services as part of the demonstration project for an integrated services network in Bois-Francs, with service coordination by case management]

It is this study that gave rise to the PRISMA-Estrie project. The study sought to determine the impact of an integrated services network on frail elders and their support network, as well as on the use of health and social services. The impact examined, however, was strictly on public financing. Based on a quasi-experimental study design that included pre- and post-measurements, the study followed 482 subjects for 3 years, some of whom used the RISPA developed in the experimental zone. The costs estimated relate essentially to services delivered by public institutions: hospitalization, surgery, placement in a CHSLD, day-center visits, day-hospital visits, and use of the intensive functional rehabilitation unit (URFI; *unité de réadaptation fonctionnelle intensive*). Audited AS-471 financial statements, statistical reports, administrative files from computer applications (for instance, Med-echo), and calculations using activity-based accounting methods provided the database needed in calculating the costs of human resources for nursing and assistance care and associated costs specific to each type of service (diagnostic and therapeutic services, administrative and technical services, prostheses).

Unit-Cost Determination Methodology

In what follows, we present the approach we used to estimate the cost of each type of service examined in our study. Tables 21.1 to 21.9 provide an overview of the unit costs calculated by our assessment process for some categories of service; while tables 21.10 and 21.11, at the end of the chapter, provide details about the way our methodology was tailored to the specifics of the elders' life settings or the different types of services.

It should not be forgotten that our methodology relied on the use of constant 2002 dollars. When it was necessary to index in order to respect this requirement, we used Statistics Canada rates or rates provided by the Estrie health and social services agency, according to circumstance.

Residential Placement/Housing

Infrastructure and operations come under residential placement / housing costs. The infrastructure that serves to house the subjects of our study includes lot, building, furnishings, and equipment, as well as adjustments made to a home. The values used for lots and buildings were their municipal appraisal values, augmented in certain cases to take account of major renovations and adjustments to homes. For furnishings and equipment, we first drew up an inventory and then estimated values based on price lists provided by merchant groups or the MSSS. Amortization for all of these assets was calculated for a period ranging from 15 to 40 years in order to reduce the cost to a yearly basis and then to a daily, per-person basis.

In order to take advantage of the broadest possible data pool, we turned to numerous sources of information in determining the cost of residential placement. These included Hébert et al. (1997), Dubuc et al. (2002), and our own survey of the owners of private residential facilities. Within each of these studies, the methodology is the same for all types of life setting, with adjustments to take account specific features of each type[2].

"Operating costs" was understood to refer to all expenditures for maintenance intended to keep infrastructure in good condition; municipal taxes; insurance; electricity; heating; grounds maintenance; the purchase of various accessories; and telephone expenses. Data on operating expenditures were drawn from Statistics Canada sources and the financial statements of the residential facilities or health institutions, as appropriate. Daily placement/housing costs according to life setting and type of zone (urban or rural) are presented in Table 21.1.

It proved relevant to differentiate between public and private financing strictly for subjects living in intermediate-type facilities or institutions. Housing in other settings was considered to be wholly privately financed. Data drawn from Hébert et al. (1997) were used to calculate the proportion of financing that was public or private for each type of setting.

Table 21.1
Daily Cost of Housing, by Type of Setting

Milieu de vieSetting		Urban Zone	Rural Zone
1 to 3	Single-family dwelling	$14.74	$13.17
4A	Licensed interm. facility – 9 res. or fewer	$6.76	$6.62
4B	Unlicensed interm. facility – 9 res. or fewer	$7.13	$7.13
5A	Licensed interm. facility – 10 res. or more	$7.04	$5.05
5B	Unlicensed interm. facility – 10 res. or more	$6.60	$6.04
6	CHSLD – private, under agreement	$14.75	$9.48
7	CHSLD – private, not under agreement	$8.75	$8.90
8	CHSLD – public	$13.39	$13.14

Administrative Support

Administrative support refers to expenditures inherent in the management and supervision in the various types of settings. No costs of this kind are associated with residence in private dwellings. As regards family- and intermediate-type (or foster care) facilities and facilities that are part of a larger public institution, administrative support has two components: the cost of the support provided by the person responsible for running the facility, which covers various expenses (bank fees, professional honoraria); and the cost of the support provided by the institution responsible for supervising these settings[2]. In the case of CHSLDs, as in that of private residential facilities, administrative support covers general administration, the administration of care, and other related management expenses.

Daily costs, presented in Table 21.2, were calculated using statistics that varied according to the nature of the expenditure and setting (users, occupancy days, records, etc.). We had recourse to the same information sources as were used for calculating the cost of housing and the distribution of financing between the public and the private sectors[2, 8] (i.e., our surveys of owners of private residential facilities).

Administrative support also covers material and management structures that support health professionals in their work. This component was taken into consideration in calculating the cost of staffing; its assessment is described under the relevant headings.

Table 21.2
Daily Administrative-Support Costs, by Type of Setting

Setting		Urban Zone	Rural Zone
1 to 3	Single-family dwelling	—	—
4A	Licensed interm. facility – 9 res. or fewer	$3.57	$2.42
4B	Unlicensed interm. facility – 9 res. or fewer	$1.72	$1.72
5A	Licensed interm. facility – 10 res. or more	$5.29	$4.02
5B	Unlicensed interm. facility – 10 res. or more	$3.31	$3.08
6	CHSLD – private, under agreement	$16.62	$10.78
7	CHSLD – private, not under agreement	$8.96	$3.10
8	CHSLD – public	$17.86	$16.45

Support Activities

Support activities cover household maintenance, laundry, and food services. The services involved, like their providers, are many and various according to setting. For this reason, we were obliged to adopt several approaches in identifying their use and cost.

In the case of subjects who are institutionalized or living in intermediate-type facilities, all the services are provided by the host facility. We used the data in Hébert et al. (1997) and Dubuc et al. (2002) to determine the cost of these activities. The researchers identified overall costs of support activities using questionnaires or by analyzing financial statements. Then these costs were combined with various measurements, either obtained directly or determined by observation (occupancy days, meals, time invested per activity, etc.) in order to arrive at costs by occupancy day as presented in Table 21.3. Where appropriate, determining the distribution of public and private financing was done based on contributions by the individuals in residential placement, as in Hébert et al. (1997).

For subjects living in their own homes or in private residential facilities, the telephone survey allowed us to identify services provided by public and private networks, while SMAF helped us learn the frequency and duration of services provided on a volunteer basis[8]. The portion of SMAF that relates to resource-payment-frequency in the handicap section was referred to as "economic SMAF." This section covers information on resources to compensate for disabilities, payment source, and frequency of use.)[8] These costs were thus assessed based on hourly rates or cost per meal. Information on the costs of private sector services was obtained from the private agencies and the survey we conducted with the owners of private residential facilities. Community organizations' and public institutions' financial statements served in assessing the cost of their services and determining the proportions of public and private financing.

Table 21.3
Daily Cost of Total Support, by Type of Setting

Setting		Urban Zone	Rural Zone
1 to 3	Single-family dwelling	—	—
4A	Licensed interm. facility – 9 res. or fewer	$10.07	$12.21
4B	Unlicensed interm. facility – 9 res. or fewer		
	Maintenance and laundry	$2.28	$2.28
	Meals – optional	$6.16	$6.93
5A	Licensed interm. facility – 10 res. or more	$7.45	$6.40
5B	Unlicensed interm. facility – 10 res. or more		
	Maintenance and laundry	$1.33	$3.00
	Meals – optional	$6.16	$6.93
6	CHSLD – private, under agreement	$25.14	$21.65
7	CHSLD – private, not under agreement	$11.58	$11.42
8	CHSLD – public	$29.72	$33.84

Nursing and Assistance Care

Assistance care refers to hours spent with a subject assisting with personal care and activities of daily living. As in the case of support services, assistance care is given by many different providers, and this entailed methodological adjustments.

For individuals living at home or in private residential facilities, assistance services were assessed in a manner similar to that used for support services delivered in the same settings. Hourly rates are presented in Table 21.4. Nursing care is taken into account under the heading "professional consultations". Financing is classified private or public according to service provider.

Hébert et al. (2000)[10] present a regression equation that makes it possible to estimate the hours of nursing care required by elderly people in intermediate-type residential facilities or institutions. This equation is based on SMAF assessments. The same study showed that, in these settings, the level of response to need is close to 100 %, and the study differentiated between two types of service provider: professional and para-professional[2]. We therefore adopted this instrument to estimate the hours of care needed by those of our study subjects who lived in the types of settings in question. We used Hébert et al. (1997) and Dubuc et al. (2002) to calculate "mixed" professional and para-professional hourly rates as presented in Table 21.5. These rates we applied to the required care hours. When appropriate, the determination of distribution of public and private financing was based on contributions by the individuals in residential placement, as in Hébert el al. (1997).

Table 21.4
Hourly Rates for Assistance Care, by Service Provider

Service Provider		Urban Zone	Rural Zone
1	Public institution	$31.13	$31.13
2 and 4	Volunteer organization/Cooperative enterprise	$15.00	$15.00
3 and 5	Private agency/Direct benefits	$13.77	$14.12
6 and 7	Private residential facility, with services included or not	$11.27	$11.27

Table 21.5
Hourly Rate for Nursing and Assistance Care, by Setting

Setting		Urban Zone	Rural Zone
1 to 3	Single-family dwelling	—	—
4A	Licensed interm. facility – 9 res. or fewer	$6.33	$5.81
4B	Unlicensed interm. facility – 9 res. or fewer	—	—
5A	Licensed interm. facility – 10 res. or more	$11.77	$13.67
5B	Unlicensed interm. facility – 10 res. or more	—	—
6	CHSLD – private, under agreement	$27.05	$28.44
7	CHSLD – private, not under agreement	$8.59	$14.34
8	CHSLD – public	$25.75	$25.01

Surveillance

Surveillance covers the occasional minder services offered to individuals living at home, as well as the full-time service provided in other settings. To determine the cost of the occasional service, we inquired about number of hours by telephone survey and obtained hourly rates from various sources (MSSS circulars, cooperative financial statements, etc.), depending on the service provider.

For the full-time service, hours of surveillance correspond to the surveillance hours available, from which nursing- and assistance-care hours were subtracted. Hourly rates in private residential facilities were determined by the telephone survey. Those for other services were calculated based on the data in Hébert et al. (1997) and Dubuc et al. (2002).

Respite Services

The costs associated with respite service cover the costs of temporary placement, including housing; administrative support; user-support activities; nursing and assistance care; and surveillance; exactly as for residents of public CHSLDs.

Professional Consultations

Medical Consultations

The Quebec health insurance board (RAMQ; *Régie de l'assurance maladie du Québec*) publishes statistics on medical acts annually. More precisely, Table 2.12 for the year 2002 specifies the number and cost of medical acts by participant sex and age group and type of service (consultation, house call, CHSLD care, surgical act, and so on). This table gave us the information needed for calculating the cost of various types of consultations and medical acts for our study. Thus, for instance, the cost of a house call by a general practitioner corresponds to the average of the cost under "House Calls" for users aged 75 and over. The cost of a surgery corresponds to the sum of the averages of the costs under the headings "Surgical Acts," "Surgical Assistance," and "Surgical Anesthesia" for that same age group. Discussions with physicians and managers in institutions helped us to identify acts specific to each situation.

Since medical consultation is covered under the public system in Quebec, it was not necessary to calculate the distribution of financing.

Other Types of Professional Consultation

During the telephone survey, elders mentioned using services by a large variety of professionals. We retained from this only those services closely associated with people's health and functional and social autonomy. The various types of professionals concerned are presented in Table 21.6. Cost per consultation, whether consultations were in the office or in user homes, and whether they were publicly or privately funded, also appear there.

To estimate the cost of a consultation in the private sector for each professional, we placed a call to the relevant association or college, and asked the average rates and what types of services are generally offered to the elderly. We then confirmed this information by talking to a number of individual practitioners and agencies, depending on practitioner availability and the type of service. Note that the cost of a consultation covers the professional's remuneration, indirect costs related to the task (infrastructure and operating costs), and a profit share.

The situation of nurses working in private residential facilities is distinct, because nurses may have to travel to see the elderly several times a day for diverse reasons and for periods of varying lengths. Using the study by Gervais et al. (2004),[11] which enumerated and worked out the proportions of acts performed by nurses for the elderly in private residential facilities, we were able to estimate an average duration for their interventions. Further, from the survey we conducted with private residential facility owners, we were able to calculate the average hourly rate, with fringe benefits and administrative support included, for a nurse working in a private facility. Combining these two sources of information enabled us to determine a daily cost of $10.

Just as in the case of nurses working in private residential facilities, estimating the cost of consulting in the public system required two stages: estimating average time by type of consultation and determining a corresponding average hourly rate.

Information obtained from the annual AS-471 financial statements for 2002 from public institutions in the experimental and control zones enabled us to calculate hourly rates. We worked with basic salaries, increasing them to take into account contributions, fringe benefits, and expenditures associated with the activity, which included travel costs, stationary, supplies, and so on. To this, we added administrative expenditures representing a portion of infrastructure, equipment, and the administrative expenditures required to support practitioners in their work. These were calculated based on data from Dubuc et al. (2002) and using activity-based accounting, because we had available to us information on costs and relevant operational data (hours worked, surface used, etc.) for four local community services centers (CLSCs; *centre local de services communautaires*). Adding associated expenditures and administrative expenditures was done to ensure the comparability of these calculations with those for the private sector.

To estimate the duration of a consultation we referred to the same study, Dubuc et al. (2002), in which from one to six professionals (nurses, occupational therapists, physiotherapists, and social workers), depending on CLSC and type of professional, were observed over the course of two weeks. These observations made it possible to describe the various tasks performed by the professionals and link them to average durations.

The distinction between public and private financing took into account the type of professional in question and the sector (private or public), since users aged over 65 receive certain private-sector services (for example, visits to the optometrist) under the public regime.

Table 21.6
Cost per Professional Consultation, by Service Provider

Service Provider	Public Sector; in Office	Public Sector; in Home	Private Sector; in Office
Physiotherapist	$111.96	$128.99	$35.00
Psychosocial			
Social worker	$158.64	$173.34	$75.00
Psychologist	$96.73	$111.44	$80.00
Other professionals			
Optometrist	$40.50	$40.50	$40.50
Oxygen therapist	$72.45	$86.77	
Dietician / nutritionist	$101.30	$116.71	$60.00
Audiologist	$30.00	$30.00	$30.00
Chiropractor			$40.00
Dentist	$80.00		$80.00
Acupuncturist			$35.00
Chiropodist			$35.00
Orthodontist			$50.00

Medications

Depending on life setting, we distinguished between two types of medications and two distinct sources of information for determining cost. For all individuals not institutionalized and all those living in private CHSLDs, not subject to an agreement, we had access to the RAMQ database, which allowed us to determine an overall cost for all medications (understood to include pharmaceutical services) bought by each subject and to differentiate private from public financing (depending on users' health insurance plans). For institutionalized individuals, an average daily cost for pharmaceutical services and medications assumed by both private and public institutions was obtained from a report by the Estrie regional health and social services agency, which presented all the pharmacy-related costs and occupancy days for all Quebec CHSLDs. In the case of CHSLDs, the type of setting determines the source of financing.

Hospital Stays

Based on the information obtained from the telephone survey, data on hospital stays were compiled that identified the hospitalization unit, namely medicine and surgery, intensive care, geriatric acute care, intensive functional rehabilitation, emergency room, day surgery, and operating suite. Costs were calculated accordingly and covered, to differing extents for each unit, institutional infrastructure and equipment costs, staffing and related costs, diagnostic and therapeutic services, administrative and technical services, food services, medical acts, and, where appropriate, time in the operating suite and prosthesis costs.

We relied on four sources of information for these data, one of which was the study by Durand et al. (2001). In this study, which reported on an implementation project for an integrated services network in the Bois-Francs region, researchers developed and set up a cost system that enabled them to determine all the costs named above, except those for infrastructure and equipment, on one hand, and medical acts, on the other. We used these data and indexed them as constant 2002 dollars. As specified under the heading "Medical Consultations" above, the costs of medical acts were assessed using RAMQ statistics. We obtained a list of equipment and the equipment's value, as well as some operational data (relating to beds, rooms, hours of operation, gurneys) directly from the institution studied by Durand et al. (2001). In this way, we were able to determine the equipment value to assign to each hospital service. Last, infrastructure costs were estimated based on the municipal tax account for a hospital center that was of a similar kind and size and was part of our study. The value obtained in this way was pro-rated for the number of beds in each hospital department and adjusted to reflect the specificities of the emergency room and the operating suite. All the hospitalization and surgical costs (presented in Table 21.7) were publicly financed.

Table 21.7
Costs of Hospital Services

Unit of Hospitalization	Cost Unit	Cost
Medicine and surgery	Day	$404.75
Intensive care	Day	$907.10
Geriatric acute care	Day	$546.21
Intensive functional rehabilitation	Day	$513.09
Emergency room	Visit	$264.98
Day surgery	Operation	$1409.26
Surgery	Operation	$3160.98

Day Hospital and Day Center Visits

The cost of a visit to a day hospital or a day center includes health-professional salaries and related costs for their activities, facility maintenance, infrastructure value, and administrative expenditures.

The major portion of the cost of a day-hospital visit is based on data drawn from the study by Tousignant et al. (2001)[12]. Using financial information from the institution and from follow-up conducted during 1 year for 101 individuals aged over 75 admitted to various programs, Tousignant and colleagues were able to determine the cost of a day-hospital visit at the Sherbrooke University Geriatric Institute. For day-center visits, we based our calculations on the financial and operational data for four CLSCs studied by Dubuc et al. (2002) and obtained from their database.

In both cases, we added facility maintenance expenditures, infrastructure value, and administrative expenditures, since these were not included in the calculations mentioned above. We assessed these costs using the same approach as described under previous headings for other types of services and through recourse to the financial and operational data available for several institutions, including those that had been studied by Tousignant et al. (2001) and Dubuc et al. (2002).

The public system assumes all the costs of day-hospital and day-center services. These are presented in Table 21.8 below.

Table 21.8
Costs of Hospital and Day-Center Visits

Facility	Cost Unit	Cost
Day hospital	Day	$255.32
Day center	Half-day	$46.52

Travel

Under travel, we considered only travel related to the types of hospital stay and professional consultations covered by our study. As shown in Table 21.9, we compiled costs for travel by ambulance, car, and transport services provided by institutions.

To determine the cost of ambulance travel we compared costs as presented in studies and various financial statements, and we concluded by using as an average cost the budget allocated by the MSSS for this type of trip in 2002. Note that, for individuals aged over 64, these costs are assumed by the public system.

For subjects who traveled on their own, we assumed this was done by car. Our kilometrage rates correspond to those of the Canadian Automobile Association (2002)[13]. To calculate the average distance of a trip, we measured the distance between home and destination for a sample of subjects. For each territory for which these measurements were taken, destinations were grouped under one or two main locations (CLSC and hospital). Their addresses and those of subjects' places of residence were identified by postal code. MapQuest provided the kilometrage. The cost of these trips was considered to be assumed by the individual and was thus classified as privately financed.

Elders who are admitted to day hospitals and day centers have a choice of going there by their own means or using the institution's services. We used the data bank provided by Durand et al. (2001) to supplement our information and reflect this fact. This data bank cumulates the number and types of trips to a day center and the cost to the institution over a period of two years. By combining these data with the estimates obtained with MapQuest, we were able to determine the cost of an average trip for a day center or day hospital visit and differentiate the portions assumed by the public system and the user.

Table 21.9
Trip Costs

Type of Trip	Urban Zone	Rural Zone
Ambulance	$462.00	$462.00
Day center or day hospital – return trip	$11.92	$11.92
Professional consultation – return trip	$5.40	$12.53
Hospital – return trip	$5.40	$23.68

Conclusion

The health services and services for maintaining independence that are essential to the elderly vary a great deal. Type of service provider and type of life setting both influence the cost of services[2]. Determining the costs specific to each of these services was essential to allow us to measure the economic impact of RISPA as implemented in the Estrie region (see Chapter 13.) The scope and complexity of the determination of these unit costs justified developing a highly elaborate methodology. As presented above, we followed the principles of opportunity cost and replacement cost, and applied them within a societal perspective. The costs we assessed were restricted to those associated with services that RISPA could have an impact on. Moreover, we normalized costs for the experimental and control zones in order to eliminate regional and institutional disparities.

The methodology presented here could serve as the basis for other studies. The costs we have presented, determined in constant 2002 dollars, could also be of use for future economic assessments. Last, Tables 21.10 and 21.11 below provide an overview of our methodology for each type of cost and each type of setting.

Table 21.10
Service Costs: Summary of Methodology

Ten Life Settings in Both Urban and Rural Zones	Seven Types of Service-Providing Organizations
S1 Private dwelling, user-owned	1 Public organization or institution
S2 Private dwelling, user-rented	2 Volunteer organization
S3 Private dwelling, user as sole lodger	3 Privately run agency
S4A Foster home, 9 residents or fewer	4 Cooperative or collective enterprise
S4B Private residential facility, 9 residents or fewer	5 Direct benefits
S5A Facility attached to larger institution, 10 residents or more	6 Residential facility, services optional
S5B Private residential facility, 10 residents or more	7 Residential facility or foster family, services included
S6 CHLSD, private and under agreement	
S7 CHSLD private and not under agreement	
S8 Public CHSLD, including USLDs in hospital centers	

Three volunteering scenarios	Regarding usage:
Rate of zero	TS Source of info. is telephone survey/follow-up
Public-sector rates	n number/quantity
Private-sector rates at minimum wage	

Information sources on costs (adjusted to 2002 dollars)

ST-1997 Hébert et al. (1997)[2]: Services requis par les personnes âgées en perte d'autonomie – Évaluation clinique et estimation des coûts selon le milieu de vie [Services needed by frail elders – A clinical assessment and an estimate of costs according to life setting]

ST-BF Durand et al. (2001)[9]: Développement et implantation d'un système de prix de revient des soins et services à domicile dans le cadre du projet de démonstration d'un réseau intégré des services dans les Bois-Francs avec une coordination de services par gestion de cas (case-management) [Developing and implementing a system of cost assessment of in-home care and services as part of the demonstration project for an integrated services network in Bois-Francs, with service coordination by case management]

ST-Laval Dubuc et al. (2002)[8]: Services requis par les personnes âgées en perte d'autonomie – Évaluation clinique et estimation des coûts sur le territoire de la Régie régionale de la santé et des services sociaux de Laval [Services needed by frail elders – A clinical assessment and an estimate of costs in the region covered by the Laval regional health and social services board]

ST-TM Dubuc et al. (2002)[1]: Temps consacré aux différentes activités de services de soutien à domicile fournis par les CLSC de la RRSSS de Laval [Time dedicated to various in-home maintenance services provided by CLSCs under the Laval regional health and social services boards]

Information sources on costs (adjusted to 2002 dollars)

ST-PR   Survey on private residential facilities conducted by PRISMA-Estrie

ST-RIS   Study of RISPA implementation and operating costs conducted by PRISMA – Estrie (See Chapter 10)

ST-IMP   Veil, A., and Hébert, R. (2005):[2] Évaluation de l'implantation des mécanismes et outils d'intégration des services aux personnes âgées en perte d'autonomie: Résultats de mise en œuvre [An assessment of the implementation of the mechanisms and tools for integrating services for frail elders: Implementation findings]

1. Dubuc, N., Hébert, R., Buteau, M., and Coulombe, C. Temps consacré aux différentes activités de services de soutien à domicile fournis par les CLSC de la RRSSS de Laval. Research report. Centre de recherche sur le vieillissement and Régie régionale de la santé et des services sociaux de Laval: 2002.

2. Veil, A., Hébert, R., and the PRISMA-Estrie Team. Évaluation de l'implantation des mécanismes et outils d'intégration des services aux personnes âgées en perte d'autonomie. (Interim report: Étude de cas comparative entre trois MRC de l'Estrie, résultats partiels). Sherbrooke: Centre for Research on Aging of the Sherbrooke University Geriatric Institute, 2002.

Table 21.11

Service Costs – Overview Presentation of Constituent Elements

Category Description	Usage: Our Information Sources	Measurement Unit	Costs: Our Information Sources	Costs: Financing Sources
(A) Residential placement/housing: infrastructure Lot, building, equipment	TS: n days spent in setting	Day of presence	S1 to 3, urban and rural; 4A, 5A, 6 to 8, rural: ST-1997, indexed S4A, 5A, 6 to 8, urban: Weighted average ST-1997 and ST-Laval, indexed S4B and 5B: ST-PR	Depending on whether setting is private or public As necessary, private/public ratio based on contributions made by adults in placement, as per ST-1997
(B) Residential placement/housing: operations Maintenance costs	TS: n days spent in setting	Day of presence	S1 to 3, urban and rural; 4A, 5A, 6 to 8, rural: ST-1997 indexed S4A, 5A, 6 to 8, urban: Weighted average ST-1997 and ST-Laval, indexed S4B and 5B ST-PR	Depending on whether setting is private or public As necessary, private/public ration based on contributions made by adults in placement, as per ST-1997
(C) Administrative support (S4A-B, 5A-B, 6 to 8) Costs of managing facility infrastructures	TS: n days spent in setting	Day of presence	S4A, 5A 6 to 8 rural: ST-1997, indexed S4A, 5A, 6 to 8, urban: Weighted average ST-1997 and ST-Laval, indexed S4B and 5B: ST-PR	Depending on whether setting is public or private As appropriate, public/private ratio is based on contributions made by adults in placement, as per ST-1997
(S4A and 5A) Supervision of licensed residences and facilities attached to an institution	TS: n days spent in setting	Day of presence	ST-1997, indexed	Public
(D) User-support activities (S1 to 3, 4B, 5B) Housekeeping and laundry (IADL) and food services	TS: n IADL-type hrs; "economic SMAF" items to determine volunteer contribution	Service hour	Service provider TS Hourly rates: 1: See consultation subsections 2, 4, 5: Portrait des entreprises en aide domestique, produced by Industrie et Commerce Québec[1], 2000-2001, indexed 3: See consultation subsections Volunteerism: three scenarios	Depending on whether service provider is public, private, or volunteer Direct benefits considered as public financing Public financing to household-aid service providers and tax credit of 23 % for home support taken into account

Category Description	Usage: Our Information Sources	Measurement Unit	Costs: Our Information Sources	Costs: Financing Sources
	(S1 to 3, 4B, 5B) TS: n meals received; other meals determined differentially; "economic SMAF" items to determine volunteer contribution	Meal	Service provider TS / Cost per meal / 2, 4: Sercovie's financial statements as at August 31, 2001 / 6, 7: ST-PR / Other meals: ST-1997, indexed / Volunteerism: three scenarios	Depending on whether service provider is public, private, or volunteer / Other meals viewed as privately funded
	(S4A-B, 5A-B, 6 to 8) TS: n days spent in setting	Day of presence	S4A, 5A, 6 to 8, rural: ST-1997, indexed / S4A, 5A, 6 to 8, urban: Weighted average ST-1997 and ST-Laval, indexed / S4B and 5B: ST-PR	Depending on whether setting is public or private / As appropriate, public/private ratio is based on contributions made by adults in placement, as per ST-1997
(E) Nursing and assistance care Assistance with ADL	**(S1 to 3, 4B, 5B)** TS: n hrs of assistance received (ADL); "economic SMAF" items to determine contribution	Service hour	Service provider TS / Hourly rates: / 1: See consultation subsections / 2, 4: Two home services coops, 2004 rates equal to those for 2002 / 3, 5: ST-1997, indexed / 6, 7: ST-PR / Volunteerism: three scenarios	Depending on whether service provider is public, private, or volunteer / Direct benefits considered as public financing / Public contribution to funding via tax credit of 23 % for in-home maintenance taken into account
All forms of nursing and assistance care provided by setting	**(S4A, 5A, 6 to 8)** Regression equation as presented in Hébert et al. (2001) used to determine n hrs of service needed	Required-service hour	Basic hourly rates for nursing and assistance care: for urban zones, weighted average as per ST-1997 and ST-Laval, indexed; for rural zones, as per ST-1997, indexed / Hourly rates determined the service provider's weighting of professional and paraprofessional components of service	Depending on whether setting is public or private / As appropriate, public/private ratio is based on contributions made by adults in placement, as per ST-1997

Category Description	Usage: Our Information Sources	Measurement Unit	Costs: Our Information Sources	Costs: Financing Sources
(F) Surveillance Occasional minder services for users living at home	(S1 to 3) TS: n hrs of surveillance received	Service hour	Service provider TS Hourly rates: 1: 2002 rates, as per annex to MSSS circular 2003-003 2, 4: Two home services coops, 2004 rates equal to those for 2002 3: ST-1997, indexed	Depending on whether service provider is public or private Public contribution to funding via tax credit of 23 % for in-home maintenance taken into account
Surveillance that may be provided for as much as 24 hrs per day	(S1 to 3) "Economic SMAF" items to determine n hrs required and supplied by close circle	Provided-surveillance hour	Three scenarios	Volunteer
	(S4B and 5B) n hrs surveillance available less n hrs ADL assistance received by TS		ST-PR	Depending on specific private setting Public contribution to funding via tax credit of 23 % for in-home maintenance taken into account
	(S4A, 5A, 6 to 8) 24 h less n hrs of nursing and assistance care required (see Subsection E)		S4A, urban and rural: 5A, 6 to 8, rural: ST-1997, indexed. S5A, 6 to 8, urban: weighted average as per ST-1997, indexed, and ST-Laval, indexed S4B and 5B: ST-PR	Depending on whether setting is public or private As appropriate, public/private ratio is based on contributions made by adults in placement, as per ST-1997
(G) Respite services All costs associated with temporary placement, including:	TS: n days respite care	Day of presence	For S3, placement costs cumulated as per subsections A, B, C, and D	The private contribution is equivalent to $20/day, according to the Finance Department of the Sherbrooke University Geriatric Institute. This sum covers all service

Category Description	Usage: Our Information Sources	Measurement Unit	Costs: Our Information Sources	Costs: Financing Sources
Nursing and assistance care	TS: n days; calculation of hrs of services required (see Subsection E)	Required-service hour	For S8, see Subsection E	
Surveillance	TS: n days; 24 h less n hrs of nursing and assistance care required (see Subsection E)	Service hour	For S8, see Subsection E	
(H) Consultation with physician Family physicians and specialized physicians	TS: n visits per type of medical specialty	Visit	Average cost of an examination (for general practitioners) or a consultation (for specialists) in *Statistiques RAMQ*, Table 2.12, relative to users aged over 75 for the year 2002	Public
(I) Other types of consultation Health and social services professionals	TS: n visits by type of professional	Visit	Private: Rate lists provided by professional college or governing body Public: Intervention time: estimates based on ST-TM Rates for various professionals: averages of salaries, benefits, and supplies for relevant centers in experimental and control territories, as per financial statements as at March 31, 2002; plus administrative and infrastructural expenditures (based on ST-Laval)	TS: public or private

Category Description	Usage: Our Information Sources	Measurement Unit	Costs: Our Information Sources	Costs: Financing Sources
(J) Medications administered at home All prescription medications purchased over the course of the year	**S1 to 3, 4 A-B, 5 A-B, 7** User's RAMQ record	Specific total cost for each study subject	RAMQ data bank, including costs of pharmaceutical-services and medication costs	RAMQ data bank: public contribution made by RAMQ (under prescription-drug insurance plan); private contribution made by user
(K) Pharmaceutical and medication services provided by institution All prescription medications provided to study subjects	**M6 and 8** TS: n days spent in setting	Day of presence	Provincial average daily cost, calculated based on data in report 2001-2002, *Pharmacie-Médicaments seulement, Coût moyen des médicaments par jour en CHSLD*	Provincial average cost for public CHSLDs Provincial average cost for CHSLD that are private and under agreement
(L) Hospitalization Infrastructures, management, care, services, non-surgical medical acts and medication services provided by institution	TS: n nights hospitalized and emergency room visits (without overnight stay); department determined by consulting patient records	Day of presence	Average daily cost calculation based on ST-BF Addition of a cost for medical acts (see Subsection H), equipment and infrastructure	Public
(M) Day surgery All costs related to temporary hospitalization and surgery	TS: n hospital visits	Cost per surgery (including hospital stay)	Average daily cost calculation based on ST-BF Estimation of costs for surgical acts based on *Statistiques RAMQ*, Table 2.12, year 2002 Cost of equipment and infrastructure taken into account	Public

Category Description	Usage: Our Information Sources	Measurement Unit	Costs: Our Information Sources	Costs: Financing Sources
(N) Surgery with hospital stay All costs related to surgery	Hospital TS: "Yes" in "Surgery" column	Cost per surgery (excluding hospital stay)	Average daily cost calculation based on ST-BF Estimation of costs for surgical acts based on *Statistiques RAMQ*, Table 2.12, year 2002 Cost of equipment and infrastructure taken into account	Public
(O) Day hospital visit All infrastructure-, consulting-, and care-related costs	TS: n day hospital visits	Day	Average cost of a visit as per IUGS study Tousignant et al. (2001), including specialized services, indexed Cost added to reflect administrative support, maintenance, and infrastructure	Public
(P) Centre de jour All costs	TS: n day center visits	Half-day	Average cost, including cost of professional services, meals etc., administrative support, maintenance and infrastructure, determined base on data in ST-Laval	Public
(Q) Travel Travel for medical and psychosocial reasons	TS: services for which the elder did or did not travel by ambulance (hospitalization, office visit to see a health or social services worker, day center visit, day hospital visit)	Ambulance trip Trip made by means other than ambulance	Average overall cost of an ambulance trip according to MSSS budget 2001-02 Cost per km as per Canadian Automobile Club Estimated average distance from place of residence to destination (hospital, clinic, day hospital, day center) based on MapQuest applied to a sample	Pour individuals aged over 64, financing is 100 % public, with some exceptions (which were not taken into account) Viewed as being 100 % private, except for day center and day hospital services, for which the public/private ration was based on ST-BF

Category Description	Usage: Our Information Sources	Measurement Unit	Costs: Our Information Sources	Costs: Financing Sources
(R) RISPA costs				
Amortization of RISPA's implementation costs (seven years) and operating costs				
Related to coordinated action and single entry point	**(S1 to 3, 4A-B, 5A-E)** TS: n days of presence in life setting	Day of presence	ST-RIS	Public Non-material private and volunteer costs
Related to case management and SIGG use	**(S1 to 3, 4A-B, 5A-E)** n days case-management file active, as per ST-IMP	Day of presence	ST-RIS	Public Non-material private and volunteer costs

1. Industrie et Commerce Québec. Portrait des entreprises en aide domestique. Direction des coopératives, Ministère de l'Industrie et du Commerce, 2002.

References

1. Drummond, M. F., O'Brien, B. J., Stoddart, G. L., and Torrance, G. W. Méthodes d'évaluation économique des programmes de santé. Paris: Économica, 1998. Note: After this entry, I will not hilite in blue the places where I change "et" to "and" and precede the word "and" with a comma, in multiple-author entries.

2. Hébert, R., Dubuc, N., Buteau, M. Roy, C., Desrosiers, J., Bravo, G., Trottier, L., and St-Hilaire, C. Services requis par les personnes âgées en perte d'autonomie – Évaluation clinique et estimation des coûts selon le milieu de vie. Series "Études et analyse. Quebec City: Ministère de la Santé et des services sociaux, Direction de la recherche et de l'évaluation, 1997.

3. Weinstein, M., Siegel, J., Gold, M., Kamlet, M., and Russell, L. Recommendations of the Panel on Cost-Effectiveness in Health and Medicine. Journal of the American Medical Association. 1996; 276(15): 1253-1258. [Note: Here I added upper-case letters because the sequence of words in question represents the name of the panel rather than the title of the article.]

4. Robinson, R. Economic evaluation and health care: Costs and cost-minimisation analysis. British Medical Journal. 1993; 307(6906): 726-8.

5. Bourgueil, Y., Brémond, M., Develay, A., Grignon, M., Midy, F., Naiditch, M., and Polton, D. L'évaluation des réseaux de soins, enjeux et recommandations. Centre de recherche d'étude et de documentation en économie de la santé (CREDES), Groupe Image-Ensp., 2001.

6. Raikou, M., Briggs, A., Gray, A., and McGuire, A. (2000). Centre-specific or average unit costs in multi-centre studies? Some theory and simulation. Health Economics. 2000; 9: 191-198.

7. Hébert, R., Guilbeault, J., Desrosiers, J., and Dubuc, N. The functional autonomy measurement system (SMAF): A clinical-based instrument for measuring disabilities and handicaps in older people. Geriatrics Today: Journal of the Canadian Geriatrics Society. 2001; 4: 141-147.

8. Dubuc, N., Tousignant, M., Hébert, R., Buteau, M., and Coulombe, C. Services requis par les personnes âgées en perte d'autonomie – Évaluation clinique et estimation des coûts sur le territoire de la Régie régionale de la santé et des services sociaux de Laval. Rapport numéro 3. Research report submitted to the Régie régionale de la santé et des services sociaux de Laval. Sherbrooke: 2002.

9. Durand, P. J., Lemay, A., Tourigny, A., Bonin, L., and Paradis, M. Développement et implantation d'un système de prix de revient des soins et des services à domicile dans le cadre du projet de démonstration d'un réseau intégré de services dans les Bois-Francs avec une coordination des services

de gestion de cas (case-management). (Report QC123). Fonds pour l'adaptation des services de santé, 2001.

10. Hébert, R., Dubuc, N., Buteau, M., Desrosiers, J., Bravo, G., Trottier, L. St-Hilaire, C., and Roy, C. Resources and costs associated with disabilities of elderly people living at home and in institutions. Canadian Journal of Aging; 2000: 20(1): 1-21.

11. Gervais, P., Hébert, R. Tousignant, M. Profils d'autonomie fonctionnelle des personnes âgées vivant dans les résidences privées d'hébergement en Estrie. Research report. Center for Research on Aging of the Sherbrooke University Geriatric Institute. 2004.

12. Tousignant, M. Hébert, R., and Desrosiers, J. Economic evaluation of geriatric day hospital: Cost-benefit analysis based on functional autonomy changes. A report prepared for the Health Transition Fund, Health Canada. Sherbrooke: National Evaluation of the Cost-Effectiveness of Home Care and Centre de recherche en gérontologie et gériatrie de Sherbrooke, 2001.

13. Canadian Automobile Association. Coût d'utilisation d'une automobile. Ottawa: 2002.

Chapter 22
Case-Finding of Older Persons with Moderate to Severe Disabilities by means of PRISMA-7 Questionnaire: A Presentation of the Instrument, Its Implementation, and Its Use[*]

Michel Raîche, Réjean Hébert, Marie-France Dubois, Johanne Bolduc, Maryse Grégoire, Céline Bureau, and Anne Veil

Highlights

- Until now little case-finding has been done for older persons with moderate to severe disabilities.
- This article presents an overview of the topic, proposes an instrument, and describes its use and implementation.
- The PRISMA-7 questionnaire has a sensitivity of 78 % and a specificity of 75 % for case-finding individuals with a SMAF score of ≤ -15.
- Currently the questionnaire is used in the emergency room, in local community service centers, and during vaccination campaigns; it is administered by telephone, in written form, or by face-to-face interview.
- Taking an approach that is both opportunistic and systematic, it is possible to identify prevalent cases of significant disability previously unknown to the health system and maximize the potential for intervention effectiveness.

Keywords: Case-finding – Disability – Older people – Validity – Implementation

---
[*] This chapter has been translated and is reproduced here by kind permission of *La Revue de Gériatrie*, where it appeared as: Raîche M, Hébert R, Dubois M-F, Grégoire M, Bolduc J, Bureau C, Veil A. Le repérage des personnes âgées en perte d'autonomie modérée à grave avec le questionnaire PRISMA-7: présentation, implantation et utilisation. La Revue de Gériatrie, 2007; 32(3): 209-218.

Summary

A significant proportion of older adults live at home with moderate to severe disabilities. Short of completing an exhaustive assessment, the only way to identify these individuals is with a case-finding tool. The Eastern Townships region in Québec, Canada, implemented different approaches to identify these persons. The PRISMA-7 case-finding tool had previously been developed to identify older adults with moderate to severe disability who could benefit from integrated services. The tool has been used progressively in different settings and at different times, including the single entry point for accessing services for older people in Sherbrooke. Implementation began in emergency departments at the university hospital. Surgery preparatory clinics then started using the tool. The annual influenza vaccination campaign provides a good opportunity to perform quasi-systematic case-finding. Using PRISMA-7 in all these settings could be described as a mix between an opportunistic (single entry, emergency, surgery preparatory clinics) and systematic (influenza annual vaccination) approach. The persons identified by the tool should then be referred for disability assessment. The processes, approach, and logistics for assessment are discussed.

Introduction

A large proportion of elders live at home with significant disabilities[1, 2]. Some of these individuals are not known to the health system and could possibly benefit by being assessed. In an optimal health system, all elders presenting with mild, moderate, or serious disabilities would be identified and assessed, and the interventions they needed would be in place. In practice, however, not even all moderate to serious disabilities are detected by clinicians in their elderly patients. Very little work has been done on proven methods for case-finding dependent elders. Yet numerous screening instruments have been validated for identifying other health issues and events that affect elders and these are being put to varying degrees of use[3-5].

Why has disability case-finding elicited so little interest to date? In 1991, *The Lancet* published an editorial on just this topic[6] and put forward an explanation, including several factors. The list included lack of time for evaluation, under-reporting of disability problems by users, and overly long or complex questionnaires developed mainly for use in research. Other publications dating from 1999[7] and 2004[8] indicate this crucial issue was still of concern at those dates; and so it is to this day. We have only begun taking concrete steps to address it. Some authors have examined the difficulties associated with case-finding elders with specific conditions, including some disabilities and frailty[9, 10].

Failure to case-find significantly disabled elders has consequences. Clinicians and managers involved in in-home and hospital service delivery too often find themselves facing elderly users and wondering why they didn't know and hadn't seen these individuals before. How, they ask, could this person have reached such an advanced stage of disability without attracting the attention of a health and social services worker? Often these individuals are encountered in the emergency room (ER), an entry point into the Quebec health system commonly used by elders or members of their close circles who do not know where else to turn.

When family caregivers contact the health system at an advanced stage of burnout, mechanisms for stabilizing a condition of disability are few. Early intervention, especially if case-finding is used, could prevent things reaching this stage. Without it, the necessary measures consist of the emergency mobilization of many home-support workers in an effort to avoid, at least to some extent, needless extended hospital stays and repeated ER visits, which constitute the health system's costly and inappropriate responses to a fundamental problem.

But are there effective interventions to be made once disabled elders are identified? The response to disability is by nature multidisciplinary, involving numerous institutional health and social services workers, organizations, and service providers whose roles are complementary and who must coordinate their actions. Coordinated and integrated intervention appears to offer the best hope for a solution[11, 12]. The absence of coordination can itself become a risk factor for disability[13].

We would like to specify here the distinction between screening and case-finding. "Screening" refers to the identification of individuals who will be affected in the future by a particular pathology or state of dependency. It is an instrument for predicting incident cases. "Case-finding" refers to identifying individuals already affected by a given pathology or state of dependency; it deals with prevalent cases[14].

When conducting our research, we reviewed numerous publications dealing with predictors of functional decline and screening for disability. What can be observed is that very little screening is actually done on the ground. Perhaps this is because, before turning to the question of elders who will develop disabilities, we must take care of all those who are already significantly disabled and not known to the system.

In the Estrie health region of Quebec, the implementation in 2001 of an integrated services network for the elderly (RISPA; French *réseau intégré de services pour personnes âgées*) took place with involvement by the research team on a project known as PRISMA (Program on Research for Integrating Services for the Maintenance of Autonomy)[11, 12]. The need for an instrument to case-find disabled elders emerged in the course of discussions relating to coordination to implement RISPA. The health and social services workers involved wished to make the transition from a reactive to a proactive approach vis-à-vis disability, thereby avoid being required to put out fires once situations have become urgent.

In 2005, Quebec's department of health and social services (MSSS; French name *Ministère de la Santé et des Services sociaux*) published an action plan for the years 2005 to 2010[15]. Page 39 of the action plan states:

> Act early, in accordance with recognized practice standards, to reduce dependency among the elderly whose health conditions require acute care:
> Develop a disability case-finding protocol that takes account of sex-related specifics, to be used in hospital emergency rooms and at hospital admissions desks, so that physicians and other health professionals can suit all their subsequent interventions to the individual's needs profile. [translation]

Consequently, the MSSS has addressed the secondary prevention of significant (i.e., moderate to serious) disabilities. What is needed is to intervene somewhat upstream of the development of various aspects of functional decline, even if the onset of disability itself has already begun. In a **population-based public health approach**, it is highly desirable to identify elders who are becoming disabled and prevent their condition from deteriorating. This gives rise to four questions: **what instrument to use, how to use it, where to use it, and what to do when individuals are identified as positive. The following sections of this chapter** seek to answer these questions. They present the PRISMA-7 instrument, statistics on its use, and areas for exploration and discussion relative to the implementation of a case-finding procedure.

The instrument

Lacking a recognized instrument for case-finding significantly disabled elders, many clinicians have developed in-house instruments in their own work settings. These pinpoint the main and most common problems affecting the elderly, which are associated with disabilities. Often, these instruments contain questions on memory difficulties, medications, falls, and the need for housekeeping assistance.

It is often observed that these instruments gradually become longer over time. Questions are progressively added on nutrition, then mobility, because that is important too, and so on. All these questions are clinically relevant. Nevertheless, the moment comes when one must choose between a brief summary instrument that has been validated using a standard measure for disabilities and simply conducting an exhaustive disability assessment. When determining a person's disabilities entails answering an excessively time-consuming assemblage of questions, measuring the disabilities directly makes more sense. For mass case-finding, an instrument that is short, if possible simple, and validated (i.e., that has been shown to have reliable levels of sensitivity and specificity) is essential.

Existing studies on screening and case-finding among elders have mainly addressed general health problems, although they mention disabilities[16, 17]. To our knowledge, very few have actually used disabilities as a validity criterion[10, 18-25]. Some, it is true, present a procedure for detailed validation and information on sensitivity and specificity[19-25]. One study used very broad criteria (dependency on another person for a certain form of daily care a few times over the course of a year),[22] while another used a construct validity design[19]. One article describes an approach that is both prospective and prevalence based;[21] others offer a strictly prospective design;[22-24] still others present a prevalence measure alone[20, 25].

The definition of disability must be specified. Attention to the activities of daily living (ADL) and instrumental activities of daily living, i.e., domestic activities (IADL), often obscures other dimensions of disability such as cognitive and mobility function, which merit more attention[10, 23]. Many authors agree on this point, yet very few studies report validation of a case-finding method that is sensitive to multi-dimensional disabilities. Only two articles[20, 25] report on a validation process that relied on a clinical instrument that measures disabilities in a multi-dimensional manner. (The instrument was the Functional Autonomy Measurement System (SMAF; French name *Système de mesure de l'autonomie fonctionnelle*)[26]. The first of these articles presents findings for an instrument intended for use in the ER[20]. Unfortunately, the instrument had a low sensitivity (≤ 60 %) for at least one disability in each SMAF subgroup of items assessed. The second article[25] describes an instrument for identifying disabled elders (including the mildly disabled) that appears not to have seen use because it found too large a part of the aged population. Concentrating on moderate to severe disabilities seems to be more feasible and clinically realistic[11, 12].

We developed PRISMA-7 to meet the need to identify moderately to severely disabled elders. We have published elsewhere a detailed account of how the instrument was developed[27]. Briefly, from an initial list of 21 yes/no questions, we identified the 7 that proved useful for identifying elders with a SMAF score of ≤ -15 (see Figure 22.1). SMAF is a clinical independence-measurement scale comprising 29 items that assess five dimensions of disability: ADL (7 items), communication (3 items), cognitive function (5 items), mobility (6 items), and IADL (8 items). Every item is scored from 0 (independent) to -3 (dependent), and the maximum score is -87. We used clinical and epidemiological criteria[1, 12, 28] in arriving at a threshold of -15 to distinguish mild disability from moderate to serious. It should be noted that, when it was developed, SMAF underwent in-depth validation[26, 29-31] and that, since 2002, it has been designated by the MSSS for clinician use across Quebec to measure the functional independence of the elderly. It is also being used increasingly abroad. Thus, in Quebec, when clinicians refer to a SMAF score of ≤ -15, they are using a shared and familiar language.

Figure 22.1
The Seven PRISMA-7 Questions

Question	Answer	
1. Are you more than 85 years old?	Yes	No
2. Male?	Yes	No
3. In general, do you have any health problems that require you to limit your activities?	Yes	No
4. In general, do you have any health problems that require you to stay at home	Yes	No
5. Do you need someone to help you on a regular basis?	Yes	No
6. In case of need, can you count on someone close to you?	Yes	No
7. Do you regularly use a cane, a walker or a wheelchair to move about?	Yes	No

Number of Yes and No answers	____	____

We validated PRISMA-7 by obtaining responses to it from 594 individuals aged 75 and over and living at home. The same individuals were then assessed with SMAF at home. The proportion who scored ≤ -15 was 19.4 %. These people belonged to the group we wished to identify with our case-finding instrument. Two PRISMA-7 threshold scores were highly interesting with respect to sensitivity and specificity. Table 22.1 presents our results for thresholds of three or more yes answers and four or more yes answers in responding to the PRISMA-7 questionnaire.

Table 22.1
The PRISMA-7 Questionnaire's Case-Finding Properties for Elders with a SMAF Score of ≤ -15.

Critical Threshold	Positive Findings	Sensitivity	Specificity	Predictive Value	
				Positive	Negative
3 or more yes answers	35.5 %	78.3 %	74.7 %	42.7 %	93.5 %
4 or more yes answers	19.0 %	60.9 %	91.0 %	62.0 %	90.6 %

This combination of sensitivity and specificity makes the instrument extremely useful for public health purposes. The time needed to administer the questionnaire is minimal. Simple, rapid use of the instrument makes it possible to conduct mass case-finding of prevalent significant disability. As well, PRISMA-7 has the advantage of circumventing the three factors identified at the start of this article as obstacles to awareness of disability. That is, it makes it possible to identify when full assessments are needed and thus avoid the time problem associated with trying to assessing *all* elders. As well, it was validated based on elders' own perceptions on one hand and a rigorous assessment of degree of disability on the other. Therefore, we know that it is not subject to distortion by users who under-assess their own disability problems. Finally, the instrument was not developed exclusively for research purposes, so its clinical usefulness is not just potential but actual, as will be seen in the following sections of this chapter.

How to use PRISMA-7

Since PRISMA-7 consists of seven yes/no questions, it is comparatively simple to use. It is necessary merely to follow a few instructions, the main one being that the elder's answers must be considered correct. At the stage of collecting the yes/no answers, no clinical judgment must be made: The assessor is not called upon to determine the correctness of the answers. It should not be forgotten that when the instrument was developed, elders' own impressions were compared with a clinical assessment of degree of disability. To introduce answers other than the elders' own would skew the results. The instrument can be used by telephone, in written form, or in a face-to-face interview. A user guide has been developed and published in the form of a book chapter[32] available online free of charge at www.usherbrooke.ca/prisma.

The Two Threshold Scores

No case-finding instrument is 100 % sensitive and specific. It is always necessary to reach a compromise between the two parameters, depending on the problem to be detected. The two thresholds (three or more yes answers and four or more yes answers) presented in Table 22.1 represent attractive options. During implementation, some teams chose to start with the threshold of four or more yes answers and lowered it to three after the break-in period. It is up to decision-makers and clinicians to choose the preferred threshold according to their teams' processes for assessing new cases of age-related disability.

Approaches

In this kind of mass case-finding, three approaches are possible. One can begin with an opportunistic approach that uses the elder's contacts with the health system to conduct case-finding (for example, at the single entry point, in the ER, at outpatient clinics, and in physician offices). It is also possible to take a systematic or quasi-systematic approach by administering the questionnaire to all elders during annual immunization campaigns (which reach a large proportion of the elderly population) or during annual check-ups. The third approach is mixed, consisting of combining the first two to maximize the potential for detecting prevalent cases.

If the mixed case-finding approach is adopted, it is probable a significantly disabled elder will be identified more than once during different contacts with the system. An efficient online method of communication is clearly very valuable in this form of case-finding process. Depending on the point where an elder makes contact, access to clinical information about the person makes it possible to determine whether this is someone already known to the system, whether degree of disability has been recently assessed, and whether the person's condition has changed significantly since the last assessment. In this way, it is possible to decide whether case-finding is appropriate. In case of doubt, the questionnaire's minimal time requirement justifies administering it.

Where should the case-finding instrument be used?

The first stage in deciding where the instrument should be used consists of identifying the points of entry into the health and social services system (for the opportunistic approach) and health events that bring together many elderly people and place them in regular contact with the system (for the systematic approach). For example, "dead time" users spend in waiting rooms could be put to good use. By targeting locations with a high level of attendance by elderly people, we maximize the potential for detecting significant disabilities.

The Sherbrooke area in the Quebec health region of Estrie has implemented the mixed case-finding approach for those aged 75 and over. PRISMA-7 is currently being implemented in most Quebec health regions, most commonly through the single entry point in local community service centers (CLSCs; French *centre local de services communautaires*) and in some ERs. We present below a few examples of the implementation of case-finding as carried out in Estrie. The region has a population of nearly 300 000, of whom 42 000 are aged 65 and over and nearly 22 000 are 75 and over.

Ongoing Experiences with PRISMA-7

The instrument is receiving increasing use in numerous consulting venues and on different occasions. In Estrie, every CLSC territory has a single entry point for the intake and referral of elderly individuals, where referral based on PRISMA-7 is being progressively put into place. Most of the region's ERs, including those at the Coaticook hospital and Sherbrooke's university hospital (CHUS; *Centre hospitalier universitaire de Sherbrooke*), use PRISMA-7 for case-finding. The CHUS serves as the local hospital for the city of Sherbrooke (population about 150,000) and the Coaticook area (population about 16,000). It also has a mandate to the Estrie region as a whole and an extra-regional mandate for some kinds of specialized care. The CHUS's ER receives 10,000 visits per year by users aged 75 and over.

In Sherbrooke, PRISMA-7 is also administered during the annual influenza immunization campaigns for elders, which provide an exceptional opportunity to conduct quasi-systematic case-finding. As well, certain points of service delivery, for example the CHUS's surgical prep clinic (which gathers data prior to elective surgery, takes specimens, and prepares users for discharge from hospital), began implementing PRISMA-7 in 2006. Consideration is being given to administering PRISMA-7 in other outpatient clinics (e.g., the diabetes clinic), as well as in the waiting rooms of physicians with private offices. Nurses attached to family physician groups (GMFs; French *groupe de médecine de famille*) also refer elders found positive for disability by PRISMA-7 at the single entry point. This is also the case with the Centre de réadaptation Estrie (a generalist rehabilitation center that serves the whole region) and many providers of housekeeping services.

Implementing the Case-Finding Process

The Single Entry Point

Implementing a case-finding mechanism entailed considering the nature of the contacts that result in a CLSC assessment of degree of disability. Once PRISMA-7 has been administered, where will the information be compiled and which health or social service worker will be required to assess the elderly person who has been found positive for disability? When an elderly person comes into contact with the single entry point, the first step consists in determining if he or she is known to the system, being followed by home-support services, or has been recently assessed; if not, case-finding should be carried out. After three years of use of PRISMA-7, managers working in Sherbrooke deem case-finding to have been conducted with nearly 100 % of the target group.

The Emergency Room

Case-finding was implemented in the CHUS's ERs following work on functionally declined elders conducted in the region. Consensus emerged regarding priorities, including screening and case-finding. A process of reflection set in motion by the work of the *Conseil consultatif national sur les urgences* (provincial committee on emergency departments), the problem of ER bottlenecks, and the high proportion of the elderly target group that visit ERs were all conducive to exploring new avenues. ER-based case-finding and referral to CLSCs appeared to be ready for testing.

Various factors influenced the implementation of case-finding in the CHUS's ERs. The commitment shown by the institution's management and the leadership role played by its department of nursing and service quality (DSIQ; French name *Direction des soins infirmiers et de la qualité*) definitely played a role. There was hesitation among ER nurses at the outset, but subsequently they gradually subscribed to the case-finding project. Concerns had had to do with adding the case-finding process to ER protocols and the appropriateness of conducting this kind of case-finding in an emergency setting. During discussions, the questions raised focused in particular on how to proceed. With input from the DSIQ and the department of clinical operations and partnerships, the decision made was to include the PRISMA-7 questions in the internal-referral instrument, which facilitated the procedure. To monitor implementation, we tracked the extent to which the PRISMA-7 portion of the referral instrument was duly filled in.

Use of PRISMA-7 was begun in the ERs of both CHUS facilities in May 2005. At the start, the case-finding was done on a proportion of 10 % to 20 % of the clients. This rose to between 50 % and 60 %, depending on the facility (see Graph 22.1). While use is slowly increasing at both facilities, it is continuous and incremental at one site, whereas more significant fluctuations are observed at the other. Case-finding at the latter sometimes reaches 70 % of the target group. The implementation percentage appeared to level off at around 50 % during summer 2006. Of course, summer is the peak time of year for vacations and there is accordingly a larger proportion of replacement staff in place.

What target percentage should be set for penetration with case-finding? Both objectively and clinically, the goal is not to reach 100 %. It is not only when an ER case consists of confirming death that case-finding is obviously inappropriate. It is equally so in cases of stroke or fractures of the lower extremities. After all, these necessarily bring about a drastic change in the patient's disabilities; and in any event, the patient is about to be hospitalized and will be assessed for disability. There are other circumstances under which case-finding cannot be conducted, such as following head injury or in cases of paranoid hallucinations, heart attack, and users with cognitive disorders (e.g., Alzheimer's) who arrive unaccompanied. The data examined during an average period in spring 2006 shows that 12 % to 15 % of consultations take place for the reasons listed above, which means the desired penetration rate should be set at 85 % of the whole target group. So, if 50 % of the entire target group for case-finding is currently being reached, it is reasonable to say that, in fact, we have reached 59 % (50/85) of the true target penetration level.

During the same period in spring 2006, we examined whether there were differences between users who were questioned with PRISMA-7 and those who were not. Our observations were that there is no statistical age-related difference, the average age being 82.5 for users who are questioned and 81.6 for users who are not ($p = 0.198$). No sex-related difference emerges either; women represent 63.9 % of users questioned and 61.9 % of those not ($p = 0.761$). Thus no difference is observable for these two variables, which are represented in PRISMA-7 by one question each. On the other hand, in practice, elderly ER users waiting on gurneys appear to be those for whom the most case-finding is done, seemingly because the user is present in the ER for a longer time.

Graph 22.1
Change in Percentage of Clients Aged 75 and over to Whom PRISMA-7 was Administered in the CHUS ERs During the First 15 Months of Implementation

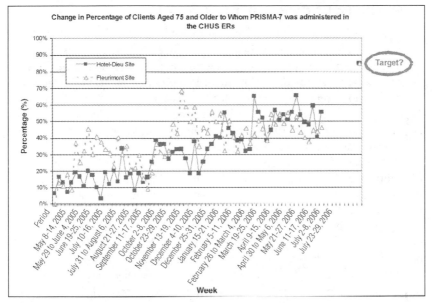

As previously mentioned, to facilitate implementation in Sherbrooke, case-finding was progressively linked to the annual influenza immunization campaign. In fall 2003, individuals aged 85 and over were targeted in Sherbrooke. Since 2004, case-finding has been done on those aged 75 and over.

In the Estrie region as a whole, a trial was made of having meals-on-wheels volunteers perform case-finding. Positive findings were conveyed to the CLSC single entry point with the elderly person's signed consent. However, volunteers were uncomfortable conveying sensitive information about the degree of disability of people they saw only occasionally. For their part, the elderly individuals tended to hesitate to sign the consent form. In the end, this approach was ruled out.

During PRISMA-7's implementation in the Estrie region in various places and on various occasions, we observed markers of case-finding's arrival at a certain degree of maturity. The process can be considered to have been more or less implemented when two positives are obtained in different settings for the same individual, even before that person has been assessed. In fact, two positives (and not the PRISMA-7 score per se) constitute a reason to prioritize assessing an individual. Similarly, when the threshold of four or more yes answers is used, clinicians realize intuitively after a time that they are allowing certain prevalent cases to slip through the net. At that point, it is deemed necessary to change the threshold, going from four to three or more yes answers. Specificity is reduced, but the instrument's sensitivity rises to 78 % (see Table 22.1).

What should be done with positives?

When a person has been found positive for disability, what is the next step? The answer is simple: Proceed to an in-depth assessment of degree of disability and of the individual's bio-psycho-social circumstances; and, as needed, refer to appropriate service providers. Note that PRISMA-7 cannot serve as an instrument for prioritizing interventions. The assessment (which should follow a positive case-finding) determines what interventions are needed, while prioritization depends on other criteria, such as the seeming urgency of the interventions needed and the resources available.

When case-finding is done in the ER, who should conduct the subsequent disability assessment and where should it be done? Naturally, in a coordinated integrated services network, these questions have already been answered. The first step is to sketch a portrait of the region's existing logistics, the organizations in place, the services concerned, and the health or social services workers involved. Who is currently assessing individuals believed to be significantly disabled? Under what criteria is an individual currently referred for assessment? Is there a waiting list? Coordinated action among service providers, institutions, and health and social services workers makes it possible to organize the logistics of assessment, follow-up, and callback.

When a person is found positive for disability, whom should the information be conveyed to? In Quebec, the CLSC single entry point plays this role for a given district. In France, could a CLIC fill the role? The logistics of assessment must obviously be organized before case-finding is begun. For example, the CHUS plays the role of regional hospital for seven CLSC districts, including that of the city of Sherbrooke itself. When an individual is found positive by the questionnaire in the ER, the information is directed to the geriatric-team nurse. If the individual is hospitalized, assessment is usually conducted by the geriatrics team before discharge. If, however, a person found positive goes home immediately after consulting in the ER, the information is conveyed by secure e-mail to the appropriate CLSC's single entry point. This approach circumvents the problem of one person receiving the information during certain hours of the day, another person in the evenings, and still another during vacation time. The recipient is the single entry point, and the health and social services worker on duty sees that, over subsequent days, the CHUS gets feedback about whether the individual is already known to home-support services and what is going to be done for the person. (For known users recently assessed, there is follow-up. For known users whose assessment was not recent, there is an assessment. For users not known to the CLSC, there is an assessment.)

A question commonly asked when the instrument's implementation is being planned is the number of elders to be assessed. The concern is whether workers will be suddenly swamped with assessment requests. The experience in Estrie suggests that this is not the case, as may be seen from Graph 22.1. Gradual implementation allows for a break-in period for the assessment team. Obviously, however, changes in practice never occur without difficulties and the need for adjustment. These are inevitable companions of change.

Conclusion

Case-finding requires that services be coordinated and integrated. Services integration itself requires case-finding, since not conducting case-finding merely postpones until a later date the handling of a problem that grows more serious in the meantime, calling for more time and energy with diminishing returns. When workers in a given territory coordinate their actions and see that nothing is to be gained by not dealing proactively with significant disability, a true population-based approach comes into effect. Such an approach ingrains a collective-responsibility approach, which consists of all parties working in their own fields and service areas while ensuring their work is linked to the efforts of others. Some authors state that service coordination, case-finding, and disability prevention are integral to the core values of geriatrics and, in fact, indicate where its future lies[33, 34].

Following the implementation of RISPA in Estrie as part of the PRISMA study, significant effects were observed that could be attributed to the introduction of case-finding. The incidence of the development of functional decline went down by 14 % (p ≤ 0.001) during the fourth year the study was in place. This consequence was unexpected and coincided with introduction of the case-finding procedure, which had not been planned on when the project was begun and which is thus currently viewed as being the most likely reason for the 14 % reduction.

One thing is certain. In the settings where case-finding is being done, a comment workers often make is that case-finding prevents their being called on mainly in emergency situations and thus facing patients whose existing disability has just been intensified by an acute health episode or family caregivers presenting with significant burnout. Case-finding increases the leeway surrounding interventions. Workers who have experience with it would not go back to doing without it.

Acknowledgements

We are grateful to all the elderly individuals who took part in the PRISMA-7 development and validation studies. We are further grateful to Lucie Bonin for her questions on case-finding and service organization, which have always been focused on the essentials and on practice. We also want to express our appreciation to the nurses in the CHUS's ERs and surgical prep clinic, as well as the single entry point nurses at the *Centre de santé et de services sociaux – Institut Universitaire de Gériatrie de Sherbrooke* (CSSS-IUGS), for their contribution in identifying elders whose degree of disability is too often unknown. We extend our thanks Carole Tardif of the CSSS-IUGS for her indispensable clarifications regarding case-finding at the single entry point. And lastly, we thank all the health and social services workers who do case-finding and who have directed relevant questions and judicious observations our way.

References

1. **Hébert, R., Brayne, C., and Spiegelhalter, D.** Incidence of functional decline and improvement in a community-dwelling, very elderly population. *Am J Epidemiol* 1997; 145: 935-44.

2. **Colin, C., and Coutton, V.** Le nombre de personnes âgées dépendantes d'après l'enquête handicaps-incapacités-dépendance. *Études et résultats – Direction de la recherche, des études, de l'évaluation et des statistiques.* Ministère de l'Emploi et de la solidarité de la France 2000; 94: 1-8.

3. **Folstein, M.F., Folstein, S.E., and McHugh, P.R.** Mini-Mental State: A practical method for grading the cognitive state of patients for the clinician. *J Psychiatr Res* 1975; 12:189-98.

4. **Raîche, M., Hébert, R., Prince, F., and Corriveau, H.** Screening older adults at risk of falling with the Tinetti balance scale. *Lancet* 2000; 356: 1001-2.

5. **Payette H.** Nutrition as a determinant of functional autonomy and quality of life in aging: A research program. *Can J Physiol Pharmacol* 2005; 83: 1061-70.

6. Recognising disability [Editorial]. *Lancet* 1991; 338: 154-5.

7. **Ebrahim, S.** Disability in older people: A mass problem requiring mass solutions. *Lancet* 1999; 353: 1990-2.

8. **Stuck, A.E., Beck, J.C., and Egger, M.** Preventing disability in elderly people. *Lancet* 2004; 364:1641-2.

9. **Ferrucci, L., Guralnik, J.M., Studenski, S., et al.** Designing randomized, controlled trials aimed at preventing or delaying functional decline and disability in frail, older persons: A consensus report. *J Am Geriatr Soc* 2004; 52: 625-34.

10. **Kasper, J.D., Shapiro, S., Guralnik, J.M., Bandeen-Roche, K.J., and Fried, L.P.** Designing a community study of moderately to severely disabled older women: The Women's Health and Aging Study. *Ann Epidemiol* 1999; 9: 498-507.

11. **Hébert, R. and the PRISMA group**. L'intégration des services aux personnes âgées: Une solution prometteuse aux problèmes de continuité. *Santé, société et solidarité – Revue de l'Observatoire franco-québécois de la santé et de la solidarité* 2003; special issue: 67-76.

12. **Hébert, R., Durand, P.J., Dubuc, N., Tourigny, A., and the PRISMA Group.** PRISMA: A new model of integrated service delivery for the frail older people in Canada. *International Journal of Integrated Care* (www.ijic.org) 2003; 3 (March): 1-10.

13. **Raîche, M. and Hébert, R.** Coordination des services aux personnes âgées en France et au Québec: Enjeux, expériences et champs de recherche traitant de leur évaluation. *Santé, société et solidarité – Revue de l'Observatoire franco-québécois de la santé et de la solidarité* 2003; special issue: 57-66.

14. **Muir Gray, J.A., Almind, G., Freer, C., and Warshaw, G.** Screening and case finding. In: Muir Gray JA, ed. Prevention of disease in the elderly. New York: Churchill Livingstone; 1985: 51-63.

15. **Ministère de la Santé et des Services Sociaux du Québec.** Plan d'action 2005-2010 – Un défi de solidarité: Les services aux aînés en perte d'autonomie. Québec; 2005. (http://msssa4.msss.gouv.qc.ca/fr/document/publication.nsf/4b1768b3f849519c852568fd0061480d/28518fb11a0a47f7852570ab00546f83?OpenDocument)

16. **Pathy, M.S., Bayer, A., Harding, K., and Dibble, A.** Randomised trial of case finding and surveillance of elderly people at home. *Lancet* 1992; 340: 890-3.

17. **Lachs, M.S., Feinstein, A.R., Cooney, L.M., Jr., et al.** A simple procedure for general screening for functional disability in elderly patients. *Ann Intern Med* 1990; 112: 699-706.

18. **Mateev, A., Gaspoz, J.M., Borst, F., Waldvogel, F., and Weber, D.** Use of a short-form screening procedure to detect unrecognized functional disability in the hospitalized elderly. *J Clin Epidemiol* 1998; 51: 309-14.

19. **Bowns, I., Challis, D., and Tong, M.S.** Case finding in elderly people: Validation of a postal questionnaire. *Brit J Gen Pract* 1991; 41: 100-4.

20. **McCusker, J., Bellavance, F., Cardin, S., and Trepanier, S.** Screening for geriatric problems in the emergency department: Reliability and validity. Identification of Seniors at Risk (ISAR) Steering Committee. *Acad Emerg Med* 1998; 5: 883-93.

21. **McCusker, J., Bellavance, F., Cardin, S., Trepanier, S., Verdon, J., and Ardman O.** Detection of older people at increased risk of adverse health outcomes after an emergency visit: The ISAR screening tool. *J Am Geriatr Soc* 1999; 47: 1229-37.

22. **Brody, K.K., Johnson, R.E., Ried, L.D., Carder, P.C., Perrin, N.** A comparison of two methods for identifying frail Medicare-aged persons. *J Am Geriatr Soc* 2002; 50: 562-9.

23. **Hébert, R., Bravo, G., Korner-Bitensky, N., and Voyer L.** Predictive validity of a postal questionnaire for screening community-dwelling elderly individuals at risk of functional decline. *Age Ageing* 1996; 25: 159-67.

24. **Dendukuri, N., McCusker, J., and Belzile, E.** The Identification of Seniors at Risk screening tool: Further evidence of concurrent and predictive validity. *J Am Geriatr Soc* 2004; 52: 290-6.

25. **Hébert, R., Bravo, G., Korner-Bitensky, N., and Voyer L.** Refusal and information bias associated with postal questionnaires and face-to-face interviews in very elderly subjects. *J Clin Epidemiol* 1996; 49: 373-81.

26. **Hébert, R., Desrosiers, J., Dubuc, N., Tousignant, M., Guilbeault, J., and Pinsonnault, E.** Le système de mesure de l'autonomie fonctionnelle (SMAF) – Mise au point. *Revue de gériatrie* 2003; 28: 323-336.

27. **Raîche, M., Hébert, R., and Dubois, M-F.** PRISMA-7: A case-finding tool to identify older adults with moderate to severe disabilities. Submitted.
   Note from the author: after publication of the text in La Revue de Gériatrie at spring 2007, this article submitted has been accepted and is in press in Archives of Gerontology and Geriatrics.

28. **Dubuc, N., Hébert, R., Desrosiers, J., Buteau, M., and Trottier, L.** Disability-based classification system for older people in integrated long-term care services: The Iso-SMAF profiles. *Arch Gerontol Geriat 2006; 42: 191-206.*

29. **Hébert, R., Carrier, R., and Bilodeau A.** Le système de mesure de l'autonomie fonctionnelle (SMAF). *Revue de gériatrie* 1988; 14: 161-167.

30. **Desrosiers, J., Bravo, G., Hébert, R., and Dubuc, N.** Reliability of the revised Functional Autonomy Measurement System (SMAF) for epidemiological research. *Age Ageing* 1995; 24: 402-6.

31. **Hébert, R., Spiegelhalter, D, and Brayne, C.** Setting the minimal metrically detectable change on disability rating scales. *Arch Phys Med Rehabil* 1997; 78: 1305-8.

32. **Raîche, M., Hébert, R., Dubois, M.-F., and the PRISMA partners.** User guide for the PRISMA-7 questionnaire to identify elderly people with severe loss of autonomy. In Hébert R, Tourigny A, Gagnon M. *Integrated service delivery to ensure persons' functional autonomy.* Québec, Edisem, 2005; pp. 147-165. ISBN 2-89130-204-4.

33. **American Geriatrics Society Core Writing Group of the Task Force on the Future of Geriatric Medicine.** Caring for older Americans: The future of geriatric medicine. *J Am Geriatr Soc* 2005; 53 Suppl 6:S245-S256.

34. **Leichsenring, K.** Developing integrated health and social care services for older persons in Europe. *International Journal of Integrated Care* (www.ijic.org) 2004; 4 (Sept.): 1-15.

Chapter 23
Estimating a Territory's Case-Management Resources

Anne Veil and Réjean Hébert

Highlights

This article describes a method for estimating the case-management resources required to respond to the needs of managers and policy-makers for establishing guidelines for allocating resources required for case management. This method takes into account case-management intervention models, organizational models for integrating the function, and the current limitations of the major population databases when attempting to develop a picture of the elderly with disabilities according to their living conditions and disability profile.

The method proposed clearly distinguishes the different case-management models, puts manager caseloads into the context of PRISMA-Estrie's experimental territories, and grounds the calculation method on empirical bases.

The results of applying this method are appropriate for clinical case-management models (direct intervention with patient and his or her caregivers) when the roles and responsibilities are shared between service coordination (main role) and certain interventions specific to the case manager's original profession (often social work or nursing). The recommended load is 40 to 45 cases and the annualized turnover rate is 25 %. The proportions of the elderly in the various living settings are established in relationship to their disability profiles, which makes it possible to estimate the number of elders living in the community who are eligible for case management and home-care services.

Introduction

Two major categories of factors must be considered in estimating the number of case managers (CMs) required in a specific territory and their caseloads. The first relates to intervention approach and the sets of elements that characterize the case-management role. Depending on preferences of the host's institution management, the CM role may be more administrative or basically clinical. CMs may serve a homogeneous target group (moderately to severely disabled, need for long-term management) or they may be called on to perform case-management activities (service coordination) and their normal clinical activities both with patients who are eligible for case management and those who are not (heterogeneous target group). How the work is arranged determines in the capacity of case managers to fulfill their expected roles. Case managers must also perform other organizational and administrative duties that require part of their time (meetings, training, committee work, statistics, etc.). Information pertaining to the time devoted to direct and indirect interventions with their patients with respect to other activities or responsibilities was not collected during the PRISMA-Estrie implementation study.

The second set embraces all of the organizational and administrative factors surrounding case management. The first of these factors that we want to call attention to is triage, which is the process for determining which target patients will have access to a given service. As eligibility criteria for case management get stricter, the proportion of the elderly with disability living in the community that could be reached specifically by the service drops. Another factor that should be considered is case-manager caseload, which should take into account the growing elderly population as well as the objective of offering quality service. Always keeping the file open in case management until the patient has been put into placement, is deceased, or moves has a direct impact on the replacement rate of managed cases. The PRISMA model implemented in Estrie planned on keeping the file open even after the elderly person recovered or his or her situation stabilized.

All of these concerns raise issues related to local and regional resource allocation, service organization, the quality of services delivered, and, ultimately, the system's capacity to serve a growing elderly population. Since these fundamental elements determine how well case management reaches its target population and the degree of resources required to achieve the objectives, we propose an estimation method that was constructed as our knowledge about the reality in the field improved. The initial version, designed from the data available yielded by the experience in Bois-Francs in Mauricie / Centre-du-Québec served to sketch the method out. Since the implementation of the integrated network in Estrie used a population approach and had to deal with the actual conditions faced by organizations, the method was revised taking into account case-management models, their organizational integration, the intervention approach, caseload, and eligibility criteria. A literature review made it possible to position the Estrie experiment with respect to the other models.

The process goal consists in establishing the target to be achieved by case management in terms of the number of elderly individuals cared for and the number of case managers required. This chapter therefore sets out the relevant data yielded by case-management implementation in Estrie and defines the method for calculating the number of full-time-equivalent (FTE) case managers needed for a given territory, based on an optimal caseload. One caveat about using this method: it cannot be applied to other territories unless the case-management models are comparable.

Objectives

This exercise responds to a need expressed repeatedly by people in the field: having guidelines for determining the case-management resources required to adequately serve an elderly population with moderate to severe loss of independence. It is the nature of innovations to have very few comparative reference points. As a result, the experiment underway is both seeking for and developing such reference points. The accelerated aging of Quebec's population provides additional impetus to complete the process, because it could be used in planning for future resource requirements. Moreover, this approach can be easily adapted to other regions and territories implementing similar models.

The estimate herein was formulated taking into account the necessity of case managers having a limited but optimal caseload and the need for better defining the case-manager function (approaches, role models, organizational integration models, caseloads). In order to achieve our objectives, we had to start by clarifying these notions pertaining to case-management models. Then, we had to establish the percentage of elderly people age 65 or older living in the community with moderate to severe disabilities, who represent the target group for case management.

Methodology

This method for estimating the required number of case managers was developed using the hybrid model of case management, which assumes that the target population is comprised of the elderly with moderate to severe disabilities and that the clinical role will consist primarily of service coordination. These conditions make it possible to achieve a standard of intervention that is specific to case management. According to our measurements and observations, this is the model that will best establish the case-manager role while ensuring greater efficacy and enhanced continuity of services.

We use two main sources of information to achieve our objectives: national and international literature on case management (approaches, models, caseloads) as well as certain relevant data taken from two implementation studies carried out in Quebec under similar conditions (Bois-Francs and Estrie). These two regions needed these innovative projects in order to resolve genuine problems in delivering services to the elderly. Additional data, beyond information about case-management models and approaches, were required to make our study feasible: 1) annually adjusted statistics on the number of people age 65 or older for each territory; 2) the case-management target among the elderly with moderate to severe disabilities living in the community (Iso-SMAF profiles); and 3) the average caseload observed in the field and that reported in the literature.

Case-management models

Survey of Case-Management Models

A number of authors have described certain aspects of how case management functions with an elderly population. That is just what prompted Long[1] to establish a typology of case-manager functions, which he broke down into two major categories: models aimed primarily at controlling traffic, costs, and gate keeping and models centered especially on the quality of care, preventing functional decline, and supporting caregivers. Scharlach[2] identified an additional category, namely, liaison, with which the various forms of brokerage are associated (brokerage model). Beyond this, he describes two other types of models that differ in their objectives. The managed-care model, also referred to *as* the gatekeeper model, aims at controlling the use of services and costs. The integrated model, *which* is clinically oriented, seeks to prevent the progression of the loss of independence through a multidisciplinary approach. It should be noted, that both involve decreasing caseloads, with the brokerage model having a high caseload and the integration models having a lighter caseload.

Typology of Case-Management Models

The study that we carried out on the different case-management models makes it possible to match a number of models to the typologies proposed by Long and Scharlach. Table 23.1 brings out their distinctiveness and positions the model implemented in Estrie among them.

Description of Certain Case-Management Models

When focusing on the literature about the elderly and mental health, it becomes apparent that there are different case-management models depending on the practice setting and problems encountered: 1) Hospital settings, in which case-management nurses must coordinate the care pathways and administrative procedures pertaining to discharge; the patients are not exclusively the elderly; 2) Case managers who work in the home of the elderly in the community who are primarily social workers and nurses, almost all of whom hold undergraduate or graduate degrees in their disciplines. 3) Case managers in the mental-health sector with highly varied backgrounds and who work in the community.

The exact definition of interventions carried out by case managers is not homogenous in the literature available in United States[5]. The first reason is that it has only recently emerged as a profession. Moreover, the specifics of the US health-insurance system must also be taken into account, since they bring out the importance of roles related to applying knowledge in the fields of economy, tax law, and negotiation and assessment strategies. This is not the case in Canada, primarily because of universal access to health care. American studies often report that nurse CMs consider that they need training in order to appro-

Table 23.1
Typology of Case-Management Models for the Elderly*

Variables	Liaison Models (*brokerage models*)	Administrative Models (*gate-keeping models*)	Clinical Models (*integrated models*)
Examples of programs described by researchers	*Centralized Individual Model* (Eggert[3]) *Brokerage Model* (Zawadski *in* Long[1])	*Financial Control Model* (Phillips[4]) *Managed Care* (Scharlach [2], Capitman *in* Scharlach [2])	*Clinical Case Management* (Scharlach[2]) Neighborhood Team Model (Eggert [3]) *Basic Case Management Model* (Phillips[4])
1. Main goal	Provide liaison between patients and service providers. Avoid impediments to access duplication of services.	Promote the use of appropriate but less costly services. Control service use and costs.	Predominantly clinical integration model that aims at preventing loss of Independence within an establish network of service providers. Counter the effects of service fragmentation.
2. Target population	Anyone with a functional disorder. No risk of institutionalization.	Anyone with medical or functional disorders who might require costly services.	Individuals with significant disabilities or with complex, progressive needs that could lead to institutionalization. Caregiver support.
3. CM authority	No authority over service delivery.	Significant authority in approving or limiting service use.	Authority shared between the CM and interdisciplinary team.
4. Approach	Logistics	Administrative	Clinic, comprehensive, patient-centered; system usability.

Table 23.1
Typology of Case-Management Models for the Elderly*

Variables	Liaison Models (*brokerage models*)	Administrative Models (*gate-keeping models*)	Clinical Models (*integrated models*)
5. CM functions	Assesses and implements the service plan through brokerage. Assessment is delegated under certain models. No home visits.	Assesses, implements service plan, ensures follow-up for a limited time. Ensures application of access criteria and regulations.	Direct, face-to-face interventions with the patient and family, indirect interventions, including counseling and others clinical tasks; coordinates multidisciplinary effort. Serves as an advocate in the patient's interest.
6. Caseload	High (60 or more). The Centralized Model has 120 to 150 cases per CM.	Higher than in clinical models; up to 60 cases per CM.	Lower. Several models indicate 40 to 50 cases per CM.
7. Service intensity	Short-term horizon for solving the problem; CM spends little time with patients.	Short-term horizon for solving the problem; services may be intensive during this time.	Long-term services depending on need progression; services deemed intensive because they require more staff time in comparison to the other models.

* Typology stemming from the work of Long[1] and Scharlach[2].

priately carry out all aspects of the CM role. Furthermore, the belief that performing these new functions comes under a new professional identity. Lastly, a number of articles from different countries[6] report on the expectations that the different actors, patients, and caregivers have of case management, which further complicates comparison.

In their recent article, Enguidanos et al.[7] described four case-management models for the elderly characterized by varying levels of follow-up and case appropriation by professionals. The first two models are of the information and referral assistance type, and the other two are of the intervention type (clinical).

1. The first model (*Information and Referral Assistance*) requires the lowest level of professional involvement: telephone interview, mailed-out information, no care plan provided. No management, therefore not caseload.
2. The second model proposes short-term telephone intervention (*Telephone Care Management*) performed by a social worker who has access to a com-

puterized database containing information about the elderly person, including services, recent diagnostic tests, and medications. Its role is to facilitate access to the required services. Patients receive an average of one hour per month. The average caseload is 30 patients, with assistance and referral provided for about an additional 80 patients each month.

3. The *Geriatric Care Management* (GCM) model is based on case management carried out by nursing or social-work professionals. Cases are assigned on a geographic basis. The case manager conducts a home assessment, which makes it possible to determine the setting's safety, among other things. The CM coordinates services and follow-up for an average of 8 months. Service plans are developed in response to the individual's medical and psychosocial problems, in cooperation with a team that includes, in particular, a geriatrician and a continuity-of-care manager. The family physician's involvement varies depending on the patient's condition. The case manager spends about 20 hours for each case during follow-up, which lasts an average of 8 months; most of the CM's interventions are carried out at the start of management. The average load per case manager is 80 patients.

4. The last model differs from the preceding in that the case manager can count financial resources that can be applied to where needed on, in addition to the infrastructure described in the GCM model (e.g. personal hygiene, home help, legal aid, money management, medical equipment not covered, transportation, caregiver respite, and any other required measure), which makes it possible to round out and personalize the offer of services based on the elderly person's needs. Case managers have a services purchase program allocating US$2000 per patient. On average, the CM spends an average of 4 to 6 hours on each patient than in the GCM model, which is the time needed to implement and follow up brokered services. The model's caseload was not specified.

These descriptions of the variable intensity of CM interventions depending on service model bring out a progression in the approach used by the case manager, moving from the primarily logistical to clinical intervention, along with enhancing the measures available and increasing control over the selection and implementation of services. There is an apparent linkage between CM degree of involvement and the growing need for assistance by patients so that they can fend for themselves and make decisions that are appropriate for their situations. Comparing the models highlights a principle: the approach must be selected in reference to patient needs and must adapt their changes in their independence.

The literature shows us that management models can vary considerably, hence the importance of selecting the one that is best suited to the targeted objectives. The outcomes of a case-management model depend on many factors, including the role to be played by the case managers and the approach advocated. Moreover, existing service structures in the community (continuum of services) and their performance (penetration rate, response time, service quality) also have an impact. The fact sheet that follows positions the case-management model implemented in Estrie among the clinical models.

Fact Sheet for the Case-Management Model Implemented in Estrie

The PRISMA model of service integration comes under the heading of integrative clinical models. In another words, its main focus is on the set of needs (often complex and changing) of the elderly with significant disabilities. It also aims at using services wisely—especially the more costly ones—and at avoiding duplication. Indeed, this model makes it possible to integrate clinical and systemic objectives in that it promotes delivering the right service at the right time by the right resource.

Its prime goal aims at preserving the patient's independence or at least slow the pace at which independence is being lost. In this sense, the model is clinical. Certain objectives related to the wise use of the continuum's costly services also demonstrates an interest in sound management promoting better use of the service network in the sense that decisions guiding the individual through the network must be based on complete, current information in order to avoid pathways that would be unproductive, especially in hospital settings and specialized services. This model is integrative for two reasons: 1) it fosters better coordination between health-care, social, and rehabilitation services; 2) it integrates patient-centered clinical objectives from a systemic perspective, which aims at countering the negative impacts resulting from service-network fragmentation affecting both patients and the network itself.

Target group: The elderly with moderate to severe disabilities with Iso-SMAF profiles of 4 or greater.

CM authority over service delivery: Shared between the CM, the family physician, specialized-care teams, and partners in the continuum of services.

Approach: Geriatric, community, proactive, centered on the needs of patients and their caregivers.

Functions: Overall assessment with a multiclientele tool. Design, planning, and implementation of the services required for the patient and caregiver, both through direct interventions (face to face with the patient and family) and indirect interventions to coordinate the interdisciplinary effort by ensuring the overall coherency of interventions; act as advocate in the patient's interest.

Caseload: 40 to 45 patients

Service intensity: Long-term horizon, intensity adjusted to changing and progressive needs of the elderly with moderate to severe disabilities.

Role Models Implemented in Estrie

The service coordination model implemented in Bois-Francs and Estrie draw directly on the *Basic Case Management* (Phillips)[4] and the *Neighborhood Team* (Eggert)[3]. When the PRISMA model was being implemented, however, it was necessary to define the various ways the model could be arranged, for example, clarifying the case manager's coordination role with respect to the CM's original profession and with respect to the caseload, which may be comprised of patients with the same or varied levels of needs. We should state that this type of arrangement relates more to the organizational insertion of the case-management function than to the intervention approach.

The case-management model implemented in Estrie was inspired from an American model designed according to an integrative clinical orientation referred to as the Neighborhood Team, which calls for greater sensitivity to the needs of patients and families. At the same time, proactive intervention (before problems occur) is fostered, with a view towards facilitating service use. Such problems can relate to patients or come under organization of the health-care system. Basic Case Management (BCM) is another model, which shares similarities with the Neighborhood Team (NT). It puts greater emphasis on the set of tasks related to follow-up as well as direct intervention support for patients and caregivers.

Comparison with the Estrie Model

The case-management model implemented in Estrie shares a common objective with the American Basic Case Management and Neighborhood Team models: early intervention along with regular follow-up that provides means for anticipating problems, which is the core of the proactive geriatrics approach. These models broaden the intervention of natural caregivers.

In such models, CMs do not set aside their past clinical professional knowledge when they become case managers. On the contrary, they maximize such knowledge. Moreover, interdisciplinarity is inherent in the model, because of the presence of several different services and professionals caring for the elderly.

The PRISMA model stands out for the place it gives to physicians, specifically the dominant role for family physicians, since the target group is already vulnerable in terms of physical and mental health. Under Quebec's system, family physicians are the professionals who must be systematically identified for each patient assigned to case management. Their participation in coordinating specialized medical services is essential. Their collaboration with case managers who can ensure that the patients can remain in their homes is equally as important.

Role of Case Managers

Case-management work in the three study territories is performed primarily by social workers (and human relations officers or HROs), as well as several psychologists and nurses. Direct clinical intervention with patients and family caregivers is an inherent part of the CM role. Indeed, CMs still perform procedures specific to their respective professions (social work or nursing), provided such procedures represent a small proportion (< 20 % of the task) with respect to the core functions of assessment, developing services plans, service negotiation and coordination, systematic follow-up, reassessment and revision of services, and support to patients and family caregivers.

Describing the case-management role solely in reference to a cycle of tasks (assessment, design of the individualized service plan or ISP, negotiation, etc.) hides and even diminishes the entire professional assistance and advisory role performed for people with impaired independence, who are often ill, anxious, or depressed. Yet, as documented by Hackstaff,[8] such patients commonly resist the introduction of services. Difficulty in accepting loss of independence and the foreseeable scenarios of disease or end of life are realities that case managers deal with on a regular basis. These phenomena are interwoven in the decisions affecting daily operations, whether for personal or home assistance, buying and using specialized equipment, budget management, transportation, and so on. Each of the formal activities guided by the CM is influenced by these human, dynamic elements that color and complicate the decision-making process.

Since negotiating and coordinating with many services is important, updating the different facets of the CM role depends on the conditions imposed on him or her, both within the employing institution and among all the organizations (primary- and secondary-care departments, physicians, community organizations and private firms, owners of private homes, etc.) with which the CM must work since the CM's responsibility is to follow the patient wherever that leads. The CM's ability to implement patient ISPs is conditional upon the relations with his or her partners and the openness in their collaboration.

The model implemented in Estrie is characterized by a clinical role that strongly emphasizes intervention and face-to-face / telephone relations with patients and their families. It also fosters contacts and negotiations with public, private, and community service providers, as well as many exposure and negotiations with public, private, and community service providers. CMs have been overall grasp of their patients' situations and can initiate implementation of ISPs and advocate their patients' interests while, at the same time, working to ensure that services are used wisely.

Organizational Integration Models

There are different case-management organizational models that can be broken down according to CM organizational integration (full or part time, homogeneous or heterogeneous patient groups, plurality of roles, caseloads), depending on patient characteristics (levels of loss of independence) and the type of role entrusted to them (clinical, administrative, logistical).

When viewed according to the principles of clinical case management, three distinct methods for inserting the CM role into organizations emerged from the territories in the PRISMA-Estrie project: exclusive model, hybrid model, and mixed model. These organizational models of the CM function represent means of combining the primary professional role (especially SW or HRO and nurse) with that of coordinating services for homogeneous or heterogeneous patient groups. Case management can be provided either concomitantly with the usual professional role by serving mixed patient groups or by a dedicated CM team (single discipline or, preferably, multidisciplinary) intervening with a homogeneous patient group comprised solely of individuals eligible for case management.

Table 23.2 below provides the original roles and organizational integration of the new case-management function as implemented at each site. Based on this experiment, the hybrid model has the greatest potential for success in Quebec, particularly when the CMs work as multidisciplinary teams comprised of social workers and health-care professionals (nurses, psychologists, occupational therapists, and physical therapists) collaborating closely with family physicians. This composition makes sharing knowledge possible.

Table 23.2
**Organizational Integration Models of Case Management in Estrie
(clinical orientation)**

Model Type	Target Group	Nature of Case-Management Role
Exclusive model	*Homogeneous patient group* (only patients in case management)	*Single role* consisting of coordination and brokering*(excluding professional services in the CM's primary discipline)
Hybrid model	*Homogeneous patient group* (only patients in case management)	*Shared role:* • Service coordination and brokering* (major) • Professional role in the CM's primary discipline solely with a homogeneous patient group (minor)
Mixed model	*Heterogeneous patient group* (elderly individuals eligible AND ineligible for case management).	*Shared role:* • Service coordination and brokering* • Professional role in the CM's discipline.

* In our description of the Estrie experience herein, the term "brokering" refers to the process of negotiating with departments in order to organize, streamline, or personalize the conditions under which different providers deliver their services in order to better meet the changing needs of patients. As a result, it is tied to the concept of advocacy. The meaning used in the United States is completely different.

In fact, the issues related to modeling the CM function relate to the CMs appropriating a new role (and not intervening as in the past or normally), which emphasizes the importance of a global, systemic approach rather than a compartmentalized one. Other issues concern assigning the patient to the "right place" and take shape through the emergence of a standard according to which different levels of coordination intensity must be offered in response to the needs of level of complexity. Efforts must be made to bring out these needs as clearly as possible in order to guide patients to the right resource. Lastly, certain issues pertaining to the lighter caseload of CMs with respect to that of other CLSC professionals are evident. The case-management model opted for in Estrie was premised on a lighter caseload for CMs (45 cases) in order to promote a more effective intervention intensity for patients. The second part of this exercise will take a closer look at the factors associated with estimating case-load.

Case-Manager Caseload

Case managers may have facilitating or demanding organizational conditions in fulfilling their expected roles. Caseload is one of these conditions. The references in the literature about the workload of case managers working with the elderly with impaired independence are not always related to the intervention model used. Moreover, even if the approaches adopted by case managers in managing their workloads is directly related to their practice conditions and the difficulties presented by patients and their families, few authors deal with these issues, let alone study or measure them. Considering the recurrent discussions elicited by case management as a theme, certain authors go as far as to qualify this exercise as "tricky business" (AHC/CMSA),[9] referring to the number of determinants, some of which, however, resulted in significant variations in caseload.

Three types of documents mentioning case-manager workload can be found in the literature: 1) scientific articles that cover pilot projects implemented under the framework of a study in order to determine if a new approach would improve patient clinical outcomes; 2) scientific articles about established projects that discuss the value of the results, sometimes involving comparisons; and 3) research reports or administrative monitoring reports that determine if the projects actually respond to the underlying objectives or that explore new aspects of a practice. We limited our references to relevant research reports and scientific articles that measure or study established projects, excluding those covering pilot projects in which the caseload was controlled. This choice is justified by our objective of accounting for actual practice conditions instead of ideal conditions.

Caseload in Services for the Elderly

We begin our discussion of literature pertaining to caseload in services for the elderly the results of a national survey conducted in the United States (AHC/CMSA)[10] that was carried out with 520 case managers working in different types of organizations. It reveals a significant variation in caseload: 36.2 % at 30 cases or less; 36.4 % have between 31 and 75 cases; and 27.4 % have 76 cases or more. With this kind of distribution, distinctions must clearly be established between practice settings and the tasks devolved to case managers in an attempt to account for them. Certain authors provide details about the intervention models by establishing a direct link to caseload. Consequently, the work carried out by Eggert and colleagues[3] in the United States describe two models of intensive case management: the Centralized Individual Model and the Neighborhood Team. Under the centralized individual model, the assessment function (medical, *nursing,* and social services) is delegated and case managers rarely conduct home visits. Linkages with caregivers are relaxed; some information is offered, but the patient must take steps on his or her own. Proactive intervention is improbable; the CM does not have much professional autonomy and little is done in the area of protecting patient rights (advocacy). CMs serve an extensive territory, with caseloads ranging from 120 to 150 cases. Under the Neighborhood Team model, the CM carries out the number of home visits required and observes actual living conditions. Reassessments should be performed by the same practitioner, making it possible to better determine how the situation has changed; counseling is more appropriate and the patient can be assisted in taking action (if required). The CM provides the patient and family with decision-making support and keeps in regular contact, making it possible to prevent problems or take action promptly. Since the territory covered is local, the CM can be very familiar with the sector's resources. In cases of hospitalization, the case manager visits the patient and makes preparations for discharge. The caseload is 40 to 45 cases per manager under the Neighborhood Team model. Other authors report similar results (Zimmer,[11] Department of Health[12]). In the United Kingdom, Challis et al.[13] became interested in the connection between a limited number of cases (fewer than 30 cases) and the intensive case-management service that they wanted to offer the elderly who were most vulnerable and at risk for placement. In particular, the investigation's results demonstrated that lighter caseloads were more frequent when the intervener carried out the roles of planning, coordination, therapy, and support for individuals with complex and changing needs.

The work carried out by B.R. Phillips et al.[4] compare two case-management models of which one—the basic case management model—is designed for the frail elderly in which the actual average caseload was 45 cases per case manager. Management quality was not assessed.

A survey conducted by Pacala et al.[14] confirmed that when the work was performed primarily on the telephone, the ratio of CM to target group was 1 per 100 people. When interventions were conducted face-to-face (in the home or elsewhere), the ratio was more on the order of 1 per 40 to 50 cases. Moreover, Quinn[15] put forward that more cases can be assigned when certain aspects of the role are delegated (e.g. diabetes education, support for nonclinical aspects, etc.).

Task delegation need not be limited to the formal services system: it can also be negotiated between the case manager and the natural caregiver. Indeed, Twigg and McCallion, cited in Noelker,[16] described case-management models according to the importance of the GC role in comparison with the caregiver's. They report that, when the caregiver can play the role of negotiator and coordinator with the various service providers, the case manager should let him or her do so. Recent research brought to light that, 61 % of caregiver seeking clinical services did so for problems related to burn out or relational tensions between the caregiver and care receiver (Diwan et al. cited in Noelker[16]). One of the CM professional roles consists in supporting the caregiver in clarifying his or her needs as well as to encourage the caregiver to accept more services. If the role devolved to the CM or the CM's workload precludes or nearly precludes the closeness needed for regularly following up the situation with caregivers, the situation could deteriorate, often at the cost of the caregiver's health, which has a direct impact on the elderly person. In this context of positioning roles, Noelker cites a study with positive results when more intensive case management is required, including a distinct clinical role. In such instances, a caseload of 35 to 40 would be ideal.

Closer to home, in Montréal, Gagnon[17] carried out a study dealing with the impact of geriatric nursing case management on functional state, quality of life, satisfaction with care, and duration of hospital stay points to a caseload ranging from 40 to 55 cases, with an average of 46 cases, based on 10 months of monitoring.

Elsewhere in Canada, Diem's study[18] on the caseloads of 89 experienced case managers working in five Canadian provinces refers to three major types of CM activities, identified in a previous study by Diwan[19]. They are 1) direct services, often the priority of case managers, which target complex cases at home and new patients; 2) indirect services, which relate to activities within the organization and with service providers; 3) lastly, program management, which affects either many patients with similar problems or other community and health-care sectors. Diem emphasizes the importance of familiarity with patient characteristics to assess caseload service availability, and actual time CMs have available. Diem's Canadian national study indicates that two thirds (66 %) of the 89 case managers in the sample were nurses and that their caseloads varied from 100 to 300 cases, without, however, specifying the case-management model or the type of organizations where the CMs were working. The qualitative data bring out complaints of lack of time and resource gaps in adequately responding to needs. These case managers are most concerned about the frail elderly with mental deterioration. Often required to react in the emergency since they do not have the means to provide the monitoring necessary for prevention, their limited availability often leads to a decision for placement. Diem therefore establishes a formal link between a discharge from placement and having a high caseload.

Massie,[20] one of the authors that Diem refers to, provides a method for determining caseload based on functional disabilities. The pilot project gave CM services to patients age 60 or over presenting with 2 or more limitations in activities of daily living as well as an average of 5.1 health problems. After sampling time and movement of a CM during a typical day and then comparing the data to the results from similar projects, the researchers recommended a caseload of between 35 and 45 cases, for an average of 40 cases per manager (FTE).

For his part, Diwan[19] focuses more on the time spent on CM core tasks and brings out the "time-consuming" determinants that go beyond the physical needs of the elderly. These determinants are 1) patient behavioral problems, 2) problems in the informal support network, and 3) new patients.

Clearly, the literature brings out that any caseload prescription must always be matched to a description of the case-management model. It is also important to take into consideration all the responsibilities assigned the case managers, since related tasks (committees, administration, training, etc.) can take up a fairly large proportion of the time available.

In concluding on the topic of caseload, we should emphasize that the number and scope of the factors influencing caseload brought out in the literature speaks to the issue's complexity. More specifically, in contemplating future research into caseload assessment, we would include the fact that the needs of vulnerable elderly patients are not uniformly easy to deal with and that community resources cannot all be mobilized at a given time. The difficulty in responding to needs (response difficulty) has been defined by mental-health researchers as the sum of clinical complications and the need for community liaison (Gournay and Birley cited in King[21]). Consequently, this working hypothesis is of interest as regards the frail elderly. While these target groups are different, as are their risk factors, the concept of a composite index based on client factors and resource availability could be applied to the elderly.

Organizational Factors Influencing Caseload

Case-Management Eligibility Criteria

From the outset of implementation of case management in the three territories taking part in the PRISMA-Estrie study, the eligibility criteria were established based on a target group of the elderly with impaired independence ranging from moderate to severe. A score of SMAF 15 or higher was used to set the loss of independence. After deployment of Iso-SMAF profiles, this criterion was replaced by an Iso-SMAF of 4 or more. There are many clinical indicators that could push a physician or practitioner in favor of referring an individual for case-management. From a systemic point of view, however, it is important to select an objective, populational indicator of affording effective use by the greatest possible number of practitioners, which is currently the case as the result of the SMAF and Iso-SMAF profiles being used in many of Quebec's regions. This criterion is more specific than the degree of loss of independence, but it fails to take into account the psychosocial situation (e.g. marginality and isolation).

The eligibility criteria for case management in the territories *monitored* are: territory of residence, age (65 or older, except for cases presenting with geriatric profiles), and an Iso-SMAF profile of 4 or greater. A criterion used initially was dropped due to problems related to interpretation and application. Elderly individuals already known to the mental-health network are not targeted by the integrated network; neither were cancer patients in the palliative phase. In contrast, an elderly person already in case management who subsequently developed mental-health disorders or cancer was allowed to keep his or her CM. Similarly, the case manager would retain responsibility for accompanying an existing patient into permanent placement.

Patient Assignment Methods

Since the case management was designed solely for the elderly with impaired independence in the moderate-to-severe range, the process for assigning patients to pivot care providers that already worked on multidisciplinary teams (CLSC) or to new case managers had to be rethought. Pivot care providers already practicing were professionals from various disciplines qualified as pivotal when the patient required a number of CLSC services calling for coordination and adjustment over time. The decision to select one practitioner as being pivotal rather than another was often based on the predominant intervention or by greater familiarity with the patient.

Assignment to case management in the territories under study was carried out in different ways. Greater organization was required when the number of patients was higher. When the assignment process was formal and organized, the procedure for discussing orientation decisions allowed for the introduction of an arbiter into the process when dealing with certain cases that were less clear and risked becoming a major issue between the CMs and the regular home-support team. When the assignment is decided informally based on individual decision, the disagreements are without recourse to arbitration. Because of its proximity to the function of home-support social workers, the introduction of case management holds the potential for disagreement. The fact that assignment to a pivot care provider is sometimes concurrent with assignment to case management militate in favor of a transparent process.

There is another consequence in that the referral, assignment, and closure processes are less organized, which affects information useful in management. For example, the length of waiting periods, the number of people waiting services, and service duration can be more or less visible. This aspect becomes a critical consideration when attempting to establish an approach for managing the quality of services in which these basic indicators are essential.

File Closure

Estrie's integrated network model is based on the principle that, once the elderly person's impaired independence has become moderate to severe, the individual must be considered fragile and should remain in case management even after his or her situation has stabilized. As a result, closing files because the "objectives have been achieved" should be a rare occurrence if the following two conditions are met: 1) the upstream case finding adequately identifies individuals targeted for case management and 2) the CM team performs preventive monitoring (or watch) for certain cases that have been stabilized but for which the files have not been closed. This leaves open a percentage of files with fewer interventions, which can reduce the caseload throughput.

Case-Management Throughput

The review of case-management literature revealed a number of elements irrelevant to patient throughput as well as the grounds for closing a file. The throughput in the Basic Case Management Model *(BCM)* and of the Financial Control Model (FCM) (Phillips et al.[4]) were comparable, that is, 37 % for the basic model and 39 % for the financial control model. In the article on the Channeling project in the United States, Philips[4] reports that the rate of file closure according to reason, depending on when the person left the project (such as prior to assessment) and depending on the case-management model *(FCM or BCM)* was similar for both models and reached 43 % within year.

In Canada, research carried out by Hadjistavropoulos et al.[22] studied guidelines related to case management specific to the brokerage model reported caseloads of 120 to 140 clients with low, moderate, or high levels of risk, as determined by the *Regina Risk Indicator Tool*. The outcomes revealed that the rate of file closure differed depending on the client level of risk and that it decreases as the loss of independence increases. Consequently, during the first six months of tracking, 37 % of individuals at low risk had their files closed, of which half (18.5 %) resulted from improved health or function. In the case of individuals at moderate or high risk during this same period, the number of file closures with respect to the number of clients served dropped to 19 %; 10 % of the individuals in the high-risk group died.

These analysts tend to confirm certain trends that were also observed in the Estrie implementation study. First of all, using a short reference period for this type of calculation can result in a period effect, then either under or overestimates. A high rate of throughput appears associated with a low level of disability and the ability to recover a major proportion of these people (about 50 %), which does not occur in groups with moderate to severe loss of independence, for which the closure rate is 19 % over 6 months. The figures appear high when the Channeling project gives a closure rate of 43 % over a year (11 % attributable to institutionalization and 16 % to death, for a total of 27 %). It must be kept in mind, however, that the level of loss of independence required for entry into the Channeling project is not known. If the level is low, a high rate of closure would be logical since, according to the rule put forward by Hadjistavropoulos, many cases of recovery would soon result in closed files.

To sum up, the factors influencing the closure rate are: 1) level of disabilities of clients upon entry into a case-management program; 2) the size of the window of time considered in calculating the closure rate (avoiding the period effect); 3) the case-management model used in the program.

In Estrie, we observed that two of the territories using a hybrid case-management model returned a rate of closure of 25 % and 26 %. Given the periods considered, it could drop to 17 % or rise to 33 %. A one-year window sometimes appears inadequate. In the case of the rural setting with a hospital, the rate of 26 % basically represents closures resulting from death and institutionalization as well as some individuals moving away. Closures due to objectives having been met were subtracted for purposes of comparison to the urban setting. Death and institutionalization represented 27 % of the closures in the *Channeling[4]* project.

We feel that these trends are adequately clear for us to assign a normalized annual closure rate of about 25 % for clinical case management using a hybrid model. As for the mixed model, the rate of closure remains around 50 % end all clients are considered, including those with mild or transitory loss of independence, according to what we observed in the rural setting without a hospital and in the Bois-Francs.

The following method was used to calculate the closure rate: a) We start with the number of active cases on a specific date and add the number of management episodes during the subsequent target period (as long as possible, such as two or three years) in order to obtain the number of clients served during this period, regardless of the duration of services; b) We calculate the number of files closed during the same period. The number of closures over the number of clients served gives the rate of closure. Although not the only alternative, this method represents a good compromise between ease of application and expected reliability.

Caseloads in Estrie

During the implementation study, we asked case managers about their caseloads and the intensity of their interventions. We learned then that intensive coordination of services and overall discharge assessments use up a substantial amount of time at the outset of management and that about 15 % of caseload files occur in this phase. When the situation stabilizes afterwards, few interventions are needed; for the most part, the CM has to monitor to intervene rapidly should deterioration occur. There would be about 15 % of cases in this preventive-monitoring mode (around one intervention per month). These data take precedence only when the caseload is mature. In other words, it must not be recently constituted because they would result in a high percentage of cases in the management phase and very few cases in preventive monitoring. Given a caseload of 40, this would equate to 6 cases in the management phase and 6 in preventive monitoring, leaving about 30 cases in intervention mode and subject to application of the service plan.

The assessment report on the implementation of the Bois-Francs model indicated that case managers deemed a load of 40 to 50 cases was acceptable in order to better carry out their role. Based on their experience, they considered that 50 to 60 cases were too many to provide follow-up appropriate to their clients' needs. The Bois-Francs region opted for a mixed model.

According to the case managers in the study carried out in the three territories in Estrie, the average caseload in the first quarter of 2005 in the two territories using a hybrid model was 36.5 cases (SD ± 7.2) in Sherbrooke and 36 cases (SD ± 2.2) in Granit, whereas the figure rose to 56.8 cases (SD ± 10.6) for the mixed model. Our continuous monitoring data, based on the I-CLSC system, reports the following results when the first year (caseloads created) is excluded. In Sherbrooke, the average was 32 cases per CM during the 2nd and the 3rd years of follow-up (January 2003 to July 2004). In Granit, the average was 39 cases, which represents a net increase in the last year of follow-up, during which the average caseload rose from 31 to 46 cases. In Coaticook, the average caseload with the mixed model was 10 cases in case management and an average of 57 cases in total. The clients not in case management can be disabled adults, individuals experiencing transitory loss of independence with a prognosis of short-term recovery, and the elderly with moderate to severe loss of independence eligible for case management who received services, but some of whom did not receive the appropriate intensity due to care provider excessive workload. Since the implementation study was supposed to monitor *case-management* clients, we do not have any data about clients who were eligible for but not under case management. We should point out that, in this case, Coaticook and Bois-Francs implemented the same model (mixed). Both regions incurred a significant caseload and experienced difficulty in serving clients according to the expectations formulated in the model.

Interviews with case managers in Estrie provided some insight into certain phenomena:

1) It is difficult to maintain a low caseload when demand is high and when regular home-care colleagues question their own caseloads in comparison to that of case managers.

2) It is impossible for case managers to develop a more intensive or proactive approach under the mixed model when the caseload can be 55 to 60 cases or more.

3) Case managers are responsible for supervising visiting homemakers, which uses up too much time in the opinion of case managers in urban settings. This is due, on the one hand, to the large number of people involved in a zone team and, on the other hand, the internal organization of tasks and responsibilities. CMs, who act as de facto pivot care providers, respond to all the demands of visiting homemakers, including those affecting issues that could be settled by the appropriate staff, such as the team leader of visiting homemakers. When responsibilities are broken down differently so that CMs can devote a greater amount of time to clinical and coordination activities, they are able to take on a few more cases.

Looking at case-management deployment compared against the initial expectations, the outcomes achieved after three years of monitoring in the territories are about 80 %, except in the territory using the mixed model, which achieved 48 % of the initial expectations, as described in the following table.

Table 23.3
Case Management: Organizational Integration and Status in Estrie after 3 Years

Description	Sherbrooke	Granit	Coaticook
Case-management model	Outset: Exclusive model Afterwards: hybrid model	Hybrid model	Mixed model
CM professional affiliation	Multidisciplinary (SW, HRO, nurse, psy.)	Single discipline, open to multidisciplinarity (SW or HRO, psy.)	Single discipline (SW or HRO)
Number of FTE* in case management after 3 years**	**15/19 FTE'S*** (79 % of expectations)	**2.8/3.5 FTE'S*** (80 % of expectations)**	**1.2/2.4 FTE'S*** (48 % of expectations)**
Caseload (average) (I-CLSC)	32 cases	39 cases	10 people in CM out of a total of 57 cases
Waiting list	150 to 175 people	None	None

* Full-time equivalents
** According to preliminary estimates of the required number of case managers, 2000

The balance between case-management service demand and resource supply varies from one territory to the next. With 80 % of the case managers required for its territory, the rural region does not have a waiting list but manages caseload primarily through the closure of files of stabilized patients. In contrast, the urban territory manages caseload by creating a waiting list assigned to a team of two case managers, who carry out telephone follow-up and ensure that certain basic services are put into place. These territories manage to maintain the caseload between 35 and 45 cases.

In the rural territory—which implanted a mixed model—about half the case-management resources had been implemented after three years. With no waiting list, but an average caseload of 57 with 15 % to 20 % in case management, the case managers deemed this proportion inadequate since they felt that a large number of their clients should have been in case management. Pressed by the pace at which demands were coming in, the practitioners lacked time to enroll clients, take steps, and make the required entries into the computerized clinical chart and the individualized service plan. The territory does not have a waiting list and basic services are normally organized promptly for large number of clients. In contrast, psychosocial workers were unable to offer the intensity of interventions that they wanted.

Estimating Caseload and Needs

In the light of the literature review and the elements yielded by the PRISMA-Estrie implementation study, we believe that a caseload of 40 to 45 cases under the hybrid model would be acceptable, once the caseload has achieved maturity. In this situation, about 15 % of cases would require a high intensity of interventions, 15 % would be in preventive monitoring, and the remainder would have a moderate level of interventions focused on achieving implementation of the services agreed on in the ISP and on the subsequent audit to ensure that the required services are indeed delivered. Taking the urban territory of Sherbrooke as an example, if the number of case managers initially foreseen had been in place at the end of the three years, the team could have resolved the waiting list. All in all, both the literature and Quebec experiences, the initial expectations for an optimal caseload appeared fairly accurate, insofar as they fell within the range of the current response to this target group by case-management services in Estrie, that is, about 5 % of people age 65 or older, in an urban center such as Sherbrooke.

Estimating the Number of Case Managers

Before the number of case managers needed in a given territory can be established, the number of potential recipients of case management (target group) must be determined. As previously stated, nearly all of the social workers (or HROs) in the Bois-Francs became case managers when the coordination mechanism was implemented. This means that they shared all of the cases, both those requiring short-term services as well as those requiring long-term services, which accounts for the high throughput. Using Iso-SMAF profiles 4 and higher as an objective criterion for access to case management in Estrie provides a measure of control over admission to case management to reserve these services for the elderly with significantly impaired independence and requiring long-term services. This represented a new element in the Estrie experiment, since the Bois-Francs mechanism did not restrict assignment of on these people only to case managers.

It was decided in Estrie to control admissions to case management reserve the service solely for people with an Iso-SMAF profile of 4 or higher, which equates to moderate to severe loss of independence. Consequently, the percentage used in establishing the target for case management must also be reassessed to determine if it is still appropriate. Faced with our objective of establishing the full-time equivalents (FTEs) needed to serve a given number of clients, it needs to be remembered that we do not take into account the number and type of interventions performed nor the CM's initial profession, because we consider current practice as an overall reality exposed to comparable opportunities and constraints within a given territory.

The Bois-Francs region opted for a mixed model under which 10 % of the elderly living in the community were reached by case-management services without recourse to a tool for selecting clients. This proportion of 10 % achieved in the Bois-Francs is confirmed in the literature, in which percentages ranging from 7 % to 10 % have been published. In the Bois-Francs study, the case-management clients were not selected or sampled because all service users were considered as potential case-management recipients. Indeed, all of the elderly with impaired independence (except in the case of mental-health problems and intellectual disability) could receive the services offered based on needs. In other words, the intensity increased as warranted by the individual's condition. Based on data from the Bois-Francs implementation study, in which the rate of SMAF scores available was 56 %, 27 % returned scores of 1 to 15, ranking them among profiles for mild loss of independence.

When adopting a case-management model specifically for individuals with moderate to severe loss of independence, the target must be brought into line with the actual number of people living with these levels of disability, whether or not they receive CLSC services. Whereas the Bois-Francs region identified the number of the elderly reached by public services on the basis of impaired independence but without regard for the impairment's duration or intensity, we need to know the real proportion of the elderly living in the community with a loss of independence ranging from moderate to severe and, eventually, the number of these people known to home-care and case-management services. According to Saucier[23] (EQLA 1999), cited by the MSSS,[24] only 11.1 % were receiving assistance from their CLSC when the survey on limitations was carried out.

Until now, it has been difficult to accurately assess to what degree a target group can be reached by services (penetration rate), because it is necessary to know how many of the elderly living in the community could have recourse to services for which they are eligible and have unfulfilled needs, yet have not applied for such services.

The major Canadian surveys inventory disability throughout the population using their own instruments and questionnaires. It is not possible to directly borrow the levels of independence they use to deliver their results (mild, moderate, severe, and very severe disability) because their disability indicators are constructed statistically. Since there is no link between SMAF and Iso-SMAF profiles and Statistics Canada indicators, the EQLA and PALS surveys cannot be used to estimate the number of people with impaired independence who would have Iso-SMAF profiles of 4 or higher.

These considerations led us to seek out other calculation methods derived from recent research using representative samples of elderly populations living in their homes and in private nursing homes in Quebec. In this regard, the reader is referred to the following documents: *Enquête québécoise sur les limitations d'activités – EQLA 1998* (Saucier et al.),[23] *Enquête sur la participation et les limitations d'activités – EPLA 2001* (Tremblay, R. and Berthelot, M., 2006)[25]. We also used two studies on individuals in private nursing homes: one in an urban setting in Laval (Hébert et al., 1997)[26] and the other in a rural setting in Estrie (Gervais et al., 2004)[27].

Quebec's EQLA populational study[23] published figures on disabilities, estimating the number of people age 65 or older living with mild, moderate, or severe disabilities. Disabilities were categorized according to the number of activities for which the individual has declared reduced capacity and the intensity of the reduction (partial or total). The EQLA sampling plan comprises people in private homes and excludes those in collective settings whose characteristic is nevertheless to group a large number of elderly with impaired independence. According to these data, the prevalence of loss of independence in people age 65 or older was 41.6 %, of which half, that is, 20.8 %, only had a mild disability. The individuals with moderate to severe loss of independence accounted for 20.8 % of individuals living in private households.

The *Participation and Activity Limitation Survey* (PALS, 2001)[25] is a more recent study, although its data are not comparable with previous studies because the questionnaires were significantly modified. In this case, the sampling plan included all individuals living in private households as well as in collective dwellings (private nursing homes, CHSLDs, RIs, and RTFs). The data are more comparable with populational studies in which the different living settings are included. The rate of self-declared disability for people age 65 years or older was 27.9 %. The 2001 PALS classified disability rates as mild, moderate, severe, and very severe. This categorization, however, is also statistically comprised (indicator based on disability frequency and intensity), which significantly limits direct comparison with the research samples in which the functional independence assessments are established on a person-per-person basis and classified into five fields of independence (activities of daily living, instrumental activities of daily living, mobility, communication, and mental functions). There are no studies on the linkage that could exist, on a case-by-case basis, between PALS and SMAF assessments. This would be very useful for subsequent assessments of the population living at home, whether or not public services are received.

Other data produced by studies specifically targeting loss of independence among the elderly living in private nursing homes reveal that 44 % of those in rural settings[27] and 57 % of those in urban settings[26] had Iso-SMAF profiles of 4 or higher, corresponding to moderate to severe loss of independence. Roughly half of the people in private nursing homes therefore experienced moderate to severe loss of independence.

We compared our calculations to data from the 1998 EQLA and 2001 PALS 2001, showing that they are equivalent to within several tenths of a percent. Since the 2001 survey is more recent and has the advantage of including the entire population living in nursing homes, residences for the elderly, and private homes, we opted for it over the 1998 edition. Table 23.4 presents the results of the exercise when the available demographic data[24] is compared with that from the 1998 EQLA and 2001 PALS in order to identify in which settings the elderly with disabilities live.

Table 23.4
Living Settings of the Elderly*

Proportion of the elderly with disabilities in QC		→	28 %*
% of elderly in **CHSLDs****	4 %	+	
% of elderly in **RIs–RTFs****	0,5 %	+	
% of elderly in **private nursing homes****	8 %	+	
% of elderly at **home with services*****	11 %	=	23,5 %
The proportion of people living **at home without services** is			4,5 %

*   Source 1 : Tremblay, R. and Berthelot, M. (2006) PALS.
**   Source 2 : MSSS, Direction générale des services sociaux, 2004 – Tableau sur la répartition des personnes aînées selon le lieu de résidence en 2004 – cited in Gouvernement du Québec, *Un défi de solidarité – les services aux aînés en perte d'autonomie – Plan d'action 2005-2010*, 2005, page 17
*** Source 3 : Saucier, A. and Lafontaine, P. (1998) EQLA.

Cross-tabulating loss of independence and living environment requires the proportion of profiles 4 and higher within the various living settings, which was done in Hébert's study[26] with a representative sample of 1977 elderly persons according to living setting. Given the sample's representativity, the results can be extrapolated to the Quebec's entire elderly population. Table 23.5 provides a summary of these results.

When the distribution of profiles 4 and higher according to living settings is known, the distribution of loss of independence can be estimated from Quebec's current elderly population. This distribution identifies the target group for case management, see the Table 23.6 following.

Once the overall target has been established, the breakdown of the elderly with Iso-SMAF profiles 4 and higher in each of Quebec's various regions can be determined. Table 23.7 indicates the estimated number of individuals directly targeted by regular home-care services in relation to demographic change in Estrie's seven territories.

Table 23.5
**Distribution of Iso-SMAF Profiles According to Living Settings
(Hébert et al., 1997)[26]**

Iso-SMAF Profiles → Living settings ↓	Mild Disabilities Profiles 1, 2, 3	Moderate Disabilities Motor: 4, 6, and 9	Mental: 5, 7, 8, 10	Severe Disabilities Profiles 11, 12, 13, and 14	Subtotal Moderate to Severe	Total N (%)
Home without services	119 (79 %)	21	10	1	32 (21 %)	151 (100 %)
Home with CLSC services	85 (57 %)	48	13	3	64 (43 %)	149 (100 %)
RTF	36 (25 %)	19	78	8	105 (75 %)	141 (100 %)
Wards	37 (28 %)	23	68	2	93 (72 %)	130 (100 %)
Private CHSLD not under agreement	42 (15 %)	95	80	62	237 (85 %)	279 (100 %)
LTCU in a CHSCD	–	29	12	138	179 (100 %)	179 (100 %)
Private CHSLD under agreement	13 (5 %)	31	72	169	272 (95 %)	285 (100 %)
Public CHSLD	13 (3 %)	159	97	220	476 (97 %)	489 (100 %)
Psychiatric hospital	–	7	117	50	174 (100 %)	174 (100 %)
Total	345 (18 %)	432	547	653	1632 (82 %)	1977 (100 %)

Table 23.6
**Method for Estimating the Elderly Population in Quebec with Profiles 4 and
Higher According to Living Settings(2001).**

Living Setting	Proportion of Profiles 4 and + According to Living Setting	% of People with Profiles 4 and +
Home without services	21 % de 4.5 % =	0.95 %
Home with services	43 % de 11 % =	4.73 %
Private home	50 % de 8 % =	4.00 %
RTFs / RIs – wards	72 % de 0.5 % =	0.36 %
CHSLD (public and private)	100 % de 4 % =	4.00 %
	TOTAL :	**14.04 %**
Less the people already placed in CHSLDs		– 4.00 %
	CASE-MANAGEMENT TARGET	**10 %**

Table 23.7
Method for Estimating the Elderly Population in Quebec with Profiles 1, 2, and 3 According to Living Setting (2001)

Living Setting	Proportion of Profiles 1, 2, and 3 According to Living Setting	% of People with Profiles 1, 2, 3
Home without services	79 % de 4.5 % =	3.55 %
Home with services	57 % de 11 % =	6.27 %
Private home	50 % de 8 % =	4.00 %
RTFs / RIs – wards	25 % de 0.5 % =	0.125 %
CHSLD (public and private)	4 % de 4 % =	0.16 %
	TOTAL :	**14.11 %**
Less the people placed in CHSLDs–RIs and RTFs		– 0.29 %
	TARGET FOR REGULAR HOME CARE	**13.82 %**

Since the case-management target is known (10 % of the elderly age 65 years or older), all that remains to be established is the number of people to be reached by case managers and the integrated-service network in each territory (Table 23.8).

Table 23.8
Target for Case Management in Estrie* Integrated-Service Network for the Elderly

Territories	FY 2003		FY 2004		FY 2005		FY 2006	
	Num. 65+ Not Plac.	CM Target (10 %)**	Num. 65+ Not Plac.	CM Target (10 %)**	Num. 65+ Not Plac.	CM Target (10 %)**	Num. 65+ Not Plac.	CM Target (10 %)*
Granit	30.186	319	30.204	320	30.276	328	30.349	335
Asbestos	20.644	264	20.588	259	20.588	259	20.603	260
Haut St-F	20.955	296	30.015	302	30.072	307	30.157	316
Val St-F	30.714	371	30.685	369	30.756	376	30.821	382
Coaticook	20.474	247	20.529	253	20.571	257	20.606	260
Memphré	60.876	688	70.046	705	70.315	732	70.611	761
Sherbr.	180.031	10.803	190.254	10.925	190.657	10.966	200.234	20.023
ESTRIE (not plac.)	390.880,	30.988	410.321	40.132	420.235	40.223	430.381,	40.338

⟶ **THREE-YEAR PROGRESSION OF 8.8 %**

* The number of people age 65 and older was taken from ISQ projections based on corrected data from the 2001 census. Source: SIISP – Direction de la Santé publique et de l'évaluation.
** The target is calculated on the basis of the population not placed in CHSLDs.

In order to find the proportion of men and women affected by long-term loss of independence (without respect to the degree of disability), we referred to Tremblay and Berthelot,[25] who mentioned that more women than men are living with long-term loss of independence. According to the Institut de la Statistique du Québec (*Perspectives démographiques, Québec et régions: 2001-2051*), there were 398,469 men (41.3 %) and 566,691 women (58.7 %) age 65 years or over in Quebec in 2001. Twenty-six percent of these men live with a long-term disability, which corresponds to 10.7 % of the total population age 65 years and over. In the case of women, 30.8 % live with a long-term disability, representing 18.1 % of the entire elderly population.

Given the preceeding, estimating the number of case managers required is based on the number of elderly individuals in each territory not in a placement setting and the estimated number of elderly people with Iso-SMAF profiles of 4 or higher in this population. With this as a starting point and given an average caseload of 40 individuals for each case manager and an average annualized throughput of 25 % with the hybrid model, we can estimate the number of case managers needed in the territory to achieve its objective.

Territory of Sherbrooke

In Sherbrooke in 2006, the number of people age 65 or older not placed in a CHSLD but having a profile of 4 or higher was 2023 people, representing 10 % of the total population age 65 and older. Some of these individuals received CLSC services (home care or case management); others did not. The number of elderly persons who must fall under case management at any time during the year can be determined by subtracting the number of files closed (on average, 25 %), which, in this example, equates to 505 files. As a result, 1518 files must be active at any time during the year, that is, if variations in caseloads are not taken into account. If the average caseload per manager is 40, 38 FTEs in case management are required in this territory to achieve the 2006 objectives.

In 2005–2006 in Sherbrooke, where the case-management target group was restricted to people with Iso-SMAF profiles of 4 or higher, 1100 individuals were reached (54.4 % of the target figure). This was achieved with 19 FTEs and tends to confirm the populational data that we obtained. This means there for that, even with a strategy for finding cases of individuals with impaired independence, only half of the people with significant loss of independence would receive CLSC services (5 %).

Territory of Granit

In 2006 in Granit, there were 3349 people age 65 and older living in the community. Of these, 10 % had Iso-SMAF profiles of 4 or higher (with or without services), equating to 335 individuals. Using a throughput of 25 % attributable to CHSLD placement and death, there would be 84 files closed during the year, so that 251 would be active at any given moment. Given an average caseload of

40, 6.7 FTEs would be required to meet the region's case-management needs according to the hybrid model.

Territory of Coaticook

In 2006 in Coaticook, there were 2606 people age 65 years or older living in the community, of which 10 % had Iso-SMAF profiles of 4 or higher. This equates to 260 individuals. This territory opted for the mixed model, which means that its real throughput is higher. It also means that the target of 10 % is not exact, because people receiving long-term services with a mild disability profile must be included as well as those receiving short-term services for transitory loss of independence (such as after surgery). When calculating the resources needed for profiles of 4 or higher requiring long-term services, the formula used for the hybrid model must also be applied. It must be remembered that the throughput is appreciably higher with mild disability profiles. Determining the number of psychosocial resources needed solely for transitory, low-demand clients would require assessing individuals served to but not eligible for case management. This was not done as part of the follow-up when case management was implemented.

Accordingly, calculating with a throughput of 25 % (only those clients with moderate to severe loss of independence) would yield 65 files closed during the year, leaving 195 active in any given moment. If an average caseload of 40 is used for each full-time equivalent, 4.9 FTEs would be needed in the Coaticook region only for profiles of 4 or higher.

In conclusion, we reiterate that we would like to be able to calculate a penetration rate for case management in the real target population. Despite its importance, this consideration has been largely neglected up until now. This rate would make it possible to establish a link between the number of clients reached with respect to the objective, the actual caseload during the same period, and the number of case managers (in FTEs). An evaluation of the actual time available for direct and indirect case-management interventions would be useful in determining the real proportion of time that can be spent on this role. These indicators would facilitate studying the efficacy and efficiency of case management.

Discussion

The process for estimating the number of case managers required and the optimal caseload is hampered by the very limited availability of relevant units of comparison, since case management is relatively new in the delivery of services to the elderly in Quebec. Additional work is needed to map the progress of loss of functional independence in the population. It would be of interest to establish a link between Iso-SMAF profiles and the PALS study, which would yield the advantage of opening the way to a transversal populational assessment of loss of independence in the elderly and to assessing the changes occurring in successive cohorts of the elderly. Such studies would make it possible to adapt services based on the characteristics of these cohorts, which would enhance the relevance of public-sector interventions. Substudies on the progression of the loss of independence and handicap based on the residential stream of individuals would definitely be useful in determining if people are "at the right place."

As typically seen in studying the loss of independence associated with aging, the complexity of these issues in response to realities that change over time (in terms of demography, disability, and management methods) is an impediment since our study subjects are not confined in laboratories, but rather live and interact with systems that are also complex. We are also faced by the main limitations of this process, which are listed below. 1) Initially, the organizational models for integrating the case-management function were not consistent across the regions, (exclusive role, mixed, and hybrid). As things progressed, the exclusive model was dropped in favor of the hybrid model in one region and the mixed model in another. For the purposes of our estimation, we opted for a single model: the hybrid. 2) The process for determining the caseload does not take into account case-management practice standards. We do not presume that similar practice standards were used in the study territories. 3) Ideally, the caseload must be matched to an intervention approach that is, in turn, supported by certain administrative methods set on the organizational level. The caseloads were not identical in the three territories and the work time spent on activities other than direct and indirect service to clients was not monitored. Any standard set should ideally take into account actual practice conditions. Our mandate under the implementation study was not that broad. 4) We built on an implementation in which none of the regions achieved the required number of case managers. The immediate effect of this variability between territories is that it becomes impossible to formally validate theoretical data with tangible experience. 5) Lastly, the composition of the case-management changed during implementation: leaves, departures, and replacements had repercussions on caseloads over periods of varying lengths. We did not take these variations into account, because they convey a reality in the setting.

In attempting to summarize all this information in relation to the models given preference in Quebec, we adopted three major kinds of factors to consider:

1. Make sure that the integrated service network reaches its target group and, specifically, it is important to distinguish clients targeted by case management from the others.
2. Make sure that the interventions performed by case managers are indeed those expected, i.e. overall and continuing management based in the community and supported by an interdisciplinary team whose total expertise contribute to maintaining independence, which is necessary for clients to continue living in the community rather than in an institution. All parts of

the network created in this way should be connected by a clinical information system.

3. Ensure the sustainability of a management system whose philosophy and methods are shared by all the local and regional stakeholders that could serve the elderly with impaired independence. This system should be supported by leadership resolutely dedicated to a network approach (rather than a silo approach), which includes the implementation and *monitoring* measures for interorganizational and interprofessional coordination (health-care institutions, social services, and rehabilitation, family physicians, specialists, community pharmacies, community organizations, private nursing homes, subsidized housing and cooperatives, social-economy agencies). Moreover, the offer of services should be broadened (availability of a range of services, accessibility, continuity, and quality of services).

References

1. Long, M.J. Case management model or case manager type? That is the question. Health Care Manager, 2002, 20 (4): 53-65.

2. Scharlach, A.E., Giunta, N., Mills-Dick, K. Case management in long-term care integration: an overview of current programs and evaluations. Paperwork written for California Center for Long-Term Care Integration, 2001, 84 p.

3. Eggert, G.M., Friedman, B., Zimmer, J.G. Models of intensive case management. Journal of Gerontological Social Work, 1990, 15 (3): 75-101.

4. Phillips, B. R., Kemper, P., Applebaum, R.A. The evaluation of the national long term care demonstration. - Chap. 4 – Case management under channeling. Health Services Research, 1988, 23 (1): 67-81.

5. Genrich, S.J., Neatherlin, J.S. Case manager role – a content analysis of published literature. Care Management Journals, 2001, 3 (1), 14-19.

6. Yau, D.C.N., Leung, A.C.T., Yeoh, C, Chow N.W.S. Global case management: Hong Kong – Care for the hospital-discharged frail elders by nurse case managers: a process evaluation of a longitudinal case management service project. Lippincott's Case Management, 2005, 10 (4), 203-212.

7. Enguidanos, S.M., Gibbs, N.E., Simmons, W.J., Savoni, K.J., Jamison, P.M., Hackstaff, L., Griffin, A.M., Cherin, D.A. Models and systems of geriatric care – Kaiser Permanente community partners project: improving geriatric care management practices. American Geriatrics Society, 2003, 51 (5): 710-714.

8. Hackstaff, L., Davis, C., Katz, L. The case for integrating behavior change, client-centered practice and other evidence-based models into geriatric care management. Social Work in Health Care. 2004, 38 (3): 1-19.

9. American Health Consultants/Case Management Society of America – AHC/CMSA Setting case management caseloads remains tricky business. Case Manager. July-Aug 2001, 12 (4): 53.

10. American Health Consultants. Job responsibilities should determine case managers' caseload. Hospital Case Management, 2000, 8 (7): 97-100.

11. Zimmer, J.G., Eggert, G.M., Chiverton, P. Individual versus team case management in optimizing community care for chronically ill patients with dementia. Journal of Aging and Health, 1990, 2 (3): 357-372.

12. Department of Health in United Kingdom. Supporting people with long term conditions: liberating the talents of nurses who care for people with long term conditions, 2005, 30 pages.

13. Challis D., Darton, R., Hughes, J., Stewart, K., Weiner, K. Intensive care-management at home: an alternative to institutional care? Age and Ageing, 2001, 30: 409-413.

14. Pacala, J.T., Boult, C. Factors influencing the effectiveness of case management - managed care organizations. The Journal of Care Management, 1996, 2:27-33.

15. Quinn, J. Case management in home and community care. New developments in home care services for the elderly: innovations in policy, program, and practice. Ed. LW Kaye, Hayworth Press, 1995, 233-248.

16. Noelker, L.S. Case management for caregivers. Care Management Journal, 2002, 3 (4): 199-204.

17. Gagnon, A.J, Schein, C., McVey, L., Bergman, H. Randomized controlled trial of nurse case management of frail older people. Journal of American Geriatrics Society, 1999, 47 (9): 1118- 1124.

18. Diem E., Alcock, D., Gallagher, E., Angus, D., Medves, J. Looking beyond casclaod numbers for long-term home-care case managers. Care Management Journals, 2001, 3 (1): 2-7.

19. Diwan, S. Allocation of case management resources in long-term care: predicting high use of case management time. The Gerontologist, 1999, 39 (5): 580-590

20. Massie, C.Z. A method to determine case manager caseloads in long-term care. Journal of Case Management, 1996, 5 (1): 25-31.

21. King, R., Meadows, G., LeBas, J. Compiling a caseload index for mental health case management. Australian & New-Zealand Journal of Psychiatry, 2004, 38 (6): 455-462.

22. Hadjistavropoulos, H., Bierlein, C., Neville, S., McNeil, D., Bremner, C., Ell, G.L., Jacobs, T., Sagan, M., Quine, A., White, T., Bourgault, M. Managing continuity of care through case co-ordination. Research report. Cana-

dian Health Services Research Foundation, Ottawa, Ontario, 2003, 48 pages.

23. Saucier, A., Lafontaine, P – Institut de la statistique du Québec – Gouvernement du Québec. Enquête québécoise sur les limitations d'activités. Chapitre 2 – Prévalence et gravité de l'incapacité dans la population québécoise, 1998, 73-87.

24. Ministère de la santé et des services sociaux. Un défi de solidarité – les services aux aînés en perte d'autonomie – Plan d'action 2005-2010, 2005.

25. Tremblay, R. et Berthelot, M. - Institut de la statistique du Québec – Gouvernement du Québec. L'incapacité et les limitations d'activités au Québec – un portrait statistique à partir des données de l'Enquête sur la participation et les limitations d'activités 2001 (EPLA), 2006, 27-79.

26. Hébert, R., Dubuc, N., Buteau, M., Roy, C., Desrosiers, J., Bravo, G., Trottier, L., St-Hilaire, C. Services requis par les personnes âgées en perte d'autonomie. Évaluation clinique et estimation des coûts selon le milieu de vie. Rapport de recherche. Ministère de la santé et des services sociaux du Québec, Direction de l'évaluation, Québec, 1997.

27. Gervais, P., Hébert, R., Tousignant, M. Profils d'autonomie fonctionnelle des personnes âgées vivant dans les résidences privées d'hébergement en Estrie. Master's thesis in gerontology, 2004.

Suggested Reading

Challis, D. Case management: problems and possibilities. PSSRU, University of Kent, Canterbury, 1989: 9-22 .

Denis, J.-L, Beaulieu, M.-D., Hébert, Y, Langley, A., Lozeau, D., Pineault, R., Trottier, L-H. L'innovation clinico-organisationnelle dans les organisations de santé. FCRSS report, 2001, 22 pages.

Eggert, G.M., Zimmer, J.G., Hall, W.J., Friedman, B. Case management: a randomized controlled study comparing a neighborhood team and a centralized individual model. Health Services Research. 1991, 26 (4): 471-507.

HMO Workgroup on Care Management. Geriatric case management: challenges and potential solutions in managed care organisations, Jan 1999, 37 pages.

Hromco, J.G., Moore, M.W., Nikkel, R.E. How managed care has affected mental health case management activities, caseloads and tenure. Community Mental Health Journal, 2003, 39 (6): 501- 509.

Issakidis, C., Sanderson, K., Teesson, M., Johnston, S., Buhrich, N. Intensive case management in Australia: a randomized controlled trial. Acta Psychiatrica Scandinavica. 1999, 99 (5): 360-367.

Jeandel, C., Pfitzenmeyer, P. and Vigouroux, P. Un programme pour la gériatrie. Rapport commandé par le ministre de la santé et des solidarités et le ministre délégué à la sécurité sociale, aux personnes âgées, aux personnes handicapées et à la famille en France, 2006.

Johri, M., Béland, F. et Bergman, H. International experiments in integrated care for the elderly: a synthesis of the evidence. International Journal of Geriatric Psychiatry, 2003, 18: 222-235.

King, R., LeBas, J., Spooner, D. The impact of caseload on the personal efficacy of mental health case managers. Psychiatric Services. 2000, 51 (3): 364-368.

Leutz, Walter N. Five laws for integrating medical and social services: lessons from the United States and the United Kingdom. The Milbank Quarterly, 1999, 77 (1): 77-110.

Meldrum, l , Yellowlees, P. The measurement of a case manager's workload burden. Australian and New Zealand Journal of Psychiatry, 2000, 34: 658-663.

Ministère de la Santé et des Services sociaux du Québec. Les orientations ministérielles sur les services offerts aux personnes âgées en perte d'autonomie, 2001, 47 pages.

Mollica, R. Coordinating services across the continuum of health, housing and supportive services. Journal of Aging and Health, 2003, 15 (1): 165-188.

NHS Institute for Innovation and Improvement. Supporting people with long-term conditions, a NHS and Social Care model to support local innovation and integration, 2006, 38 pages.

NHS Institute for Innovation and Improvement. Improving care for people with long-term conditions – a review of UK and international frameworks, University of Birmingham, 2006, 35 pages.

Paradis, M., Bonin, L., Tourigny, A., Durand, P.J. Réseau de services intégrés aux aînés des Bois-Francs – Mécanisme de coordination des services géronto-gériatriques. Process and implementation report, CQRS and FASS, 2001, 164 pages.

Reed, J., Cook, G., Childs, S., McCormack, B. A literature review to explore integrated care for older people. International Journal of Integrated Care, 2005, 5: 1-10. Source: http://www.ijic.org/

Reese, D. J., Sontag, M.-A. Successful interprofessional collaboration on the hospice team. Health and Social Work, 2001, 26 (3): 167-175.

Vanchieri, C. Eye on the elderly. Hospitals & Health Networks, 1998, 72 (12): 54.

Warner, M. and Gould, N. Integrated care networks and quality of life: linking research and practice. International Journal of Integrated Care, 2003, (3): 1-9. Source: http://www.ijic.org/

Chapter 24
The Use of Research Data for Management Purposes

Linda Dieleman, Pierre Richard, Céline Bureau, and Johanne Bolduc

---

Highlights

- This chapter presents the conditions for implementing integrated service delivery networks in Estrie, implementation history, and the way things stood before the start of the PRISMA-Estrie project.
- The chapter discusses the usefulness of the research project's data and instruments:
  - The contribution of Iso-SMAF profiles is discussed. The role of case management is presented, as is the implementation of single entry points and PRISMA-7. Coordination and partnerships are discussed. The subject of the costs of services networking, including the cost of the case management component, is broached.
- Lastly, the chapter presents possible topics for further research.

Introduction

As part of the implementation of integrated service delivery networks for the elderly, managers are called upon to make a transition from managing resources within an institution to managing a network of services. This represents a challenge that demands new management skills and calls for using new clinical and management data.

Making this shift gives rise to many questions about the best practices to put into place and the organizational approaches that can support them. Moreover, as the system undergoes transformation and new operating methods are tried out, managers, in their concern to exercise true leadership in the system's transformation, need feedback on the implementation of the new practices and their effects. Such feedback enables managers and health and social service professionals to evaluate the progress of the changes, make adjustments where necessary, and look for new solutions in order to obtain the desired outcomes.

Sometimes, however, the questions that emerge have no answers, and it becomes very difficult, indeed impossible, to measure the effects of the new program's implementation on the elders ability to retain their independence. In a context of experimentation and rapid change in which rapid adjustment, flexibility, responsiveness to the need for innovation, and networking are the keys to success, partnership with researchers conducting a research project emerged as a winning solution.

The Context

Work to convert services for the frail elderly into a network has been ongoing in Estrie since 1996. Managers were able to draw lessons from the experience of restructuring the system in 1995. At that time, in each of six of Estrie's seven health territories, health and social services institutions were merged to form a single institution. Local community service centers (CLSCs: French *centres locaux de services communautaires*), residential and long-term care centers (CHSLDs: French *centres d'hébergement et de soins de longue durée*), and acute-care hospital centers (CHCDs: French *centres hospitaliers de courte durée*) formed a single entity. This shift prepared the ground for services integration. Over subsequent years, in the remaining territory of Sherbrooke, CLSCs and CHSLDs underwent a similar transformation, while the territory's CHCDs were merged horizontally.

As recently as 1996, Estrie's regional service organization plan (PROS: French *plan régional d'organisation des services*)[1] for the elderly had called on managers and health and social service professionals to set up continuous and complementary services and to view the elderly as users of a network of services rather than as constituting individual institutions' captive clientele. The PROS was transformed concretely into local service organization plans (PLOSs: French *plan local d'organisation des services*) developed by CLSCs and their partners, all operating as members of local joint-action committees.

In 1998, the Estrie regional health board's guidelines on services to the elderly[2] recommended implementing integrated networks, which were to include a joint triage system, a case-management approach, and the use of individualized service plans (ISPs). As of 1999–2000, coordinating activities began to intensify within territories and this contributed to the emergence of services networks. Work on the system's transformation continued following dissemination of the departmental (MSSS) guidelines on services to the frail elderly[3] issued by Quebec's department of health and social services (MSSS) in 2001. The Estrie region forged ahead.

The various components of a networked set of services were gradually put into place. In 1998, implementation of the use of the Multiclientele Assessment Tool (OEMC: French *Outil d'évaluation multi-clientèle*) in CLSCs got underway. This was followed in 2000–2001 by its adoption in CHSLDs for use as an information transmission instrument and by intermediate-type placement facilities, family-type placement facilities, and institutions that serve the Estrie region as a whole.

In institutions other than CLSCs, use initially centered on the Functional Autonomy Measurement System (SMAF: French *Système de mesure de l'autonomie fonctionnelle*) and the OEMC during applications for placement. The mechanism for accessing placement was decentralized to the seven territories in 2000 in order to promote progress towards a single entry-point system. Single entry points were in turn put in place in 2001. Work on the system for using Iso-SMAF profiles to classify the needs of clients in placement began in 2000. From 2001 on, the region applied a method for determining financial benefits for CHSLD clients based on Iso-SMAF profiles and using the equity framework.[4] Implementation of the case manager role commenced in 2001-2002; in 2002, PRISMA-7 (see Chapter 22)[5] was put in place as an instrument for finding individuals at risk of frailty. From 2002 on, the computerized clinical chart (CCC) known as SIGG (*Système d'information géronto-gériatrique*) was in use in the seven CLSCs and three regional institutions concerned. Work is ongoing to make this CCC available to all family medicine groups (GMFs: French *groupe de médecine familiale*) in the region. On the regional level, other work relating to ISPs has been done at various times over the past few years in all the relevant target-group-based programs; the work continues to this day.

Given a context of ongoing change, managers have been required to manage change and display leadership within their services networks, regardless of lack of clarity in the situation or any management-related conundrums they may face. The vision was clear: those involved knew the desired destination but did not always know how to get there and had more questions than answers about how to manage the innovations being put into place. Managers were ready to give their commitment and a partnership with members of the PRISMA-Estrie research team was set up early in 2000.

Research Data and Instruments

The partners in the research project agreed at the outset to use the PRISMA model to define the integrated network, as recommended by the researchers. The model was designed with six components: coordination, a single entry point, case management, ISPs, a single assessment instrument (incorporating a classification system), and an information system. The study generated data on each component of the model. The population study portion of the research had to be tailored to the actual conditions in the field. All the partners, local players, policy makers, and researchers joined forces so that instruments for supporting the implementation of the integrated networks could be devised.

Although all the data generated by the study were useful to managers at the local and regional levels, the research data relating to implementing Iso-SMAF profiles, the case-manager role, the PRISMA-7 case-finding instrument, coordinated action, and the calculation of the cost of implementing services networking stood out.

Implementation of other components, such as SMAF (as part of the OEMC) and the SIGG CCC, was speeded up because their contents often provided the research project's raw materials. In many cases, SIGG functioned as a lever for implementing services networking.

In our view, the research-related work made rigor second nature to us, which we employed in choosing and producing quality clinical data to underpin our management-monitoring operations. Since good decision-making rests on accurate information, managers took measures to ensure the quality of the clinical data entered in OEMCs, the I-CLSC information system, and SIGG. Research supported clinical work, which, in turn, was useful in the managers' work.

Iso- SMAF Profiles

The research data relating to Iso-SMAF profiles enabled managers to better manage the placement mechanisms that had been decentralized to the seven territories; support service organization in residential facilities; and update the method for allocating placement benefits. The data provided in interim reports made it possible to evaluate the effects of services networking on elder independence, as determined by Iso-SMAF profiles. The results of research on in-home services in the Montérégie region[6] led us to introduce the use of data on the index of level of required care (ILRC) in residential facilities.

Implementing the use of Iso-SMAF profiles as a management device for classifying user needs by paradigm functional-autonomy profiles proved to be among the most useful changes on several levels. First, these profiles made it possible to draw portraits of the populations placed in CHSLDs and non-institutional facilities; determine various intake profiles; allocate benefits in line with the equity framework's CHSLD placement dimension; determine eligibility criteria for the various types of placement facility and for case management; and support-service organization according to user needs in intermediate-type placement facilities, family-type placement facilities, and certain other kinds of facility such as day centers. Research on ILRCs was also introduced, so that changes in the clientele could be monitored. Note that ILRCs measure the scope of needs exclusively in connection with nursing care, assistance, and support services for instrumental activities of daily living (IADL).

The experience and benefits of using Iso-SMAF profiles proved so successful that the region is implementing their use in connection with in-home services, including those delivered to clients in private homes. Work is also ongoing to make information on the needs of PALV clients (a program for people with age-related frailty: French *Perte d'autonomie liée au viellissement*) available to the whole service continuum and also to adjust the organization of home-support services so that in-home resources are optimized in line with the departmental home-support policy[7].

Iso-SMAF profiles are also being used regionally in management agreements on targets for placement rates and for compliance rates respecting the profiles of users admitted to placement.

We should also note that the use of Iso-SMAF profiles in determining financial benefits functions as a lever when senior managers, managers, and health and social service professionals engage in the yearly exercise of measuring the needs of placement clienteles, as well as in implementing the procedures needed to produce high-quality data. Operationally, this classification system is very useful to committees on access to local placement, who use Iso-SMAF results as guidelines to enhance their clinical judgments when making decisions about how to refer users.

Lastly, health and social service professionals approve of this system because it uses data from the OEMCs and SMAFs as filled in by clinicians. In other words, management data are derived from clinical data. This is an important organizational asset: professionals and managers are working with the same instruments as they make their decisions, which can be shared or made separately according to their levels of responsibility.

The Case-Manager Role

Case management occupies a central position in services networking. The case-manager function, consisting of assessing user needs, coordinating and implementing ISPs, and acting as a broker on behalf of individuals and their families in dealings with the services network, makes all the difference to users and is a core part of integrated service delivery networks.

The research data made it possible for each territory to choose the case-management model that best suited its needs, all within the context of a regional agreement. Some territories preferred to first implement the single-role model (homogeneous caseload consisting of users being case managed; coordinating role that excludes the delivery of services specific to the case manager's profes-sional background) and then shift gradually towards other models, such as the hybrid one (homogeneous caseload consisting only of case managed individuals, with the coordination component playing the major role and interventions in his or her profession a minor one). Four territories currently operate with the hybrid model, while one has opted for the single-role model and two use a mixed model (mixed caseload comprising some clients eligible for case management and some not, with the CM role being divided between coordination and profession-based activities).

The research data provided organizational information that could serve to guide the local networks in implementing the case-manager role. This included information such as a definition of the target population (moderately to severely frail individuals); eligibility criteria (Iso-SMAF profile of four or higher, i.e., significantly frail and in need of long-term services); and criteria for closing files (placement, death, moving out of the territory).

The research project yielded another concrete result, specifically a method for calculating the number of case managers needed according to target population (see Chapter 23)[8]. This method was used by the *Agence de la santé et des services sociaux de l'Estrie* (regional health agency; hereafter the Agency) in assigning budgets for implementing case management. In response to a request from the Agency, the method was revised in 2006. Following an agreement with the relevant institutions, the Agency plans to draw inspiration again from the method to adjust the number of case managers needed to reach the target group. Regionally, management agreements between the Agency and institutions deal with management indicators for the number of case managers to put in place according to budgets spent and annualized, as well as for the number of users to target.

Updating the method also makes it possible to step back and ask questions about how case management has progressed since being implemented, looked at in relation to the role's definition. Institution managers in the different territories can use this information in reviewing practices and making needed adjustments.

Research data yielded by a mail survey of family physicians[9] drew attention to physician lack of information about the case-manager role and CM clientele, and prompted the *Centres de santé et de services sociaux* (health and social services centers or CSSS) to identify steps that can be taken:

1. How can physicians be reached?
   - Mail, fax, GMF nurse, physician's secretary.
2. What should be communicated and when?
   - When a case manager takes on a case.
   - If a user's biological, psychological, or social condition is unstable or deteriorating.
   - On discharge from hospital, by sending the physician the summary sheet.
   - When a reassessment is done, even if the situation is stable.
   - When the ISP reaches completion or is altered.
   - When a significant visit has been made to the emergency room.
   - On the user's death.
3. Other needs expressed by the physicians surveyed:
   - Having case manager's details.
   - Being acquainted with the process for accessing in-home services.
   - Receiving follow-up information after a referral has been made.
   - Being aware of the kinds of service available.
   - Having direct access to case managers.

Single Entry Points and PRISMA-7

Institutions implemented single entry points based on local service organization and in collaboration with the partners represented on each territory's coordinating committee. The various models underwent change over time, but the function of the single entry point for the vulnerable elderly and their families needing home-support services or placement was retained by all territories.

In general, the single entry point was set up at the entrance to the CSSS facility. There, an interdisciplinary team sees to intake, assessment, follow-up, and call back in relation to service requests. Elderly individuals may refer themselves or partners in the network (hospital centers, rehabilitation centers, community groups, GMFs, medical clinics, etc.) may refer individuals at risk of frailty who have made contact with them. In this respect, the single entry point may be likened to a network of entry points. Users thus never feel they have knocked at the wrong door. The single entry point is a component of the integrated service delivery network that contributes to service accessibility and continuity. It becomes the reference point for the different players in the local services network.

The research team developed PRISMA-7 to bring the case-finding function up-to-date in response to a request from managers. This extremely useful instrument may be employed by all the partners in the local services network (emergency rooms, family physicians and GMFs, surgical prep clinics and other care units, community groups, community pharmacies, collective and cooperative businesses, private residences for the elderly, etc.).

Note that the research project's impact is apparent in the sustained recognition of the importance of case finding.

Coordination and Partnership

Once the PLOSs were set in motion, partners in several territories began to coordinate their activities around local target groups in line with departmental and regional guidelines promoting home care. The research project gave strong support to this approach. It provided the instruments required for measuring coordinated action and the collaborative activities carried out as part of the partnership process: topics discussed; meeting frequency; meeting attendance rates; relevance of issues; participant satisfaction; and recognition for leadership. These instruments, which were developed by the research team, provided managers with criteria for measuring degrees of implementation and the appropriateness of their joint-action structures. Local partners at the joint-action table accomplished these things:

- They got to know each other and drew up a list of the resources they had at their disposal for the region's population (network put into place).
- They reached service agreements that made each institution's services complementary to those of the other institutions (ISP updated).
- They made a list of the needs of users who had not yet received a response, for whom the local services network needed to find solutions. Such solutions could include finding new private residential facilities to work with, sharing training activities, and so on.

- They drew up a concrete plan of work to improve services to the frail elderly in their communities, including workshops, seminars, training for family caregivers, developing specific approaches for Alzheimer patients, and so on.

The Costs Associated with Services Networking

At the request of managers, the matter of the costs associated with implementing and operating the integrated service delivery network's components was incorporated into the research protocol. The question to be answered was, "Do the sums allotted to setting up and operating the network components represent a wise way of meeting the needs of the elderly?" When our project began in Estrie, we took the work done by the SIPA project[10] and the Bois-Francs experience[11] as models, importing several of their concepts and work methods into our own approach. At that time, the implementation costs of these two experiments diverged significantly. It was hard for Estrie to determine, at the start of implementation, just how high implementation and operating costs would be. All the sums invested were drawn from the regional budget for services to the frail elderly, namely the PALV program mentioned above. In other words, Estrie did not have a supplementary budget to carry the project out. The limited financial resources available at precisely the time when the vulnerable elderly are becoming more numerous forced Estrie, like other Quebec regions, to make difficult choices and reach certain decisions. Given that services networking had been pinpointed as a winning solution in ensuring service continuity, we opted to invest in it at the expense of other services. That said, regional and local managers wished to have a clearer idea of the costs of services networking.

At the time, the Agency had already allocated budgets to support the work of joint-action committees in different territories. There followed budgets intended for setting up case managers and regional-level sums were freed up for the SIGG partnership fund. The aim was to enhance the solution developed in the Bois-Francs region, pending the development of a province-wide solution. Lastly, sums were assigned to support the use of SIGG in CLSCs and the regional institutions concerned in order to support services networking.

Research data on cost calculations showed that we had set out on the right road and the sums allotted were enabling us to make a significant contribution to implementing those components essential to services integration. We opted for a blended scenario for budget distribution converging on real integration by approaches such as coordination, the single entry point, case management, and so on.

Thus, the research data prove that the choices made in Estrie were wise ones. However, there are other research data, including those relating to the number of case managers needed based on target population that reveal a conspicuous gap between available resources and the number of individuals to be reached. We are on the point of completing work to set attainable targets between now and 2011.

Conclusion

Managers were supported in their work by research data throughout the implementation period. The data continue to be useful to the network's operations: They contribute to better concept definition and a clearer sense of expected results.

It is our belief that, as this project unfolded, manager influence on researchers and researcher influence on managers allowed all parties to go much further in fulfilling their roles and enhanced the quality of the product delivered, to the benefit of the vulnerable elderly and their families. Moreover, the criteria developed by PRISMA for drawing a portrait of the implementation of the components of integrated services significantly influenced the development by the provincial department of health and social services of an instrument for monitoring the implementation of integrated service delivery networks for the elderly (OSIRSIPA: French *Outil de suivi de l'implantation des réseaux de services intégrés aux personnes âgées*), soon to be disseminated.

Possible Topics for Further Research

If we were to continue our research, we would find it interesting to pursue efforts at understanding context-based changes in professional practice. It would also be useful to try to describe how setting up or building new social networks emerging from local efforts at coordination to meet the needs of people with age-related frailty: How do these networks support families and members of the close circle and to what extent will they replace them? Will members of the close circle be the services network's clients or its partners?

As regards the service-planning component, it would be desirable to develop, test, and monitor an online ISP instrument linked to the OEMC and to further the incorporation of systematic chronic-disease monitoring into ISPs.

1) Regarding service planning: Develop instruments to determine the model used and make a link with empowerment.
2) Regarding the strengthening of support networks for family members: How does the case manager's role support the contribution of the family (empower the family) with a view to maintaining the independence of the sick?
3) Regarding services integration: The concept of integrated service delivery networks underpins the development of local services networks. The sharing of clinical instruments (OEMC, ISP) characterizes all local services networks. Why?

As for case management, it might be useful to develop instruments to identify what models are used and link them to empowerment. Certain aspects of the joint-action component could be scrutinized, for instance, how mergers of management structures either support or hinder clinical integration.

Other questions that have emerged relate to the usefulness of transdisciplinary practices in an integrated service delivery network and how to optimize structures so that they promote interaction across service programs (as well as the systematic monitoring of users with ISPs). Lastly, needs have emerged that relate to adapting Iso-SMAF profiles to the traits of emerging aging target groups (individuals with physical disabilities, intellectual disabilities, and mental-health problems) and to adjusting the acute-care service supply for the elderly to bring it into line with services networking.

Many questions therefore remain unanswered. It is our hope they will be addressed by a partnership of researchers, policy makers, and local players.

References

1. Régie régionale de la santé et des services sociaux de l'Estrie, *Plan régional d'organisation de services aux personnes aînées*, Québec, 1996, 166 p.

2. Régie régionale de la santé et des services sociaux de l'Estrie, *Orientations concernant les services aux personnes âgées*, Québec, 1998, 105 p.

3. Québec (Department), Ministère de la Santé et des Services sociaux, *Orientations ministérielles sur les services offerts aux personnes âgées en perte d'autonomie*, Québec, 2001, 47 p.

4. Tousignant, M. et al., Application of a case-mix classification based on the functional autonomy of the residents for funding long-term care facilities. *Age and Ageing*, 2003, 32: 60-66.

5. Raîche, M. et al., Case-finding of older persons with moderate to severe disabilities by means of PRISMA-7 questionnaire: a presentation of the instrument, its implementation, and its use. In Hébert R., A. Tourigny and M. Raîche, *Integration of services for disabled people: Research leading to action*. Edisem, Québec, 2008.

6. Tousignant, M. et al., Home-care programmes for older adults with disabilities in Canada: How can we assess the adequacy of services provided compared with the needs of users? *Health & Social Care in the Community*, 2007, 15 (1), 1–7.

7. Québec (Department), Ministère de la Santé et des Services sociaux, *Chez soi: Le premier choix – La politique de soutien à domicile*, Québec, 2003, 43 p.

8. Veil, A. and R. Hébert, Estimating a Territory's Case-Management Resources, in Hébert, R., A. Tourigny, and M. Raîche, *Integration of Services for Disabled People: Research Leading to Action*. Edisem, 2008.

9.   Milette, L., R. Hébert, and A. Veil, Early perceptions of family physicians regarding the introduction of integrated service delivery networks for older people. *Canadian Family Physician Journal*, 2005, 51: 1104-1105.

10. Béland, F. et al., A system of integrated care for older persons with disabilities in Canada: Results from a randomized controlled trial. *Journal of Gerontology* – A Biological Sciences and Medical Sciences series, 2006, 61 (4): 367-73.

11. Tourigny, A. et al., Quasi-experimental study of the effectiveness of an integrated service delivery network for the frail elderly, *Canadian Journal on Aging*, 2004, 23 (3): 231-46.

Chapter 25
Physically and Intellectually Disabled Target Groups Served by CLSCs: Representing Their Functional-Autonomy Needs Using Classification by Iso-SMAF Profiles

Nicole Dubuc, Michel Tousignant, Danielle Benoit, Guylaine Allard, Myriam Bergeron, Lise Trottier, and Réjean Hébert

Highlights

In organizing services in the home-support program (SAD; French *soutien à domicile*) that are suited to, and of the level of intensity required by, the diverse needs of the program's various target groups, individual needs assessments are a vital step.

In this study, data produced by the Functional Autonomy Measurement System (SMAF; French title *Système de mesure d'autonomie fonctionnelle*) were drawn from 8251 patient records of clients in the program for age-related disability (ARLI; French *perte d'autonomie liée au viellissement*) as well as for 1762 patient records for physically and intellectually disabled clients. These data were used to classify the clients under the 14 Iso-SMAF functional-autonomy profiles.

The Iso-SMAF classification instrument, which was originally designed for use with the frail elderly target group, was used without modification and accurately represented the functional-autonomy needs of 87 % of the physically and intellectually disabled clients.

The rate of accurate classification was higher for clients aged 19 or older. For individuals 18 and under, the deviation can be accounted for clinically when factors such as age are taken into account and the data associated with each specific SMAF assessment item are more closely examined.

Introduction

In Quebec, the agencies that govern health and social services at the regional level (French *agences de la santé et des services sociaux*), together with local authorities, are responsible for organizing service supply, including home-support services, which form a part of the services provided to the public as a whole. Home-support services are intended for individuals who are temporarily incapacitated and for specific groups who need the services for the medium and long term (Ministère de la Santé et des Services sociaux, hereafter MSSS, 2004a). These specific groups are frail individuals; individuals with chronic diseases, including cancer; individuals reaching the end of life; those with a physical or intellectual disability or an invasive developmental disorder; individuals with mental-health problems; and some others. In organizing services suited to, and of the level of intensity required by, these groups' diverse needs, individual needs assessments are a vital step (MSSS, 2004b).

In this context, in 2002, the Montérégie regional health agency (hereafter the Montérégie Agency) and the region's coordinating committee for CLSC executive directors decided to undertake research, in collaboration with the Research Centre on Aging, to develop a method to measure the goodness of fit between services and the needs of the target groups served by the home-support program (SAD; French *soutien à domicile*) (Tousignant et al., 2007). As part of this research effort, the Multiclientele Assessment Tool (OEMC; French title *Outil d'évaluation multi clientèle*), which includes the Functional Autonomy Measurement System (SMAF; French title *Système de mesure de l'autonomie fonctionnelle*), was systematically used to assess all individuals receiving SAD services, with assessments updated yearly (MSSS, 2000). The method of measuring goodness of fit relies on a profile-based classification system called Iso-SMAF. This is the basic instrument for drawing a portrait of clients in the program for age-related disability (ARLI; French *perte d'autonomie liée au viellissement*) and for measuring service adequacy (Dubuc et al., 2006). A classification system is a practical way to organize and summarize a large number of facts and characteristics under subgroups so that the information can be grasped easily and rapidly (Everitt et al., 2001). Clinically, this way of organizing information is often used to better pinpoint and differentiate the characteristics of individuals presenting with various health problems (Dilts et al., 1995). The information is then of use in setting up treatment plans or service-organization plans specific to subgroups.

Iso-SMAF profiles were designed using rigorous scientific methodology to represent the functional-autonomy needs of individuals experiencing age-related disability. The SAD program targets other groups besides frail elders, including physically and intellectually disabled people. So far, no clinical-administrative system has been devised that is similar to Iso-SMAF but tailored to support the management of services provided to these target groups. In the absence of such a system, the Montérégie Agency decided to verify the extent to which Iso-SMAF profiles could serve the purpose.

The general objective of this study, then, was to explore how well suited Iso-SMAF profiles are to representing the functional-autonomy needs of the physically and intellectually disabled target groups.

The study's specific objectives were:

1. Determine the Iso-SMAF profiles of the physically and intellectually disabled clients for home-support services delivered by CLSCs in the Montérégie region;
2. Analyse what proportion of individuals were correctly classified by the instrument;
3. Identify what factors might account for the differences in individuals whose actual profiles diverged from their assigned Iso-SMAF profiles (referred to herein as having "distant profiles").

Methodology

Study Population

The study population consisted of all the long-term clients of the SAD program in Montérégie's 19 CLSCs. Eligible individuals were long-term clients with care profiles for physical and intellectual disabilities who qualified as "active" users; that is, they had been recipients of at least one CLSC service or one direct benefit during the study's observation period of September 29, 2002 to December 21, 2002.

Data Collection

To determine an individual's Iso-SMAF profile, scores for 29 SMAF items are used (Hébert et al., 2003). Since 2001, SMAF has been incorporated into the OEMC, the instrument chosen by Quebec's department of health and social services (MSSS) to assess users both at home and for purposes of placement and follow-up in a residential facility (MSSS, 2000). In this study, existing data in clients' patient records were used. When this information was lacking, an assessment was conducted by SAD staff. Since the OEMC is not available in online form, the data were input locally and transmitted to a research officer at the Centre for Research on Aging. A rigorous validation process was set up to ensure data quality.

Measurement Instruments

SMAF: The Functional Autonomy Measurement System

SMAF assesses 29 functions in the areas of activities of daily living (ADL), mobility, communications, cognitive function, and domestic tasks (instrumental activities of daily living, or IADL). Every function is assigned a score according to precise criteria based on information obtained by questioning the subject, by observation, or by questioning a third party. The score indicates what the individuals can do in everyday situations: on their own (0); on their own but with difficulty (0.5); with assistance (1); with partial assistance (2); or with full assistance (3). The maximum disability score obtainable is 87. SMAF also allows for gathering information on available resources (the client's close circle and public, private, or community-based resources) that provide help, partial assistance, or full assistance. In this way, it is possible to arrive at a disability score that indicates how far services are falling short of needs (Hébert et al., 2003).

Iso-SMAF Profiles

Iso-SMAF's reliability as a method of classification was originally determined by using the 29 SMAF items as classification variables and conducting a sequence of steps including automated classification-analysis procedures, validation according to various parameters, and the formulation of an opinion by a committee of experts (Dubuc et al., 2006). Iso-SMAF profiles are characterized from the first to the last profile by an increase in the mean level of disability ranging from 9.4 to 73.8 out of a potential 87. Figure 25.1 presents a summary of the main features of the 14 Iso-SMAF profiles. For clearer presentation, the profiles can be categorized under five headings based on predominant impairment. Category 1 comprises profiles 1, 2, and 3 and covers subjects who present with impairment relating principally to IADL. At the other extreme, Category 5 comprises profiles 13 and 14 and covers the least independent subjects, generally individuals who are bedridden and dependent with respect to ADL. The area between these two extremes is a progression in the degree of disability with respect to IADL and ADL, usually accompanied by more significant disability in mobility and cognitive function. Category 2 comprises profiles 4, 6, and 9 and covers individuals with predominantly motor impairment and comparatively well preserved cognitive function. Category three comprises profiles 5, 7, 8, and 10, covering individuals with predominant cognitive impairment. Category 4 comprises profiles 11 and 12, covering individuals presenting with substantial motor and cognitive impairment.

Analysis

An elderly person's Iso-SMAF profile is determined with a computer program that uses Euclidean distance to classify the subject under one of the 14 profiles. Euclidean distance indicates the degree of similarity between two individuals. Besides its usefulness for classification purposes, it can be used to determine how similar an individual's characteristics are to the mean of characteristics of other individuals under the same profile (Everitt et al., 2001). Distance is expressed as a six-digit number, of which five digits are to the right of the decimal point, e.g., 2.77904. Every decimal place is relevant to profile assignment. The threshold value of 5 was determined to indicate when an individual was sig-

Figure 25.1
Chart of the 14 Iso-SMAF profiles

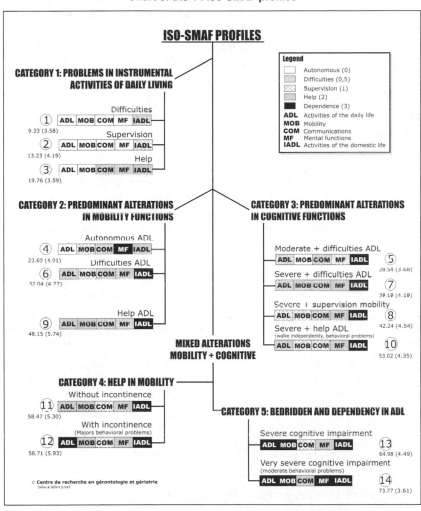

nificantly distant from the others grouped under the same profile and was therefore less sure of truly belonging under that profile. With this criterion, we were able to determine whether a physically or intellectually disabled person had been properly classified or whether instead the individual's true profile was far from the one assigned, which we referred to as having a distant profile. It was thus possible to determine the proportion of individuals who had been correctly classified using the Iso-SMAF instrument. For each of the two samples (i.e., physically disabled and intellectually disabled individuals), the data relating to each specific SMAF assessment item were then reviewed in order to identify the possible influence of scores for certain items on the assignment of profiles. The data from the population sample originally used in developing Iso-SMAF served as a basis for comparison. That sample, drawn from three Quebec health regions, consisted of 1977 frail elders, all of whom were assessed by research nurses trained for the purpose (Hébert et al., 2001; Dubuc et al., 2006). Of that original sample, 99.3 % had been correctly classified by Iso-SMAF.

Findings

During the recruiting period, SMAF data were gathered from the patient records of 1 762 physically and intellectually disabled clients. Since the clinical characteristics of physically and intellectually disabled individuals are distinct, we present the findings for the two groups separately. For comparison purposes, the records of 8251 ARLI program clients in the same CLSC territories were examined over the course of the same period. These individuals, whose mean age was 81 ± 7.6 years, proved to have been correctly classified in 98 % of cases (see Table 25.1). They were assessed by some 950 health and social service workers in the course of regular practice.

Table 25.1
Proportion of clients in ARLI, PD, and ID correctly classified according to Iso-SMAF profiles

Age category	ARLI Sample		Physically Disabled Sample		Intellectually Disabled Sample	
	Correctly classified	Distant profiles	Correctly classified	Distant profiles	Correctly classified	Distant profiles
0- 18 yrs	Nil	Nil	101 (80 %)*	26 (20 %)	175 (79 %)	48 (21 %)
19-64 yrs	185 (96 %)	7 (4 %)	841 (87 %)	126 (13 %)	198 (95 %)	10 (5 %)
65-74 yrs	1596 (96 %)	64 (4 %)	147 (89 %)	18 (11 %)	10 (100 %)	0
75 yrs or older	6455 (98 %)	136 (2 %)	58 (98 %)	1 (2 %)	3 (100 %)	0
Total	8236 (98 %)	207 (2 %)	1147 (87 %)	171 (13 %)	386 (87 %)	58 (13 %)

* n and % of subjects

Physically Disabled Sample

The sample of individuals with physical disabilities numbered 1 318; 60 % were women. The mean age was 49.4 ± 18.3 (range: 3 to 93 years). Applying the Iso-SMAF profile classification to the whole sample, we found that 87 % of individuals were correctly classified. On the other hand, when the results are broken down by age group (see Table 25.1), it becomes clear that the proportion of correctly classified clients varies from group to group. For example, 98 % of those aged 75 or older were correctly classified, while the figures are 89 % for those aged 65 or older, 87 % for those aged 19 to 64, and 80 % for those aged 18 and under.

Furthermore, 35 % of this sample fell into the Iso-SMAF category comprising profiles 1, 2, and 3, with IADL impairment predominant; 51 % into the category comprising profiles 4, 6, and 9, with mobility impairment predominant; 7 % in the category comprising profiles associated with cognitive impairment; and 7 % in the two categories comprising profiles 11 to 14, which cover individuals with mixed cognitive and motor impairment and are associated with the highest level of required care. Individuals with distant profiles (Euclidian distance > 5) accounted for 13 % of the physically disabled sample, with the majority (78 %) coming under profiles 4 and 9. A proportion of 89 % of these were less than 65 years old. Figures 25.2 and 25.3 show the differences between physically disabled individuals with distant profiles and the original sample of frail elders. The curves show the mean/3 for the various SMAF subsections (IADL, mobility, communication, cognitive function, and ADL). Careful examination of individual SMAF-item results for profiles 4 and 9 shows that individuals with more distant profiles are slightly more impaired in their mobility

Figure 25.2
**Comparison of individuals in PD presenting with profile 4
in the original MSSS sample**

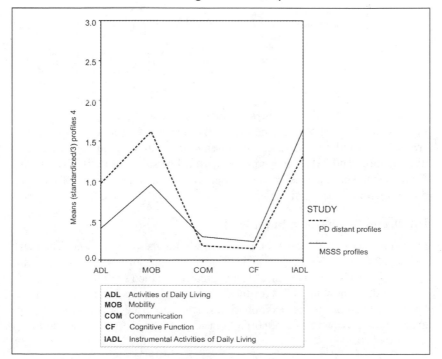

Figure 25.3
**Comparison of individuals in PD presenting with profile 9
in the original MSSS sample**

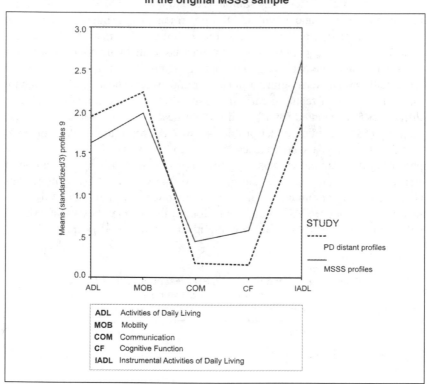

ADL   Activities of Daily Living
MOB   Mobility
COM   Communication
CF   Cognitive Function
IADL   Instrumental Activities of Daily Living

function and such daily activities as washing, dressing, and personal grooming. Incontinence should not be overlooked, either. On the other hand, they are less impaired than ARLI clients when it comes to communication, cognitive function, and IADL. In summary, it could be said that individuals with a distant profile have curves similar to, but slightly displaced from, ARLI client profiles with motor impairment.

Intellectually Disabled Sample

In the intellectually disabled sample, 444 individuals were assessed. The mean age was 24.6 ± 18.3 (range: 1 to 83 years). The proportion of women in this sample (44 %) is smaller than in the physically disabled sample.

The data show that 87 % of these individuals were assigned the correct Iso-SMAF profiles. Close examination of the age effect reveals that the age group with the lowest rate of correct classification (21 %) was 18 and under (see Table 25.1).

In this sample, profiles 1, 2, and 3 accounted for 24 % of clients; profiles 5, 7, and 8, which cover clients with predominant cognitive impairment, accounted for 10 %; and 12 % came under profiles 11 to 14, characterized by mixed impairments. A proportion of 13 % of the sample had distant profiles (Euclidian distance > 5. Of these, a majority (74 %) were assigned profiles 7 or 12 (see Figures 25.4 and 25.5). Note that 83 % (n = 48) of those with distant profiles were in the 18 and under group.

As seen in figures 25.4 and 25.5, for profiles 7 and 12 differences in mobility impairment can be observed between the ARLI sample and the intellectually disabled sample: Especially for Profile 12, impaired mobility is less significant in intellectually disabled individuals than in ARLI clients. The disabled sample also shows less IADL-related impairment than the ARLI sample (2 points less on /24). On the other hand, clients in this sample are impaired to a far higher degree than clients in the ARLI sample in communicative function and ADL. Cognitive impairment tends to be similar to that for ARLI clients, except for the lower-level profiles 1, 2, and 5: Here, disabled individuals with distant profiles

Figure 25.4
**Comparison of individuals in ID presenting with profile 7
in the original MSSS sample**

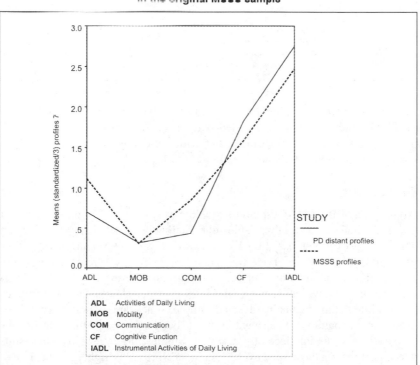

ADL	Activities of Daily Living
MOB	Mobility
COM	Communication
CF	Cognitive Function
IADL	Instrumental Activities of Daily Living

Figure 25.5
**Comparison of individuals in ID presenting with profile 12
in the original MSSS sample**

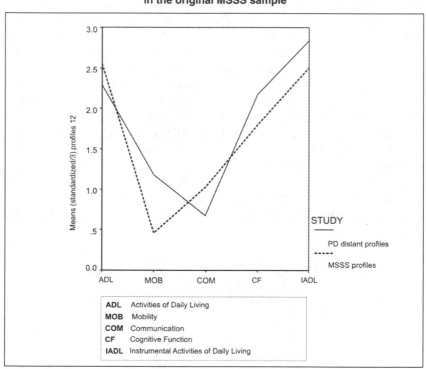

(n = 7) presented with a higher degree of cognitive impairment. In summary, profiles for the intellectually disabled sample are similar to ARLI profiles with predominant cognitive impairment, but with the curve slightly displaced for some individuals who fall under profiles 7 and 12.

Discussion

Application of Iso-SMAF (unmodified in any way) resulted in classification of physically and intellectually disabled client target groups that are 87 % correct. The concise overview based on 14 profiles that this instrument provides thus offers health and social service workers a simple means of representing these clients' functional-autonomy needs. Not surprisingly, the majority of physically disabled individuals come under profiles for predominant motor impairment, while the intellectually disabled sample comes largely under profiles for predominant cognitive impairment. It should be noted, though, that, for both the physically and the intellectually disabled samples, the rate of correct results was higher among those aged over 18; in other words, it is higher for the time of life when chronic health problems quietly make their appearance over time. Note too that, in the Mauricie-et-Centre-du-Québec region, in a cohort of 230 intellectually disabled individuals aged 55 or older, only 2 % had distant profiles. This classification system appears to be less useful for individuals aged 18 and younger, probably because the years until 18 are the time of life most closely associated with learning. When they are used, SMAF scores tend on the whole to provide something like a snapshot of the individual's functional autonomy at a given moment in time.

For individuals whose profile was distant (13 % of the physically and intellectually disabled samples), visual inspection suggested their true profiles are similar in structure to those assigned by Iso-SMAF but the extent of impairment for some SMAF sub-dimensions varies slightly, thereby causing these individuals' distance from the base profiles. The deviations can easily be accounted for clinically when factors such as age are taken into account or the data for individual SMAF items are closely examined. For example, the mean age of the physically disabled individuals is 49, as compared with the sample used in developing the Iso-SMAF profiles, whose mean age was around 80. Certain disabilities associated with the onset of chronic health problems are thus not yet represented among the physically disabled sample. Note too that mobility impairment is more significant than for ARLI clients, especially in the case of profiles with a lower total number of disabilities. This finding is consistent with the medical diagnoses most commonly occurring in the physically disabled target group: muscular dystrophy, multiple sclerosis, cerebral palsy, or spina bifida. Cognitive impairment is less present, and this is normal for a sample with a lower mean age. Last, we observed slightly less difficulty with IADL, which can be explained by the adaptive strategies employed by members of the physically disabled target group. These include assistive technologies and devices for organizing adjusting the physical setting, which are less often resorted to by the ARLI target group.

Age and learning factors also account at least in part for the deviations found among the younger members of the intellectually disabled sample. The mean age of this sample was 24, with 50 % aged 18 or less. Clinically, members of this sample had more difficulty with communicative function, while their mobility function was better preserved. This is consistent with the kinds of health problems experienced by the target group the sample represents.

In Quebec, recent reports have suggested that needs assessment is often conducted as a function of service supply rather than the individual's needs. As well, certain kinds of inequity exist as regards access to assessment and services and the way needs are determined to be urgent or priority (MSSS, 2004a; MSSS, 2006). According to Quebec's bureau for disabled people (OPHQ: French name *Office des personnes handicapées du Québec*), the home-support needs of the disabled are being only partially met even though more funding has been assigned to this area (OPHQ, 2006). No data exist, however, on which an estimate of the scope of these unmet needs could be based. It would appear this situation is not unique to Quebec. Judging by a Canada-wide study conducted in 2002, things are more or less the same across Canada (Naderson et al., 2002).

The findings of our study show that, for the majority of physically and intellectually disabled clients, we can certainly consider meeting this information need at least in part by using a classification system based on Iso-SMAF profiles. A much larger sample would be needed to determine more specifically the way in which clients like the 13 % of our sample with distant profiles present with functional limitations. It would then be possible to determine whether it is necessary to create new versions of profile 4 or 9 specifically tailored to physical impairment and a new version of 7 or 12 tailored for intellectual disability. Such new profiles would complement the original ones. As things stand at present, the partners who participated in this assessment acknowledge that Iso-SMAF profiles serve to pinpoint only a portion of physically and intellectually disabled individuals' needs. We believe that, in line with departmental policy on services to the physically and intellectually disabled, other needs associated with individual, residential, social, and professional independence must be considered if members of these target groups are to take a real part in community life (MSSS, 2003; MSSS, 2001a). Of course, this is equally true of the frail elderly. But given an ongoing climate of financial restraint, both the regional health agencies local authorities and service providers need to consider equity among different target groups, primacy of needs, the principle of neutrality, and the principle of user's choice when organizing and delivering services (MSSS, 2001b; MSSS, 2003; MSSS, 2004b). It would seem that the data generated by Iso-SMAF profiles could be used in taking a step in the right direction. Transversally, the same information could help in drawing portraits of the target groups, showing their distribution in different settings and making possible a review of how appropriately services are organized. Monitoring the data in an ongoing manner could help determine what functional-autonomy needs are shared by the different target groups—ARLI, physically disabled, and intellectually disabled clients—and, based on specific realities, identify necessary differences related to scope, partnerships, and inter-sectorial action in service-delivery methods and ways of meeting needs.

Acknowledgements

We wish to thank Robert Johnson, member of the executive director's office of network coordination at the Montérégie Agency (Agence de la santé et des services sociaux de la Montérégie) and member of the research committee; Jean-Pierre Beaudry; Céline Charest; Chantal Arsenault; Murielle Savignac; Marie-Christine LeTellier; Nathalie Delli-Colli; and all the health and social service workers, managers, and policy makers who contributed to this undertaking.

References

Dilts, D., Khamalah, J. and Plotkin, A. (1995). Using cluster analysis for medical resource decision making. *Medical Decision Making*, 15(4), 333-347.

Dubuc, N., Hébert, R., Desrosiers, J., Buteau, M. and Trottier, L. (2006). Disability-based classification system for older people in integrated long-term care services: The Iso-SMAF profiles. *Archives of Gerontology and Geriatrics*, 42, 191-206.

Everitt, B.S., Landau, S. and Leese, M. (2001). *Cluster Analysis*, 4th ed., Edward Arnold Publisher, London, 224 p.

Hébert, R., Desrosiers, J., Dubuc, N., Tousignant, M., Guilbault, J. and Pinsonnault, E. (2003). Le système de mesure de l'autonomie fonctionnelle (SMAF) – Mise au point. *La Revue de Gériatrie*, 28(4), 323-336.

Hébert, R., Dubuc, N., Buteau, M., Desrosiers, J., Bravo, G., Trottier, L., St-Hilaire, C. and Roy, M.A. (2001). Resources and costs associated with disabilities of elderly people living at home and in institutions. *The Canadian Journal on Aging*, 20 (1), 1-22.

Ministère de la Santé et des Services sociaux (2003). *Orientations ministérielles «Pour une véritable participation à la vie de la communauté: Un continuum intégré de services en déficience physique. Objectifs 2004-2009.»* Services des personnes handicapées, Gouvernement du Québec, 93 p.

Ministère de la Santé et des Services sociaux (2000). *Comité aviseur sur l'adoption d'un outil d'évaluation intégré des besoins des personnes en perte d'autonomie et de détermination des services requis notamment en institution ou à domicile* Gouvernement du Québec, 84 p.

Ministère de la Santé et des Services sociaux (2001a). *De l'intégration sociale à la participation sociale. Politique de soutien aux personnes présentant une déficience intellectuelle, à leurs familles et aux autres proches.* Gouvernement du Québec, 109 p.

Ministère de la Santé et des Services sociaux (2001b). *Orientations ministérielles sur les services offerts aux personnes âgées en perte d'autonomie*, Direction générale de la planification stratégique et de l'évaluation, Gouvernement du Québec, 47 p.

Ministère de la Santé et des Services sociaux (2003). *Chez soi le premier choix: La politique de soutien à domicile.* Gouvernement du Québec, 41 p.

Ministère de la Santé et des Services sociaux (2004a). *Chez soi le premier choix: Précisions pour favoriser l'implantation de la politique de soutien à domicile.* Gouvernement du Québec, 39 p.

Ministère de la Santé et des Services sociaux (2004b). *L'architecture des services de santé et des services sociaux. Les programmes-services et les programmes-soutien.* Gouvernement du Québec, 30 p.

Office des personnes handicapées du Québec (2006). *Revue de l'année 2005-2006: Actions gouvernementales et personnes handicapées.* Direction de la recherche et de l'intervention nationale, Office, 139 p.

Ministère de la Santé et des Services sociaux (2006). Sous comité personne en quête d'autonomie du comité scientifique pour l'évolution de l'outil d'évaluation multiclientèle (2006). *Piloter son projet de vie et participer socialement: Les finalités attendues de l'OEMC pour les personnes en quête d'autonomie.* Québec, February, 56 p.

Naderson, M., Parent, K., MacLellan, M. and Keefe, J. (2002). *Analysis of Interfaces Along the Continuum of Care. Technical report 3: Adults with physical disabilities.* Hollander Analytical Services Ltd, Victoria.

Tousignant, M., Dubuc, N., Hébert, R. and Coulombe, C. (2007). Home care programmes for disabled older adults: How can we assess the adequacy of services provided compared with the needs of users? *Health and Social Care in the Community,* 15(1), 1-7.

Chapter 26
PRISMA France: Adapting the PRISMA Integration Model to the French Health and Social Services System

Dominique Somme, Hélène Trouvé, Yves Couturier,
Sébastien Carrier, Dominique Gagnon, Benoît Lavallart,
Réjean Hébert, Carole Crétin, and Olivier St-Jean

Highlights

PRISMA is an integration model that has significantly impacted on public health.

Based on these convincing results, the French government is currently funding experimental implementation of this model in France.

This chapter presents how the model was adapted to take into account France's distinctiveness and analyzes the conditions for implementing this innovative integration model in France.

The authors thank Catherine Périsset, project manager for Prisma France, Laurence Leneveut, project pilot for Prisma France and Sylvie Lemonnier, local pilot for PRISMA Paris 20 for their involvement in the implementation of the project described in this article. The authors thank all their partners in the various committees of partnership in all three sites. Finally, the authors are grateful to the clinical research unit at the Georges Pompidou European hospital (HEGP) for its constant support, efforts in data management, statistical assistance, value commitment, and expertise.

The PRISMA study in France is funded by the Direction Générale de la Santé (general directorate for health) of the Ministère de la Santé et des Solidarités (ministry of health and solidarity), the Caisse Nationale de Solidarité pour l'Autonomie (national solidarity fund for autonomy), and the Régime social des Indépendants (social programs branch).

Complexity of the Service Offering in France

Home-support services for the frail elderly in France have significantly stepped up their activities. This is the result of demographic changes and recent regulatory dispositions (in particular, the personalized independence allocation, known under the French acronym of APA), which has increased the capacity of the targeted individuals to contribute to the cost of services. At the same time, needs have multiplied and the types of assistance have increased, occasionally making coordination rather complex. As a result, on average, recipients of a home-support service receive care or assistance from three providers (professional or informal) and 25 % of the most dependent recipients receive assistance from six or more caregivers[1]. Moreover, the constantly growing number of APA beneficiaries (+7 %/year since 2003) is outstripping the total number of individuals aged 75 or over (+3 % in 2005)[2]. This has an impact on the average number of APA cases handled by sociomedical teams (or more often, the social assistant alone) and therefore on their ability to provide attentive follow-up for the most difficult home-support situations.

Beyond these demographic and epidemiological data, the area of home support for the frail elderly is subject to a semantic difficulty in that there is no precise definition of the area of competence of health and social assistants, as pointed out by the French Court of Account[3]. This lack of a definition is strikingly illustrated by the confusion about the territorial boundaries for interventions: while regulatory dispositions are primarily managed on the departmental level, assistance is usually delivered locally by providers from the community sector. It is also evidenced by a barrier between the providers primarily giving health care (such as home nursing care) and those primarily from the social or sociomedical sector. This vague definition of the spheres of jurisdiction and intervention for health-care, social, and sociomedical providers results in a multiplicity of actors that may be governed by a variety of potentially conflicting criteria for accessing to services. Given the fragmentation in the procedures regulating the service offer, each actor has only partial control over coordination, which leads to multiple assessments responding to many different clinical and administrative tracks. Dispersal of the management system has been all the greater since there has been no compelling consensus on or distribution of a standardized assessment instrument.

Many dispositions have been put into practice in France over the last two decades in response to the lack of coordination, including local information and coordination centers (referred under the acronym of CLIC) and geriatric care networks. The CLICs and care networks have yielded significant progress in coordinating care and services for the frail elderly through the use of communication means that provide a more complete listing of health and social services. This enhances access to information and therefore delivery. Yet the areas of intervention of the CLICs and geriatric care networks remain compartmentalized. The former are mainly social in nature; the latter mostly health-related, especially independent of APA sociomedical teams and with nonsystematic links to all other actors, including attending physicians, hospitals, and home hospitalization services (French acronym: HAD). While these two dispositions hold significant potential for coordination, they encounter a certain number of constraints, which include low levels of resources, the fact that neither consistently covers the same territory (which hampers the adoption of a strong territorial approach), lack of common assessment instruments, and absence of a shared information system. On a more fundamental level, this difficulty results from the fact while all the institutional actors recognize the added value of these two measures, it has yet to lead to coordination being given precedence.

PRISMA: Assessing an Innovative Model for Integrating Care and Services for the Frail Elderly based on Case Management

PRISMA (Program of Research on the Integration of Services for the Maintenance of Autonomy) has provided means for analyzing the implementation and impact of the most typical coordination model as defined by Leutz[4]. According to this model, integration occurs when the following integration mechanisms and tools are put into place[5]: coordination between institutions at every levels (strategic, tactical and clinical); case-management process; single entry point to the care and services continuum; use of a single standardized assessment instrument with classification system; use of individualized service plans and deployment of a continuous information system.

These integration mechanisms and instruments are viewed as reference points. Their operational implementation must be adapted to the territorial reality to ensure that implementation actually takes place. This flexibility in applying the integration mechanisms and instruments referred to above allows the model to be implemented in various health and services contexts[6]. This model's convincing results in frailty prevention, satisfaction, empowerment of individuals, and economic efficiency are addressed in other chapters in this book.

Implementing PRISMA in France: Adapting the Integration Model

The convincing results from implementing the PRISMA model and its flexibility in terms of practical implementation made it possible to conduct an experimental project in three geographic areas, referred to hereafter as "experimental sites," that roughly correspond to the French legal concept of catchment area. The entire array of integration mechanisms and instruments had to be specifically adapted to France's care and assistance context and, as was done in Quebec, adapted even more precisely to the local context.

This experimental project, which began in January 2006, was made possible through the joint efforts of a certain number of actors at the highest levels of policymaking. This joint effort, which focused on the conditions required for continuity—including those needed for adaptation to local contexts—led to appropriation of the integration mechanisms and principles.

The *Coordination*: Implementing Partnership Procedures

Coordination refers to the existence of partnerships between the actors:

1. Strategists and funding providers (on the national and departmental levels)
2. "Operational," corresponding to a tactical management level (local)
3. Service and care providers (with the person on a clinical level).

Joint-action mechanisms—in particular, meetings, formal partnership mechanisms, and collective decision-making—aim at jointly defining the organizational and financial conditions for implementing the integration system.

In France, the level of political and financial responsibility for services for people with impaired independence rests with the department. Since the general councils (elected policy-making bodies for French departments) implement their policy for services to the frail elderly with the various operational actors, they must also be associated with it. Implementing a strategic partnership of this type at each experimental site is a mandatory condition for implementation. This partnership takes the shape of a Comité Départemental Stratégique (CDS for departmental strategic committee), bringing together at least representatives of the general council, the mayor's office, regional and department government bodies (Direction Régionale et Départementale de l'Action Sanitaire et Sociale – DRASS and DDASS, Agence Régionale de l'Hospitalisation – ARH), health insurance (Union Régionale des Caisses d'Assurances Maladie – URCAM), retirement funds, users, health-care professionals in private practice, and, depending on local configurations, other policy (or financial) actors from the health and social services sector.

While necessary, this condition is not enough to ensure the success of model implementation. Its meaning can be seen through partnership-strategic functions:

1. Define an overall management policy for the frail elderly within the territory.
2. Define partnership conditions between the structures and actors, and specify the process through which these conditions can be modified.
3. Define the financing mechanisms for case managers.
4. Give legitimacy within the territory to the actions of case managers.
5. Monitor development of case-manager actions and identify impediments and service needs.

The partnership structure required at experimental site plays a dual role. On one hand, the actors at each site needed to carry out locally the directions decided on at the strategic level. It also provides a means to feed overall information back to the strategic level, instead of simply fragmented information from the services provided under the jurisdiction of each decision maker. The composition of the Comité Local Opérationnel (French acronym: CLO for local operational committee) varied from site to site, but could include representatives of the CLIC, health networks, the departmental center for the disabled, APA sociomedical teams, varied social services (municipal, departmental, etc.), home nursing care, home hospitalization, home-help services, volunteer associations, local associations of general practitioners and nurses in private practice, the concerned hospital services and psychiatric sectors, social services in Centres Communaux de l'Action Sociale (municipal social-action centers), and any other local actor in a position to offer services or care, according to local characteristics.

Partnering at this level and aims at:

1. Defining the integrated health and services system's operating means and methods.
2. Implementing single entry point access to case management, specific admissions criteria, and eventually case-management closure.
3. Identify individuals who could be case managers.
4. Define the procedures for sharing information.
5. Give local legitimacy to case-manager intervention.

Case-Management Process

Even more than organizational mechanisms, consistency between care provided by the different health-care practitioners (physicians, nurses, kinesiotherapists, occupational therapists), how they work in conjunction with social actors (social assistants, home helpers for activities of daily living), and continuity of delivered care and services have a major relational dimension[7]. For this reason, the French Court of Account[3] proposed that a system with a single representative to coordinate the patient's care and services be promoted. Indeed, the concept of case management arises from this observation that frail individuals should be paired with a single person who would be responsible for organizing their care and assistance plans.

The case manager is the sole provider representative involved in coordinating social and health care and services. For anyone under their management, case managers:

1. Perform, in the home, an exhaustive assessment of the individual's health and social needs in order to determine if case management is appropriate and, if so, define the assistance plan.
2. Play the role of coordinating a resource person for the frail individual.
3. Plan the necessary services.
4. Take steps to admit the individual to the services.
5. Ensure that the planned services are provided.
6. Organize support and coordinate the various providers involved.
7. Ensure periodic review of the individualized service plan.

The relevance of limiting the number of cases in carrying out these tasks has been demonstrated[8]. The findings of past studies have revealed that the maximum number of active cases per case manager is 40[9]. In other words, the level of intervention is intensive, requiring triage to ensure the most appropriate access possible. The case managers under the PRISMA model implemented in

Quebec came from different health and social services structures[5]. Their initial competencies were both social and health care in nature. While becoming a case manager required specific training, the candidate's professional background added value to the case-management team by contributing an interprofessional or even trans-professional perspective[10]. In France, this is a new professional field and appears to correspond to social workers or nurse–coordinators. Regardless of their background, complimentary training appears necessary insofar as this professional field calls for competencies related to both social work and health.

Single Entry Point

The single entry point is defined as convergence point of requests for access to case management. It provides significant leverage in implementing the model, particularly because of its visibility among the elderly and their families, because it relieves them of having to locate the services they require for their conditions at multiple access points. This single access point also facilitates the work of many professionals. Implementing the access point is also an equity issue because all requests are processed according to the same procedures. Intake and information complete the access point's missions, whether the individual is eligible or not for case management. The access point's efficiency is premised on request centralization, access coordination, updating of knowledge about the service and care offer, and a common, standardized assessment system. Consequently, the creation of this access point can only be viewed as a result of the operational partnership (CLO), supported by the strategic partnership (CDS). In France, strengthening the CLICs could eventually make it possible to institute this kind of single entry point.

Use of a *Standardized Multidimensional Assessment Instrument* with Classification System

Using a standardized multidimensional assessment instrument yields a diagnosis that can shared and understood by the various caregivers of the frail population. The resultant classification system must help practitioners develop a common language. France's regulatory instrument for measuring the degree of dependency is the AGGIR grid (Iso-Ressource group-based Assessment of Geriatric Independence). It can be used to classify the elderly into six significantly close profiles of dependency and use of resources: GIRs (for "Groupes Iso-Ressources" or Iso-ressource groups). Yet, as stated by the Inspection Générale des Affaires Sociales (IGAS for general inspector for social affairs)[11], the AGGIR grid appears inadequate when it comes to producing a satisfactory sociomedical assessment. This is true for a number of reasons: doubtful validity conditions and reproducibility, underestimation of cognitive dependence, lack of correlation with the need for assistance, and the problematic linkage between the grouping and the plan. AGGIR is also difficult to configure to take into account social and environmental compensations for dependency issues. Moreover, it is often used to assess service eligibility and to identify the payer, rather than as a clinical tool that serves first and foremost the clinical continuity of services. Consequently, IGAS advocates combining and/or integrating AGGIR with other instruments. Whatever more complete analysis instrument is developed:

1. It must produce GIR group information.
2. It must not be limited solely to activities of daily living.
3. There must be specific rules for using the instrument to produce individualized plans.
4. It must have been previously validated, tested for reproducibility, and adapted for people with cognitive impairment.

It would also appear useful if the instrument could provide more information than the GIR group. In this context, the Système de mesure de l'autonomie fonctionnelle (SMAF or functional independence measurement system) seems to respond fully to the need for independence assessment and compatibility with GIR groups (see Chapter 27 herein). In addition, a comprehensive instrument close to the Outil d'Évaluation Multiclientèle (multiple client-group assessment instrument) but containing SMAF could be adopted by care providers as a whole.

Use of the *Individualized Service Plan*

After multidimensional assessment of the situation, the case manager's task consists in developing an individualized service plan (ISP), in partnership with the person concerned, along with social-services and medical professionals and non-professionals (family, friends, neighbors, *etc.*), whatever their position in the offer of services. Consequently, the ISP aims at sketching a portrait of the person's needs, whether or not social-services and medical professionals respond to these needs. Once the ISP has been produced, its implementation is subject to monitoring and regular based on changes in needs and the offer of services. It allows for analysis of the possible discrepancies between the person's needs and the services currently offered. The ISP is revised with each reassessment. Case managers view the ISP as a kind of an evolving logbook of services and needs, primarily from a clinical viewpoint. At the institutional level, the ISP provides a means of monitoring the service provider's performance in meeting the needs of the recipient client group[12, 13]. This corresponds to the "assistance plan" as provided for statutorily by APA legislation, but is not limited to use of the APA allocation, which is too often the case with the assistance plan.

Use of a *Computerized System* (computerized clinical chart)

Like the ISP, assessment can only be a clinical integration insofar as the various clinical practitioners have access to it. This underscores the importance of having a shared information system when aiming for integration. The use of shared computerized clinical charts during Quebec's PRISMA program proved to be a factor in the successful implementation of integrated care and services networks. Public authorities in France are currently developing a single patient record (Dossier Médical Personnel or DMP), which will probably require a sociomedical component. Pending completion of this single record, integration requires that procedures for sharing information be defined. All such procedures must be presented to and adopted by the various levels involved.

Innovation in France: Analysis of Implementation Conditions

Based on the theoretical model developed recently from a systematic analysis of scientific literature[14], we have mapped out the factors for and against implementation of this innovation as well as the issues involved. Table 26.1 provides an analysis of the factors that depend on the innovation's inherent characteristics. It appears that the difficulties incurred when implementing innovations in the systems for managing loss of independence relate to the diversity of payers, organizations, competition between these organizations, and the actors that might be affected by or use the innovation in question. This shows up in the perception of such people as a high level of innovation complexity, in particular, because of integration problems at the operational level. It would be unrealistic to attempt to implement an innovation in a fragmented system unless the innovation had significant flexibility and a high level of reinvention. This would also hold true if its integration would restrain their capacity for initiative and independence. According to Greenhalgh,[14] the perception that an innovation would be beneficial is a sine qua non condition for its implementation. The PRISMA model's known benefits have been discussed earlier. They are based on the PRISMA study carried out in Quebec and dealt with in detail elsewhere in this book. Nevertheless, there is currently some doubt that the impact can be reproduced in the French system, which accounts for the model's homophilia (its adaptability to potential new users) being perceived ambiguously. The cooperation of a research team yields observable results, making it a major condition during the "experimental" implementation phase. It also promotes dissemination of knowledge between current users of the model in Quebec and its potential users in France, while providing a means for training the potential users. We should also point out that, according to PRISMA assessment data in Quebec, there is no perceived risk in implementing the integration model[15] Moreover, this perception is shared by the actors. All these factors, which are attributes of the innovation, are not completely stable throughout the entire implementation process. This tends to complicate identification of the adoption determinants and even assimilation of the innovation at this level, given their variability in time and space[14].

Table 26.1

Analysis of factors influencing a priori probability of implementing the innovation represented by an integration model in the French health care and services system based on innovation characteristics

Innovation Characteristics	Favorable to Implementation	Objective	Unfavorable to Implementation
Advantage for users	Existence of scientific evidence of the model's impact on quality and efficiency		Various perceptions related to homophilia
Compatibility with organizational and professional standards			Diversity of standards
Complexity	Existence of evidence of implomontation in various organizational contexts Simplification by breaking down into elements		High initial perception of complexity. Many organizational or regulatory obstacles to overcome.
Field of application	Progressive implementation starting with "complex cases"		
Observation of the benefits of implementation		Expectations of the research team	
Flexibility	Choosing a flexible model		
Hierarchization of elements	Selection of a element-based model		
Risk for individuals	Perceived as low or inexistent		
Direct utility in tasks	Perceived as high (single entry point, sharing of information, shared plan)		
Knowledge to be mobilized	Significance of collaboration with professionals from other countries that have implemented the model	Expectations of the training team	
Technical support	Collaboration with a center of expertise in Sherbrooke	Expectations of the change agency	

Table 26.2
Analysis of factors influencing a priori probability of implementing the innovation represented by an integration model in the French health care and services system based on the characteristics of potential users of the innovation

Characteristics of potential users	Favorable to Implementation	Objective	Unfavorable to Implementation
Psychological	High motivation, need for change		Diversity and destabilization through a proactive process (low tolerance of ambiguity)
Meaning for the elderly		Expectations of the research team	
Adherence to decision-making processes	Involvement of all levels, two-way process, authorization/collective		
Information lag time between the various policy levels	Involvement of all levels		Diversity in needs for information, the time available for information, communication methods
Coaching during the initial implementation phase	Role of the change agency		
User feedback			Innovation in France: no users set up
Concern about the unfinalized aspects of the project		Major concern	

The criteria dependent upon potential users and the context itself are often overdeterminants. Indeed, it would be simplistic to assume that potential users would be passive in the adoption process. To the contrary, they tend to study the innovation, try it out, assess it, see sense in it (or fail to find any), learn from the experience, and modify it. They often seek out discussions with other users. In these regards, as well (see Table 26.2), implementation of the intervention is made more complex by the diversity of the professional cultures involved and the experiences of the actors. While flexibility is the model's main strength, it is also destabilizing for the actors if they have to do any reengineering. Respecting the decisional process of individual agencies is very important in the French system, which is highly fragmented. Lastly, Table 26.3 provides an overview of the factors dependent upon organizational context. On this level, the varied influences that can affect the implementation process range from diffusion (in which the professionals appropriate the innovation, mainly through a horizontal

Table 26.3

Analysis of factors influencing a priori probability of implementing the innovation represented by an integration model in the French health care and services system based on the characteristics of the implementation context

Characteristics of the organizational context	Favorable to Implementation	Objective	Unfavorable to Implementation
Structure of the social networks involved			Varied, many, and uncontrollable social networks
Model homophilia			Varied perceptions
Leader involvement			Presence of various leaders (people authorized to give an opinion without necessarily being a potential user), many, uncontrollable
Champions	Presence of champion (future users defending the innovation on the different discussion tables on the local and strategic levels about utility)		
Experimental implementation program	Presence of a change agency whose credibility relates to linkages with the international research network on integration		
Structural aspects			Quite varied in size, levels of independence, specialization, and adaptation to change
Intra- and interorganizational communication			No new means: strategic arbitration to be carried out
Financial means			Pas de nouveau moyen : arbitrage stratégique à faire
Tension towards change	Very important at all levels (increased)		

process between peers that is often informal) to dissemination (in which implementation is planned, formalized, and produced by centralized mechanisms that are often hierarchal). Currently, the organizational context is characterized by tension towards change. This occurs on the strategic level, given the anticipated increase in demand for means and, on the operational level, because of saturation in the system's current operations. Dynamic analysis of implementation led Greenhalgh to develop a scale broken down into three categories of actor strategies whether in supervisory or funding capacities. At one end of the scale is the "Let it happen" position. The middle position is labeled "Help it happen." The "Make it happen" strategy is located at the far end of the scale[14]. Adopting this scale provides a means for determining that the policy that French authorities have followed up to now is close to the "Let it happen" strategy (e.g., implementing the CLICs and gerontology networks with limited means). In the case of the trial attempt to integrate care and services, public officials developed a policy that falls between "Let it happen" and "Make it happen." They funded both an experiment and the evaluative research accompanying it (see below) and had a presence on the strategic committee. The reason for this intermediary position appears to lie with a desire to have recourse to technical expertise (through a change agency) to benefit from knowledge transfer.

Overall, French attempts to integrate services have been characterized by:

1. Complex funding methods, giving rise to assessment focused on determining right rather than need.
2. System open to a certain amount of competition, making the offer of services more complex, while leading to strategies of discrimination and protection of individual interests.
3. Conceptual confusion between integration, coordination, and liaison.
4. Low concern with service integration, at least on the operational level.
5. Strong partiality for sustaining many centers of interorganizational coordination so as to increase continuity in the offer of services without spontaneously leading to a restrictive form of systematization.
6. Clinical continuity issues are recognized, but the response seems to be interinstitutional coordination rather than clinical in nature.

A Research Protocol Assessing Implementation of the Plan

A number of questions face researchers organizing systems for managing loss of independence when implementing an experimental integration plan is involved.

- Can an integration plan based on case management be implemented in France?
- Can the experiment yield the elements needed to develop a more general policy, if successful?
- Does the plan really modify professional practices?
- What do the individuals managed under the plan experience?

Consequently, the authors developed an implementation study with longitudinal assessment without control group. The methodology is based on action research. This means that the members of the research team interact constantly with the project team and upon occasion with the strategic and operational actors. More specifically:

- The research team coaches the project team.
- The project team members closely involve operational actors in their process.
- Project team members support operational and strategic actors in implementing the integration model.
- The operational and strategic actors give rise to questions for the research team.

The study's more general objective is to provide information to national policy-makers. This means that the project must be conducted concurrently at three sites differing in care and services (rural, urban and megalopolis). The overall assessment of implementation breaks down into three main research thrusts.

1) Thrust 1: Studying model implementation
The objective of this thrust is to estimate to what degree the six model elements have been implemented as planned using and adapting the method mix used for the PRISMA project[9]. This thrust should make it possible to identify the factors shedding light on the successes or failures observed in the implementation phases (particularly by comparing the three zones) and to identify any adjustments needed to ensure the best fit possible between integration instruments and mechanisms and the target environment.

2) Thrust 2: Analyze and state the modifications in professional practices related to case management
This thrust aims at documenting changes in perception in how the various actors perceive case management and other objectives (integration, continuity, etc.) during the implementation process. It consists in identifying the changes experienced by professionals resulting from case management with respect to two dimensions (their working conditions and professional identity) and modeling interprofessional relations around case-manager practice. The study also focuses on understanding the case manager's report on using the information and assessment instruments in order to document adjustment needs. Special attention will be paid to characterizing initial training and identifying the ongoing training needs of case managers. As a whole, this should bring out the conditions underlying successful implementation.

3) Thrust 3: Study how the concerned populations view case management
This thrust aims at understanding the experience of individuals and their informal networks with respect to the practice of case management, understanding how case management modifies the quality of services received from the point of view of the patient and natural caregiver, and identifying the elements that

the patient and natural caregiver feel impact on the three levels of continuity (informational, approach, and relational).

The research associated with the experimental implementation of PRISMA case management in France is an evaluative implementation study. The assessment method is of the "before-during-after" type without comparison group. The assessment is ongoing, based on multiple action-research methods that are basically qualitative.

The action-research process implies that the research team, project team, and strategic/operational actors work interactively:

- Research-team members took part in the various steps of the implementation process and were involved in decision-making.
- Research-team members supported operational and strategic actors in implementing the integration model with the interim results they produced, and the actors questioned research-team members to clarify some of the results.

No impact study has been carried out at this stage of the project. The proposed model is supported by a sound level of proof (see the other chapters in this book). Therefore, it remains to determine to what degree this kind of approach could be meaningful within France's health and social services system. An impact study could be undertaken subsequently if the findings indicate that the approach could be implemented in France.

Conclusion

Integration results from a set of mechanisms that can be modeled and that are flexible. They provide for improvements in taking into account the changing and complex needs of individuals with impaired independence, regardless of its origin. Current conditions appear largely favorable to implementing integration. Yet this innovation in organizing health care and services appears to be complex.

Implementing the model in France requires partnering for a consensus on a common terminology for diagnostics and solutions. Consequently, a group of researchers and policymakers in the fields of health care and services was formed and finalized the project to demonstrate implementation of integration in three experimental sites in France (rural, urban, and megacity). The findings of this project should provide the means to define the factors for and against achieving integration on a per-site basis (contrasted analysis) and systematically (linked to the specific context of Frances health care and services system as a whole.

References

1. Bressé, S. Les bénéficiaires des services d'aide aux personnes à domicile en 2000, D.r.e.e.s, Editor. 2004, Ministère des affaires sociales, du travail et de la solidarité et Ministère de la santé, de la famille et des personnes handicapées. Paris. 1-8.

2. Perben, M. L'allocation personnalisée d'autonomie au 31 mars 2006, in Etudes et Résultats, D.r.e.e.s, Editor. Paris: Ministère de l'Emploi, de la cohésion sociale et du logement et Ministère de la Santé et des Solidarités, 2006: 1-4.

3. Collectif. Les personnes âgées dépendantes. Paris: La cour des comptes, 2005. Available from: http://www.ccomptes.fr/FramePrinc/frame-rapports.htm.

4. Leutz, WN. Five laws for integrating medical and social services: lessons from the United States and the United Kingdom. Milbank Q. 1999; 77: 77-110, iv-v.

5. Hébert, R., Durand, P.J., Dubuc, N., and Tourigny, A. PRISMA: a new model of integrated service delivery for the frail older people in Canada. Int J Integr Care. 2003; 3: e08.

6. Carrier, S., Couturier, Y., Gagnon, D., and Chouinard, I. L'expérience des gestionnaires de cas est-elle concluante? Élucider une pratique émergeante pour en comprendre les conditions de succès, in Enjeux et controverses dans les soins aux personnes âgées en grande perte d'autonomie, Jacques Allard and Arcand Marcel, Editors. Sainte Hyacinte, (QC): Edisem, 2005: 295-302.

7. Reid, R., Haggerty, J., and McKendry, R. Dissiper la confusion: concepts et mesures de la continuité des soins. 2002, Fondation canadienne de la recherche sur les services de santé: Ottawa, (ON).

8. Eggert, G.M., Zimmer, J.G., Hall, W.J., and Friedman, B. Case management: a randomized controlled study comparing a neighborhood team and a centralized individual model. Health Serv Res. 1991; 26: 471-507.

9. Hébert, R. and Veil, A. Monitoring the degree of implementation of an integrated delivery system. Int J Integr Care. 2004; 4: e05.

10. Hébert, R. Travailler ensemble: des théories aux pratiques, in Interprofessionnalité en gérontologie, D Manière, Aubert F, and Ouata S, Editors. Ramonville Saint Agne: Eres, 2005: 9-12.

11. Rousille, B. L'évaluation du handicap dans la perspective de la nouvelle prestation de compensation, La documentation française, Editor: I.G.A.S, 2004: 109. Available from: http://www.ladocumentationfrancaise.fr/rapports-publics/054000098/index.shtml.

12. Collectif. Cadre de référence sur la planification des services. Rapport du Groupe de travail sur la planification des services. Québec, 2005.

13. Somme, D., Hébert, R., Bravo, G., and Blanchard, F. Le plan de services individualisé (PSI). Concept et utilisation à travers les expériences québécoises et internationales d'intégration des services aux personnes âgées, in Intégrer les services pour le maintien de l'autonomie des personnes, Réjean Hébert, Tourigny André, and Gagnon Maxime, Editors. Québec (QC): Edisem, 2004: 281-299.

14. Greenhalgh, T., Robert, G., Macfarlane, F., Bate, P., and Kyriakidou, O. Diffusion of innovations in service organizations: systematic review and recommendations. Milbank Q. 2004; 82: 581-629.

15. Hébert, R. and Raîche, M. Résultats de l'étude d'impact de PRISMA-Estrie. in 4ᵉ Colloque PRISMA: L'intégration des services: les fruits de la recherche pour nourrir l'action. 2006. Sherbrooke, (QC), Canada: Centre d'expertise en Santé de Sherbrooke.

Chapter 27
Classifying the Frail Elderly: A Comparison of Iso-SMAF Profile Assignment with AGGIR-based Classification into GIRs (Iso-Ressources Groups)

Pauline Gervais, Michel Tousignant, Réjean Hébert, Sylvain Connangle

Highlights

In France, the frail elderly are assessed with an instrument known as AGGIR. Those thus assessed are assigned "Iso-ressource" groups, or GIRs, a process that determines eligibility for certain benefits. AGGIR does not allow, however, for the multidimensional assessment of functional independence. One French residential facility for the elderly opted to use SMAF and Iso-SMAF profiles to meet this need. In May 2006, 207 residents in a residential and care facility for the elderly were assessed using SMAF and assigned Iso-SMAF profiles. The results revealed the study group's heterogeneousness. Although GIR classification, based on assessment with AGGIR, and Iso-SMAF profile assignment, based on assessment with SMAF, correlated very highly (r = 0.86), disparities were observed between the results of the two methods of classification.

Introduction

In 2006, the population of those aged 65 and over in France was estimated to be 10,208,421, i.e., 16.3 % of the country's population as a whole[1]. Life expectancy at birth has continued to rise; in 2006, it reached 83.8 for women and 76.8 for men[2]. Given the aging of the population and the increase in the number of elderly with disabilities, policy makers and managers must implement measures for providing this target group with effective and efficient care.

In the sphere of residential care in France, the passage of Bill 97-60 mandated a shift towards a process of quality enhancement in services to residents and a reform of the billing structure for residential and care facilities for the elderly (EHPADs, for "établissements d'hébergement pour personnes âgées dépendantes"). This shift took concrete form through tripartite agreements reached between each EHPAD, the Conseil général départemental (department general council), and the Caisse régionale d'assurance-maladie (regional health insurance fund), as well as through the establishment of three levels of funding: a) a fee linked to housing, borne by the resident; b) a fee linked to degree of dependency, assumed by the Conseil général départemental; and c) a fee linked to care, assumed by the Direction départementale des Affaires sanitaires et sociales (DDASS or departmental branch for health and social services).

Since their implementation, Bill 2001-647 [on responsibility for care of the frail elderly and the creation of the personalized independence benefit (APA, for "allocation personnalisée d'autonomie")] and Bill 2002-2 (which over-hauled social and medical-social services)[3] have spurred service providers to develop individualized assistance plans and ensure their interventions take account of the needs of the frail elderly. The instrument used to assess the degree of dependency is called AGGIR (for "Autonomie Gérontologique Groupe Iso-Ressources", or Iso-Ressource-group-based Assessment of Geria-tric Independence)[4]. It can be used to classify the elderly into six groupings known as GIRs (for "groupes Iso-ressources"), which, in turn, determine the elderly person's access to APA benefits. Several weaknesses in the instrument's validity and sensitivity have been identified. It is said to overlook the influence of the person's environment, the complexity of psychological factors, lifestyles, and compensatory devices; to underassess disabilities related to mental and sensory function; and to neglect certain variables (e.g., mental function and communication) in assigning individuals to GIRs[5]. Moreover, the degrees of need for assistance vary widely among the persons grouped in any given GIR[6-7]. Finally, AGGIR is said not to yield a multidimensional assessment allowing for an individualized assistance plan, thus opening the door to concerns about the practices professionals use in assessing needs.

As a result, the EHPAD La Madeleine de Bergerac, which had adopted a process approach to quality enhancement, sought a multidimensional assess-ment procedure that would allow for developing individualized assistance plans, as had been proposed in the report of the scientific committee set up by France's Department of Health, the Family, and Handicapped People at the time of the vote on Bill 2001-647[5]. As well, La Madeleine de Bergerac undertook to cultivate a geriatric approach among staff. To this end, the Functional indepen-dence Measurement System (SMAF, for "Système de mesure de l'autonomie fonctionnelle"), used to assess frail adults in Quebec, was adopted. This ins-trument allows for exhaustive assessment of an individual's abilities. It serves to assign individuals to one of 14 functional independence profiles ("Iso-SMAF profiles"), comparable to being placed in the GIRs that determine APA eligibility.

Implementing use of the SMAF in an EHPAD made it possible to carry out a study with these objectives: 1) to determine residents' Iso-SMAF functional independence profile and 2) to compare Iso-SMAF profile assignment with classification in GIRs.

Methodology

Implementing SMAF Use

Full implementation of the SMAF-based assessment process was spread out over a year. First, an implementation committee was formed. On it sat a nurse who was a department head, who was given the task of conducting SMAF assessments; the nurse in charge of quality control and admissions; the manager of the temporary intake facility; the coordinating physician; and the institution's managing director. Committee members received 28 hours of training on SMAF, Iso-SMAF profiles[8], and use of the eSMAF software for compiling data[9]. The training was given in house in May 2005 by the Centre d'expertise en santé de Sherbrooke (the Sherbrooke Health Expertise Centre), or CESS. Over the following three months, committee members consolidated their learning by performing several assessments in situ. Skill in using the instrument was then monitored in September 2005 by the CESS trainer. Next, all the residents of the EHPAD (n = 211) and its temporary intake facility (n = 29) were assessed between October 3, 2005 and November 18, 2005. The nurse in charge of conducting the SMAF assessments did so in consultation with each department's care team. Forms were used to record the information, and the data were then entered by the same nurse in cSMAF. The whole assessment procedure was conducted under ongoing supervision.

Research Protocol

Population

The population consisted of residents occupying an EHPAD bed (n = 211). The criteria for inclusion in the study were: 1) permanent EHPAD residency, which excluded residents in the temporary intake facility; and 2) having been at the EHPAD for at least a month, in order to ensure that subjects had adjusted to their setting and the staff knew them well.

Measurement instruments

The variables under study were: 1) degree of functional independence and 2) degree of dependency. They were measured using both SMAF [10] and AGGIR.

SMAF had already been the subject of several studies confirming its metrological reliability[11-14]. It had been adopted by Quebec's Department of Health and Social Services to assess adults receiving home support services or referred to a public residential facility[15]. SMAF is based on the World Health Organization's conception of functional independence[16] and assesses 29 functions grouped under five headings: activities of daily living, or ADL (7); mobility (6); communication (3); mental function (5); and instrumental activities of daily living, or IADL (8). Functions are scored on a scale of five: 0 (independent); −1 (surveillance or stimulation required); -2 (partial assistance required); −3 (full assistance required). An intermediate score of −0.5 or −1.5 indicates a given activity is carried out independently but with difficulty. The maximum score is −87. SMAF makes it possible to measure the gap between services needed and services provided, and evaluate resource stability.

SMAF also allows for generating a portrait of care and for classifying those assessed under 14 graduated clinical profiles (Iso-SMAF profiles), each of which covers similar subjects needing similar services at a similar level of cost[17-18]. Unlike with GIRs, every SMAF item contributes to establishing an individual's Iso-SMAF profile. Furthermore, SMAF profiles provide the basis for determining facility intake profiles and for arriving at an index of level of required care (ILRC), which makes it possible to compare different analytic units[19]. The 14 Iso-SMAF profiles are, in turn, clustered into 4 groupings. The first of these consists of profiles 1, 2, and 3, assigned to individuals whose disabilities relate strictly to domestic tasks. The second consists of profiles 4, 6, and 9, associated with individuals who have motor impairment but comparatively intact mental function. The third consists of profiles 5, 7, 8, and 10, which are associated with individuals in whom mental disability is predominant. Last, the fourth grouping consists of profiles 11, 12, 13, and 14, associated with individuals with impaired mobility and ADL dependency, or with cognitive deficits and almost total communicative disability. Table 27.1 presents SMAF items opposite their corresponding AGGIR variables.

In France, AGGIR is the legislated instrument for assessing dependency (Bill 97-60, January 24, 1997; order-in-council 97-427, April 28, 1997). The general councils use it to assign APA benefits, but the DDASS also uses it to determine the budget for care delivered in EHPADs and some insurers do likewise for dependency insurance. AGGIR was derived from the Géronte clinical instrument[20]. It comprises ten discriminant variables and seven descriptive variables. In EHPADs, only the discriminant variables are considered when conducting an assessment. Each variable can take three forms, based on the function of four adverbs[21].

Only the first 8 discriminant variables are taken into account in the algorithm used to determine the GIR for a person. The classification system has six levels, each of which covers individuals with similar degrees of need for assistance in carrying out activities essential to daily life[22]. The ordering of GIRs is the inverse of that for Iso-SMAF profiles: GIR 6 corresponds to Iso-SMAF profile 1 and GIR 1 to Iso-SMAF profile 14. Only individuals falling in GIRs that correspond to a moderate to significant degree of service needs, i.e., GIRs 1 to 4, are eligible for APA benefits.

Table 27.1
AGGIR Variables and SMAF Items

	AGGIR	SMAF	
Discriminant variables (in care facility and at home)	Eating and drinking*	Eating and drinking	Items used to assign Iso-SMAF profile
	Dressing*	Dressing	
	Personal hygiene*	Washing	
		Personal hygiene	
	Urinary and fecal elimination*	Bladder function	
		Rectal function	
		Toilet use	
	Transfers*	Transferts	
	Moving around indoors*	Walking indoors	
		Putting on prostheses or ortheses	
		Moving around indoors using wheelchair	
		Using stairs	
	Moving around outdoors (at home)	Circulating outdoors	
		Vision	
		Hearing	
	Coherence*	Speech	
		Judgment	
		Behaviour	
	Orientation*	Orientation	
		Memory	
		Comprehension	
	Ability to raise alarm	Use of phone at home	
Descriptive variables (at home)	Housekeeping	Housekeeping	
		Laundry	
	Cooking	Meal preparation	
	Errands	Errands	
	Transportation	Use of methods of transportation	
	Treatment follow up	Taking medication	
	Management	Budget management	
	Leisure		

Table 27.1
AGGIR Variables and SMAF Items

10 discriminant variables and 8 descriptive variables 4 – ADL 3 – Mobility 1 – Ability to raise alarm 2 – Cognitive function 7 – IADL 1 – Social	29 items 7 – ADL 6 – Mobility 3 – Communication 5 – Cognitive function 8 – IADL
Scores	A – Performs independently (spontaneously), in full, habitually (over time), and correctly B – Performs partially or not habitually or not correctly C – Does not perform	0 – Independent −0.5 – With difficulty −1 –Stimulation or supervision required −2 – Partial assistance required −3 – Dependent
GIR	**Iso-SMAF Profile**
* 8 discriminant variables considered	29 items considered

Data Collection

The data were collected from April 10, 2006 to May 5, 2006, that is, a year into implementation of the SMAF procedure. SMAF assessments were conducted in alternation with AGGIR ones. A calendar of meetings was set up with the care teams for the EHPAD's eight departments, ensuring that each team's meetings with the nurse conducting SMAF assessments and the coordinating physician conducting AGGIR assessments were two weeks apart. Residents in all of the facility's eight departments were thus assessed using both instruments.

Data Analysis

Based on descriptive statistics and the relative distribution of Iso-SMAF Profiles in the EHPAD, we present a portrait of the population studied. Then, we use ILRCs to compare workloads across EHPAD units. The ILRC is calculated as follows: The median of the hours needed daily to meet nursing care, assistance, and support needs for each Iso-SMAF Profile[11] is divided by the median of the total number of hours required for the most demanding profile, 14. Each coefficient thus obtained is multiplied by the number of individuals assigned the profile in question. The sum of the coefficients is divided by the total number of subjects.[19] Lastly, we present descriptive statistics, including a Pearson correlation, to arrive at a comparison between the two classification systems.

Findings

Portrait of the Facility's Clientele

The 211 beds in La Madeleine de Bergerac were all filled when the study began. Three residents died before the intended date of their assessment; one resident, who had been admitted less than a month previously, was excluded. Thus, 207 subjects were assessed. The overall average age of residents was 86, more specifically 87 for the women, who numbered 152 (73 %), and 84 for the men, who numbered 55 (27 %).

Figure 27.1 presents the break down of study subjects into the 14 Iso-SMAF profiles and the 6 GIRs. More than half the study subjects (52 %) falls into GIRs 1 and 2. These are the groups associated with the highest levels of required care; they comprise individuals entitled to receive the most substantial APA benefits. GIRs 5 and 6 cover 28 % of subjects. Individuals falling into these groups are ineligible for benefits. GIRs 3 and 4, the intermediate groups, cover 20 % of subjects. Within each group, needs are undifferentiated.

The distribution of Iso-SMAF profiles reveals the heterogeneousness of the clientele. Close to 1 subject in 4 (24 %) presents with disabilities related to IADL only (profiles 1, 2, and 3), a proportion slightly lower than that for GIRs 5 and 6. The profiles associated with disability cover 24 % of the clientele, while 22 % have been assigned a profile associated with mental disability (5, 7, 8, or 10), which corresponds to the proportion classified in GIRs 2, 3, and 4. Lastly, 30 % of subjects are seriously frail, with significant motor and mental disabilities (profiles 11, 12, 13, and 14).

Figure 27.2 shows how the distribution of Iso-SMAF profiles and ILRCs varies from one department of the EHPAD to another. Taken together, the departments' intake profiles and ILRCs provide a portrait of the nature and intensity of residents' needs.

The average time needed to conduct a SMAF assessment was 20 minutes and 30 minutes for AGGIR. We believe the difference in duration is accounted for by the time needed to interpret the meaning of AGGIR questions.

Comparison of Iso-SMAF Classification and GIR Classification

The degree of alignment between Iso-SMAF profile assignment and GIR classification is presented in Table 27.2. The correspondence is very good for Iso-SMAF profiles 1 and 2, as it is for the profiles associated with higher care levels, 9 to 14. With the intermediate profiles, divergence is observable. Figure 27.3 presents GIR prediction on the basis of Iso-SMAF profiles (r = 0.86, p < 0.001). Generally speaking, GIR levels are overestimated when predicted on the basis of SMAF.

There is a perfect correspondence between classification in Iso-SMAF profile 1 and GIR 6. At the other end, 93.4 % of Iso-SMAF profile 14 assignments

Figure 27.1
Distribution of Iso-SMAF Profiles and GIRs at La Madeleine de Bergerac EHPAD

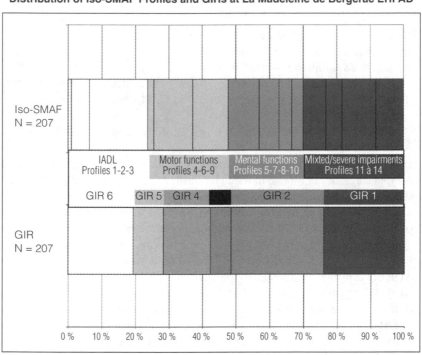

Figure 27.2
Distribution of Iso-SMAF Profiles in Different Departments of the EHPAD

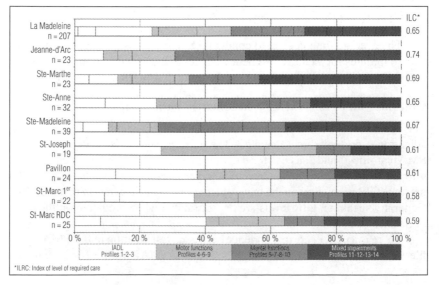

Table 27.2
Correspondences between GIR Membership and Iso-SMAF Profile Assignment

	GIR 1	GIR2	GIR 3	GIR 4	GIR 5	GIR 6	n
Profile 1	0	0	0	0	0	2 100 %	2
Profile 2	0	0	0	0	3 27.3 %	8 72.7 %	11
Profile 3	0	0	1 2.8 %	9 25.0 %	3 8.3 %	23 63.9 %	36
Profile 4	0	1 33.3 %	0	2 66.7 %	0	0	3
Profile 5	0	2 10.5 %	2 10.5 %	7 6.8 %	5 26.3 %	3 15.8 %	19
Profiel 6	0	2 8.3 %	2 8.3 %	10 41.7 %	6 25.0 %	4 16.7 %	24
Profile 7	1 8.3 %	7 58.3 %	3 25.0 %	0	1 8.3 %	0	12
Profile 8	0	5 62.5 %	2 25.0 %	1 12.5 %	0	0	8
Profile 9	0 26.1 %	14 60.9 %	2 8.7 %	0	1 4.3 %	0	23
Profile 10	1 14.3 %	6 85.7 %	0	0	0	0	7
Profile 11	8 57.1 %	6 42.9 %	0	0	0	0	14
Profile 12	8 61.5 %	5 38.5 %	0	0	0	0	13
Profile 13	12 60.0 %	8 40.0 %	0	0	0	0	20
Profile 14	14 93.3 %	1 6.7 %	0	0	0	0	15

correspond to classification in GIR 1. It's another matter for the remaining profiles, which are distributed unequally among the intermediate GIRs, from 2 to 5. The distribution of Iso-SMAF profiles across GIRs is illuminating. In trying to predict GIR classification on the basis of groupings of Iso-SMAF profiles, we observe that 67 % of subjects assigned profiles 1 to 3 were classified in GIR 6, while the remaining third of these cases were classified in GIRs 5 (profile 2) and 4 (and profile 3). Of those assigned profiles 4 and 6, 44 % were classified in GIR 4; but the remainder were grouped in GIRs 2 (profile 4) and 5 (profile 6). For 70 % of subjects assigned profiles 7 to 10, this corresponded to being classified

Figure 27.3
Distribution of Iso-SMAF Profiles and GIRs

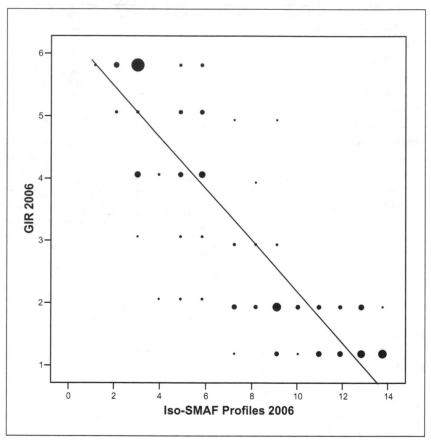

as GIR 2, while the remaining 30 % are distributed over GIRs 3 (profiles 7 and 8) and 1 (profiles 9 and 10). Finally, 68 % of subjects assigned profiles 11 to 14 were classified in GIR 1, with the remainder falling into GIR 2 (profiles 11, 12, and 13).

Discussion

The objectives of this study were to determine the functional independence profiles of residents of EHPAD La Madeleine de Bergerac and compare the results of classification using Iso-SMAF profiles and classification using GIRs. To our knowledge, our study is unique in this respect.

At La Madeleine de Bergerac, there are two-and-a-half times as many women (73 %) as men. One senses the range of degrees of frailty is very broad.

Figure 27.4
Distribution of Iso-SMAF Profiles across GIRs

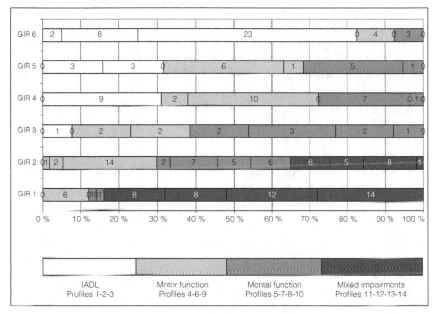

This is confirmed by residents' Iso-SMAF profiles. Unlike the GIRs, which only indicate level of dependency and do not allow for a description of the complexity of the circumstances,[6] residents' Iso-SMAF profiles reveal the diversity of their needs. Further, calculating the ILRC makes it possible to assess the level of need and make comparisons among different groupings within the facility's clientele.

Twenty-eight percent of subjects fall into GIRs 6 and 5, two groups intended to cover independent individuals and those who require only occasional help with IADL and hygiene. The classification based on SMAF yields a smaller proportion of individuals identified as needing only supervision or partial assistance with IADL. The GIR associated with the highest level of dependency, GIR 1, covers 24 % of the EHPAD'S clientele, a lower proportion than that associated with Iso-SMAF profiles 11 to 14, which correspond to mixed and serious impairments. These differences between the results obtained with the two classification systems support observations from other studies, which have shown that AGGIR underestimates the extent of need.[24] The distribution of Iso-SMAF profiles across GIRs also shows that use of AGGIR results in classification errors.[22] Thus, 10 % of frail residents are classed in a GIR for independent individuals and therefore receive no financial benefits, even though they actually meet the threshold of need. The inverse is also true: 5 % of residents receive benefits for which they do not really meet the threshold of need.

What's more, 10 % receive an amount that does not correspond to their degree of independence.

The internal validity of this study derives from a set of measures worth presenting here. The fact that the survey was carried out in a large EHPAD (n = 211) is one of the study's strengths. Doing so prevented selection bias and optimized the study's applicability to similar settings within the French administrative department. Moreover, we strove to minimize information bias. The data were collected by two trained assessors familiar with the use of the instruments they administered. In every case, both the SMAF and AGGIR assessments were conducted with the same care team with a lapse of two weeks between assessments. The SMAF data were input during the assessment procedure, while the AGGIR data were entered on a form and then verified and recorded electronically the same day. Without claiming perfect control for biases, we are confident of the quality of the study data.

Conclusion

The primary objective of this study was to determine the functional independence profiles (Iso-SMAF profiles) of residents of a French residential and care facility for the frail elderly or EHPAD. The study represents a departure in the field of the assessment of the frail elderly in France. Under legislative changes made over the past few years, care of the elderly and the development of individualized assistance plans are required to be based on multidimensional assessments. SMAF tangibly responds to this requirement.

The study made it possible to compare the classifications resulting from use of the SMAF and AGGIR instruments. To our knowledge, no similar study had been carried out in the past. The comparison revealed divergences between classification in GIRs and Iso-SMAF profile assignment. Residents may find themselves classified in a GIR that does not correspond to their degree of frailty and therefore fail to receive financial benefits their degree of frailty qualifies them for. By the same token, a resident may be assigned a GIR that confers entitlement to benefits when, in fact, she or he does not meet the eligibility threshold. These initial findings suggest it would be worth continuing the study and including the whole range of residential and care settings in order to arrive at an informed judgment regarding equity in the assignment of financial benefits.

Note: Despite a high correlation ($r = 0.86$), prediction of GIR assignment using SMAF shows up as weak, because of the low number of subjects in many cells. A study should be conducted with a broader and more diversified group to validate these preliminary results.

References

1. Institut national de la statistique et des études économiques (2005). Population totale par sexe et âge au 1er janvier 2006, France entière. INSEE (www.insee.fr/fr/ffc/chifcle_fiche.asp?ref_id=NATCCF02120&tab_id=5).

2. Institut national de la statistique et des études économiques (2006). Espérance de vie à la naissance et taux de mortalité infantile. INSEE (www.insee.fr/fr/ffc/chifcle_fiche.asp?ref_id=NATTEF02221&tab_id=434).

3. République française. Loi 2002-02 du 2 janvier 2002 rénovant l'action sociale et médico-sociale.

4. République française. Order-in-council 97-427, April 1997.

5. Colvez, A. (2003). Rapport du comité scientifique pour l'évaluation de l'autonomie. Ministre de la Santé, de la Famille et des Personnes handicapées.

6. Coutton, V. (2000). Les mécanismes de la grille AGGIR. INSERM Démographie et Santé.

7. Roussille, B. (2004). L'évaluation du handicap dans la perspective de la nouvelle prestation de compensation.

8. Guilbeault, J., & Delli-Colli, N. (2005). Formation utilisation du système de mesure de l'autonomie fonctionnelle (SMAF) & utilisation des profils Iso-SMAF. Centre d'expertise en santé de Sherbrooke.

9. Boissy P, Brière S, Tousignant M, Rousseau E. (2007). The eSMAF: A software for the assessment and follow-up of functional independence in geriatrics. BMC Geriatrics (www.biomedcentral.com/1471-2318/7/2); 7:2, 1-14.

10. Hébert, R., Desrosiers, J., Dubuc, N., Tousignant, M., Guilbeault, J., & Pinsonnault, E. (2003). Le système de mesure de l'autonomie fonctionnelle (SMAF) – Mise au point. La Revue De Gériatrie; 28: 323-36.

11. Hébert, R., Dubuc, N., Buteau, Roy, M., Desrosiers, J., Bravo, G., Trottier, L., & St-Hilaire, C. (1997). Services requis par les personnes âgées en perte d'autonomie – Évaluation clinique et estimation des coûts selon le milieu de vie. Direction de la recherche et de l'évaluation, Ministère de la santé et des services sociaux, Gouvernement du Québec.

12. Desrosiers J, Bravo G, Hébert R, Dubuc N. (1995). Reliability of the revised Functional Autonomy Measurement System (SMAF) for epidemiological research. Age and Ageing; 24: 402-6.

13. Hébert, R. Carrier C. R, Bilodeau A. (1988). Le système de mesure de l'autonomie fonctionnelle (SMAF). Revue de gériatrie; 14:161-7.

14. Hébert, R., Spiegelhalter, D. J., & Brayne, C. (1997). Setting the minimal metrically detectable change on disability rating scales. Archives of Physical Medecine and Rehabilitation, 78: 1305-8.

15. Ministère de la santé et des services sociaux (2000). Comité aviseur sur l'adoption d'un outil d'évaluation intégré des besoins des personnes en perte d'autonomie et de détermination des services requis notamment en institution et domicile. Gouvernement du Québec.

16. World Health Organization. (1980). International classification of impairments, disabilities, and handicaps: A manual of classification relating to the consequences of disease.

17. Dubuc, N., & Hébert, R. (2002). Les profils Iso-SMAF: Un système de gestion clinico-administratif pour la planification des services de longue durée dans un système de soins intégrés. SMAF: Quoi de neuf? Expertise Centre of the Sherbrooke Geriatric University Institute.

18. Dubuc, N., Hébert, R., & Desrosiers, J. (2004). Les soins de longue durée aux personnes âgées: Choix d'un système clinico-administratif dans le contexte d'un réseau de soins intégrés. Revue Canadienne du Vieillissement, 23(1): 35-45.

19. Tousignant, M., Hébert, R., Dubuc, N., & Coulombe, C. (2003). Détermination du profil d'autonomie fonctionnelle et du taux de réponse aux besoins de la clientèle long-terme du programme soutien à domicile des CLSC de la Montérégie. Centre for Research on Aging, Sherbrooke Geriatric University Institute.

20. Besso, M., Saos, J., & Attalli, G. (1989). Méthodologie d'évaluation de l'autonomie des personnes âgées (en France). Échanges Santé, (55): 23-26.

21. Caisse nationale d'assurance maladie des travailleurs salariés (2004). Propositions pour améliorer l'utilisation du modèle AGGIR. République française.

22. Coutton, V. (2000). La grille AGGIR. INSERM, Démographie et Santé.

23. Caillot, L., & Mesrine, A. (2003). Présentation des enquêtes EHPA et SAPAD. Dossiers Solidarité et Santé, (1): 9-16.

24. Kerhuel, N. (2001). Vieillissement et habitat. Recherche comparée sur les politiques de l'habitat en direction des personnes vieillissantes et en perte d'autonomie. Ministère de l'Équipement, des Transports et du Logement, République française.

Assistance in Publishing this Book

This book's publication was facilitated by financial support from various organizations and a grant:

- On November 22, 2005, the **Canadian Institutes of Health Research (CIHR) Regional Knowledge Translation Award** was given to Réjean Hébert and the PRISMA Group. Recipients must use the award to further their knowledge-application activities. The entire award was used to produce the French- and English-language versions of this book.
- The publication of this book was also made possible with the support of the Réseau québécois de recherche sur le vieillissement (RQRV) under its 2006-2007 competition for publication assistance.
- The Canadian Health Services Research Foundation (CHSRF) defrayed part of the translation costs for the English-language version of this book.

Funding of the PRISMA Program

The PRISMA program was funded by:
Granting agencies:

- Canadian Health Services Research Foundation (CHSRF)
- Canadian Institutes of Health Research (CIHR)
- Fonds de la recherche en santé du Québec (FRSQ)
- Réseau québécois de recherche sur le vieillissement (RQRV)

Public health and social services organizations:

- Ministère de la Santé et des Services sociaux
- Health and Social Services Agencies
  - Estrie
  - Montérégie
  - Mauricie-Centre-du-Québec
  - Laval
  - Québec
- Centre de santé et de services sociaux – Institut Universitaire de Gériatrie de Sherbrooke
- Institut national de santé publique du Québec (INSPQ)

Université de Sherbrooke

The various projects presented in this book may be funded by other sources that are identified in each chapter.

Acknowledgments

We cordially thank all of the elderly people who took part in the studies recounted in this book. We are also grateful to the secretarial teams for their assistance in smoothing our work and the drafting processes that precede (grant applications) and follow (articles and reports) the research. Lastly, we want to thank everyone involved in entering and compiling the data in the enormous databases that we will analyze for years to come.

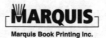

Marquis Book Printing Inc.

Québec, Canada
2008